The Complete 4-in-1 Kidney Disease Diet & Food List Guide for 60+ CKD Stages 3-4

Essential resource for avoiding dialysis and managing CKD with comprehensive renal diet plan, detailed low potassium, and low sodium food lists for Kidney Health

Janeth Kingston, BSN RN

© Copyright 2025
All rights reserved
Janeth Kingston, BSN RN
BINNOVATE PUBLISHERS

The content contained within this book may not be reproduced, duplicated or transmitted without direct written permission from the author or the publisher.

Under no circumstances will any blame or legal responsibility be held against the publisher, or author, for any damages, reparation, or monetary loss due to the information contained within this book. Either directly or indirectly. You are responsible for your own choices, actions, and results.

Legal Notice:

This book is copyright protected. This book is only for personal use. You cannot amend, distribute, sell, use, quote or paraphrase any part, or the content within this book, without the consent of the author or publisher.

Disclaimer Notice:

Please note the information contained within this document is for educational and entertainment purposes only. All effort has been executed to present accurate, up to date, and reliable, complete information. No warranties of any kind are declared or implied. Readers acknowledge that the author is not engaging in the rendering of legal, financial, medical or professional advice. The content within this book has been derived from various sources. Please consult a licensed professional before attempting any techniques outlined in this book.

By reading this document, the reader agrees that under no circumstances is the author responsible for any losses, direct or indirect, which are incurred as a result of the use of the information contained within this document, including, but not limited to, — errors, omissions, or inaccuracies.

Table of Contents

BOOK 1: Avoid Dialysis Diet Plan for Kidney Disease

INTRODUCTION 1

The Need for a CKD-Specific Diet 1

Overcoming Your Barriers To Healthy Eating 2

The Role of Diet in CKD Progression 5

How This Book Can Help 6

Understanding CKD 6

Importance of Age-Based Diet 10

Chapter 1: The CKD-Diet Connection 14

What Does Food Do to Your Kidneys? 14

The Impact of Overworking Your Kidneys 16

Foods That Put Extra Strain on Your Kidneys 17

How Diet Can Slow CKD Progression 18

The Connection Between Diet and Dialysis 20

Research on Diet and CKD 20

The Importance of Controlling Blood Sugar and Blood Pressure 21

Chapter 2: The Basics of a CKD-Friendly Diet 23

What Makes a Diet CKD-Friendly? 23

The Role of Macronutrients and Micronutrients 24

Importance of Individual Dietary Requirements 25

The Role of Different Food Groups 27

The Right Kind of Carbohydrates 29

The Importance of Healthy Fats 30

Fluids and CKD - Hydration and Fluid Restrictions 30

Choosing the Right Beverages 31

Chapter 3: The Role of Protein, Potassium, Phosphorus, and Sodium in CKD 33

Protein and CKD 34

Potassium's Impact on CKD 40

Sodium and CKD 43

Phosphorus and Your Kidneys 46

Chapter 4: Translating Diet into Daily Meals 51

Importance of Meal Planning 51

Meal Planning Tips for Success 55

Creating a CKD-Friendly Meal Plan 56

Understanding Portion Sizes 60

CKD-Friendly Recipes 65

Lunch and Dinner Ideas 73

Snack Ideas and Healthy Desserts 86

Chapter 5: Adapting Your Diet to Your Lifestyle 91

Working with a Dietitian 91

Maximizing Your Dietician Appointments 92

Diet Adjustments for Common Comorbidities 94

High Blood Pressure and CKD 101

Chapter 6: Handling Special Occasions and Dining Out 106

Navigating Different Eating Situations 106

Strategies on Staying On-Track 110

Chapter 7: Exercise and CKD Management 112

The Benefits of Exercise 114

Personalizing Your Exercise Plan 115

Types of Exercises That Should Be In Your Plan 117

Duration, Frequency, and Intensity: Tips and Tricks 120

Making Sense of the Whole Package: Integrating Nutrition, Diet and Exercise
.... 122

Your Diet and Activity Plan 123

Chapter 8: Stress, Mental Health, and CKD 124
Understanding the Mental Impact of CKD 125
Mental Health Journey of a CKD Patient 128
Strategies for Managing Stress 129

Chapter 9: The Importance of Sleep in CKD Management 131
Understanding Sleep and CKD 133
The Role of Sleep in Health 133
Sleep-Friendly Environment 134
When to Seek Help for Sleep Problems 135
Results of Improved Sleep Patterns 136

Chapter 10: Medication and Dietary Supplements 137
Understanding the Importance of Medication 138
Practical Things About Prescriptions 140

Chapter 11: Staying Motivated and Dealing with Setbacks 143
Ask For Help: Let's Overcome Those Support Setbacks 144
3 Motivation Movers 146
Strategies to Overcome Setbacks 149

Conclusion 155

Annex 157

References 159

BOOK 2: The Kidney Diet Food List Guide for Renal Disease

Introduction 167
About This Book 167
Purpose and Scope 167
How to Use This Book 167

Part I: Understanding Kidney Disease and Nutrition 169

Chapter 1: Understanding Kidney Disease 169

Chapter 2: The Basics of a Kidney-Friendly Diet 173

Key Nutrients to Monitor:
Potassium, Phosphorus, Sodium, and Protein 173

What Should You Eat for Your CKD? 173

Hydration and Fluid Management 175

General Fluid Guidelines Based on CKD Stages: 175

Chapter 3: The Renal Diet Food List 177

How to Use the Charts 177

A. Vegetable Proteins 179

B. Animal Protein 183

C. Milk and Cheeses 205

D. Fats 215

E. Vegetables 227

F. Fruits 245

G. Herbs and Spices 265

H. Carbohydrates 271

Part II: Kidney-Friendly Food Lists 283

Chapter 4: Foods to Avoid or Limit 283

High-Potassium Foods 283

High and Low Potassium Foods 284

High-Phosphorus Foods 287

What Should I Do If My Phosphorus Level is Too High? 288

High-Sodium Foods 289

Tips to Cut Down Sodium Intake 289

Understanding Nutrition Labels 292

Part III: Meal Planning and Recipes 295

Chapter 5: Meal Planning for Kidney Health 295

Creating a Balanced Meal Plan 295

Sample Meal Plan for Stages 1 and 2 297

Stage 3-5 Chronic Kidney Disease (CKD)
Daily Meal Plan Guidelines 298

Portion Control and Serving Sizes 304

Tips For Grocery Shopping 305

Chapter 6. Renal Diet Recipes 307

Breakfast Dishes 308

Lunch Dishes 313

Dinner Dishes 317

Snacks 321

Hydration Tips and Safe Beverages 324

Part IV: Thriving with Kidney Disease 326

Chapter 7: Living with Kidney Disease 326

Myths and Facts about CKD 326

Coping Strategies 327

Working with Your Healthcare Providers 329

Conclusion 331

Meal Planning 331

Portion Control and Nutrition Labels 332

Knowledge is Power 332

Appendix A: Glossary 333

Appendix B: Resources 337

Appendix C: Index 339

BOOK 3: Low-Potassium Food List for Kidney Disease Patients

INTRODUCTION 350
    About this Book 350
Chapter 1: Understanding Potassium and Kidney Health 352
Part 1. The Comprehensive Food List 355
    Navigating Through The Charts 355
Chapter 2: Carbohydrates 357
    Grains and Cereals 358
    Breads and Pastries 363
    Pasta 368
Chapter 3: Proteins 369
    Vegetable Proteins 370
    Poultry 373
    Meats 377
    Seafoods 383
Chapter 4: Dairy and Non-Dairy 393
Chapter 5: Fats, Oils, and Nuts 403
Chapter 6: Fruits 415
Chapter 7: Vegetables 435
Chapter 8: Herbs and Spices 453
Part 2. Meal Planning and Recipes 458
Chapter 9: Low Potassium Meal Plan 458
    Creating a Low Potassium Meal Plan 458
    5-Day Low Potassium Sample Meal Plan 460
    Low Potassium Dietary Recommendations 461

Chapter 10: Low Potassium Recipes 463

Chapter 11: Embracing the Journey 475

    Coping with Chronic Kidney Disease, ... 475

Conclusion 477

References 478

Low Potassium Food List Index 479

BOOK 4: The Kidney-Friendly Low-Sodium Diet Guide Essential Food List

Introduction 493

Chapter 1: Understanding Kidney Health 495

    Overview of Chronic Kidney Disease (CKD) 495

    The Importance of Diet in Managing Kidney Health 495

    Understanding Sodium's Role in Kidney Disease 496

    The Importance of Diet in Managing Kidney Disease 497

Chapter 2: The Basics of a Low-Sodium Diet 501

    What is a Low-Sodium Diet? 501

Chapter 3: Essential Foods for a Kidney-Friendly Diet 505

    Comprehensive Low-Sodium Food List by Category 505

    Foods to Avoid and Alternatives 507

Chapter 4: The Low-Sodium Food List Chart 509

    A. Vegetables 511

    B. Vegetable Proteins 529

    C. Fruits 533

    D. Carbohydrates 553

    E. Milk and Cheeses 565

    F. Fats 575

    G. Animal Protein 587

    H. Herbs and Spices 609

Chapter 5: Flavor Without the Pinch 614

    Low-Sodium Recipe Ideas 614

Chapter 6: Meal Planning for Success 633

    How to Create a Weekly Meal Plan 633

    Sample One-Week Low-Sodium Meal Plan 635

Chapter 7: Cooking Tips and Techniques 639

    Flavor Enhancement Without Salt 639

Chapter 8: Coping with Dietary Restrictions 643

    Navigating Social Situations with Dietary Needs 643

    Involving Family in Meal Preparation 644

Conclusion 647

    Empowering Your Kidney Health Journey 647

Reference 650

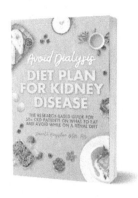

Avoid Dialysis Diet Plan for Kidney Disease

A research-based guide for 50+ CKD patients on what to eat and avoid while on a renal diet.

Janeth Kingston BSN, RN

From The Author

Hello and thank you for investing in your health with **"Avoid Dialysis Diet Plan for Kidney Disease"** I'm deeply grateful for your trust, and I'm excited to be part of your journey towards better kidney health.

My name is Janeth Kingston, BSN, RN. I have spent over a decade working as a dedicated nephrology nurse, both in the US and the EU. Throughout my career, I've been privileged to contribute to the research and development that improves the quality of life for those living with Stage 3 to 5 Chronic Kidney Disease (CKD).

This book is the culmination of years of research, patient interaction, and careful study. This book uses the same research-based background from a project we have undertaken together with numerous nephrology experts. The project has been recognized and awarded by esteemed bodies like the American Society of Nephrology, which awarded our work in their KidneyX program in 2019. You can check their website www.KidneyX.org under "Digitally Delivered Behavior Change Program to Help Patients Delay Dialysis". The success of our program has also been presented at prestigious nephrology conferences, such as Kidney Week in Washington DC and the ERA-EDTA in Europe.

Since 2017, my team and I have helped over 10,589 CKD patients navigate their dietary needs and confidently manage their condition. Each of these individual stories has further enriched our knowledge and understanding, and I'm thrilled to bring that collective wisdom to you today.

In collaboration with seasoned nephrology researchers, kidney-specialized chefs, and leading nephrologists, we have created this guide. Our goal? To provide you with a simple, accessible roadmap to managing your condition and avoiding dialysis.

As you take your first steps on this journey, remember: change is a process, not a destination. Be patient with yourself and take each day as it comes. With each page you turn, you're taking a proactive step towards better health.

I'd like to extend an invitation to ***join our FREE weekly newsletter online***, where we share:

- weekly kidney-safe recipes

- meal plans, and
- the latest research-based advice.

Follow these steps to join our online weekly newsletter:

1. Please type on your phone or pc browser **https://go.renaltracker.com/joinnewsletter** to sign up.

2. Or you can also scan the QR code below.
    a. Open your phone's camera
    b. Hover your phone over the QR code
    c. Tap on the link and enter your name and email.

It's a great way to stay informed and feel supported as you navigate your CKD journey.

Once again, thank you for your trust. Here's to a healthier, brighter future for your kidneys.

With gratitude,

Janeth Kingston, BSN,

INTRODUCTION

The Need for a CKD-Specific Diet

Taking charge of your own health can help you achieve better outcomes. This can also give you a sense of empowerment and, eventually, give you the motivation you need to be responsible with the choices you make concerning your health.

And one simple way to do this is to take an active role in your health decisions, particularly on things you can control on your own: Your Diet.

Changing your diet will require a tremendous shift in your routines. You'll need to avoid most of your favorite meals. You'll need to fit in types of food you're not particularly fond of in your diet plan. You'll also need to make changes in your grocery lists, most especially in your budget since healthy eating can quite get financially demanding. And the list goes on.

But if you were to take the right steps towards this change, it will remarkably improve your health outcomes and alter your overall lifestyle to a better one. And I assure you that throughout your journey to a better kidney health, it will be worth it.

Now, I know that change, especially when you have to replace bad habits with good ones, can be hard and may take time and patience. But if you keep practicing and stick with your new choices, **it will become part of your daily routine.**

That is why I'd like to lay a solid foundation before we get started with anything, and really pound things at the beginning of this book.

From setting your goals to getting support, it will require several steps to get to where you should be. But one of the most important steps is to **figure out what your barriers are.** By identifying your barriers and having a plan to help you get past them will help you change bad habits into good habits.

Overcoming Your Barriers To Healthy Eating

What's a barrier?

A barrier is anything that causes you to slip up in your goal to make the lifestyle changes you need, such as changing your eating habits. By figuring out what those barriers are and how you can get around them can help you reach your kidney-friendly eating goals. When you hit a certain barrier, get support, especially from your family, friends, or even your kidney doctor.

Having slip ups is normal. Chef Duane Sunwold, a dear friend turned CKD chef, once battled hard with his own Chronic Kidney Disease. In fact, the first time he was advised to change his diet by completely taking out animal protein, he slipped up and decided to eat a cheeseburger instead! But when he was committed to his goal, he managed to feel much better and improved his creatinine levels from 4.99 to 0.8! Therefore, you need to have a plan on how to get back on track for when that happens.

So, what's the best way to overcome barriers? You have to identify them ahead of time and create a backup plan on how to deal with them. There will be some barriers right away, that will keep you from trying to change a habit, while others may appear later on. When they do, get support by talking to your family and friends who are there to cheer you on. And if you have any questions or concerns about your health, talk to your doctor to make sure you're on the right track.

There are a few reasons why you will have trouble changing your eating habits. Here are some of them and how to handle each one.

"I'll never be able to change how I eat."

By not believing you are capable of doing something, especially change, is often **just a fear of failure.** This kind of barrier can keep you from even starting to make a lifestyle change. Here are two possible solutions:

1. Carefully define "success" and "failure". If your goal is to lower your nutrient intake, like Sodium, from 2,000mg to 1,200mg a day, you will probably be successful. But if your goal is to cure kidney disease or eat perfectly, it is not realistic and may lead to failure.
2. Set small, yet measurable goals. Eating a low-sodium fruit is an easy goal to reach. However, completely giving up your favorite foods is much harder, and you will be more likely to not try.

"I don't have time to make changes."

This is a very common reason not to change. It can take in the form of *"My life is just too busy right now"*, or *"I have more important things to do"*, or *"I will start next week"*. Here are four possible solutions:

1. Manage your time better. Find time-management techniques that will work best for you.
2. Ask others how they manage to fit good nutrition into their lives.
3. Don't try to make too many changes at the same time. Small changes take less time, but they add. Remember, small changes eventually add up to huge results.
4. Ask for help from family and friends when you change your eating habits.

"I don't like healthy foods"

Most people use this reason and may come in the form of, *"I don't like vegetables"*, *"I don't like low-fat foods"*, or *"I'll miss eating them"*. Here are two possible solutions:

1. Be patient and give it time. Food preferences are not easy at first, but they do change over time. Remember when you start changing by picking one habit at time, it will eventually become part of your routine. Decide to withhold your judgements about what you like or dislike in foods until you have given the new foods a chance. If you need help, be sure to discuss with your doctor and dietitian how to integrate foods into your new kidney diet.
2. Take it slow. You don't have to completely give up your favorite foods, but you may have to change how often and how much you eat them. Make your changes small, and give yourself time to adjust your diet.

"Healthy foods cost too much."

It's true that food items such as fresh produce, whole-grain breads, and other healthy food items can cost you more than purchasing cheap fast food or quick meals. Sometimes it makes you think that maybe you should just go with cheap fast food every day. But you can stay within your budget if you carefully plan your meals, know what to buy, and what to cook. The more time you invest, the more money you'll be able to save. Here's are possible solutions:

1. Save money by learning and planning. To carefully plan a week's worth of meals at a time, be sure to consult your dietitian for a meal plan that best fits your condition. This is so you are not likely to go out to eat on the spur of the moment.
2. When you're at the grocery store, save money by buying store brands instead of name brands and do shopping in bulk foods aisle.
3. If you're not used to preparing and cooking your own meals, you have to start learning.

"I'm not good at making changes."

This one actually may take the form of *"I'm too old to make changes."* Often, low self-esteem makes it hard to change. Here are possible solutions:

1. Make small and measurable changes. They are easier to make and monitor. For example, try eating a low-sodium fruit instead of the usual fruit.
2. Work on your self-esteem *(if this is an issue for you)*. Seeking help from a counselor can help with issues of self-esteem. The success that you will feel from improving your eating habits may improve your self-esteem as well. Little by little, you may begin to change the way you view yourself and your ability to change.

To help you identify your own barriers, think about the last few times you thought about changing your eating habits but didn't follow through with it.

What stopped you from doing it? Be sure to write your reasons. For each reason, write a response that will help you reconsider your choice. After which, look at your list of reasons and responses whenever you are about to make a choice on what to eat.

Why should you start small? Because...

"Success is the sum of all small efforts, repeated day in and day out" - R. Collier

The Role of Diet in CKD Progression

Now that you have gone through your need of a CKD-specific diet and identified personal areas that might keep you from achieving your goals for health, let's dive a little deeper on why diet is so important in the management of Chronic Kidney Disease and to keep it from progressing.

"Diet is one of the largest modifiable risk factors for chronic kidney disease (CKD)-related death and disability" Snelson et. al. While it is no longer a mystery that certain types of food have been linked to the development of CKD, studies have also shown that optimized diets

which include both restrictions and modifications of certain nutrients and minerals in the food that we eat help in reducing the burden of CKD.

These restrictions and modifications focus on specific micro and macronutrients such as Protein, Sodium, Potassium, and Phosphorus, as well as the intake of dietary fibers, and certain carbohydrates, and even go as intensive as involving the food preparation process to ensure that the patient only gets the preventative benefits from his/her diet.

How This Book Can Help

This is not another recipe book where you will find suggestions for your next meal. *(But I'll sure to indulge you in some recipes as we move along).* In the next few chapters, you will discover in-depth but practically applicable knowledge on how you can take an even better approach to managing your kidney disease.

From understanding the connection of diet and how it works in CKD, to learning by heart the ins and outs of nutritional modification, to handling special occasions and creating a holistically balanced wellness involving your mind and body, through exercise and stress management.

However, if you are reading this for a family or friend, this book will equip you with the right knowledge to effectively assist your loved ones and even pass the knowledge forward to whoever might need it in the future.

This book is written based on recent research and personal experiences of working with CKD Patients for the past 10 years. Thus, I too am convinced, that this book will help you in battling with CKD as with everyone who are with you in this journey.

Understanding CKD

Before we take that plunge into the amazing world of CKD management through diet, let's first do a quick recap of what this is we are dealing with in the first place.

Knowing Your CKD Stage.

You might have heard a couple dozen times, that CKD management does not come in a one-size-fits-all solution, and rightly so due to the diversity of the factors that need to be considered e.g. age, weight, lifestyle, and so on. But one thing that makes the deal here is when you understand your diagnosis to the nines, so you have a better grasp in making informed decisions about your health. Let's get to know YOU a little better, so we can both begin this journey already knowing important things for your CKD Stage.

What CKD Stage are you diagnosed in?

_____

So here's what you need to know:

An eGFR between 30 and 59 ml/min indicates that there's some damage to the kidneys and they; are not working as well as they should. As a result, you are more likely to have health complications such as high blood pressure, anemia, and bone disease.

But did you know that Stage 3 is divided into 2 stages?

Stage 3a means that you have an eGFR between 45-59 ml/min, while stage 3b means that you have an eGFR between 30 and 44 ml/min.

Symptoms might be already present at this stage, such as:

- Fatigue
- Fluid retention, swelling (edema) of extremities and shortness of breath:
- Urination changes (foamy; dark orange, brown, tea-colored or red if it contains blood; and urinating more or less than normal)
- Kidney pain felt in your back - Sleep problems due to muscle cramps or restless legs

To keep your kidneys from getting worse, you need to switch to a kidney-friendly diet that consists of:

- Limiting your nutrient intake such as sodium, protein, phosphorus, potassium, and calcium.

- Consuming some grains, fruits and vegetables (potassium and phosphorus are at normal levels).
- Cutting back carbohydrates (if you have diabetes).
- Decreasing saturated fats to help lower cholesterol.
- Take in prescribed medication from your doctor.

Disease Progression and Options

Now, as the CKD progresses, here are the following symptoms that are usually experienced at stage 4:

- Fatigue
- Fluid retention
- Urination changes (foamy; dark orange, brown, tea-colored or red if it contains blood; and urinating more or less than normal)
- Kidney pain felt in your back
- Sleep problems due to muscle cramps or restless legs
- Nausea
- Metallic taste in mouth
- Loss of appetite
- Numbness or tingling in the toes or fingers

Also known as **End Stage Kidney Disease (ESKD)**, the kidneys have already lost their ability to do their job effectively and treatment options such as hemodialysis, peritoneal dialysis, or kidney transplantation is needed to live.

Once you begin your treatment (depending on what you choose), your diet will continue to be a very big part of your treatment. Some of this would include:

- Including grains, fruits and vegetables, but limiting or avoiding whole grains and certain fruits and vegetables that are high in phosphorus or potassium
- A diet that is low in saturated fat and cholesterol and moderate in total fats, especially if cholesterol is high or if you have diabetes or heart disease
- Limiting intake of refined and processed foods high in sodium and prepare foods with less salt or high-sodium ingredients

- Limiting fluid intake

Now, I know what you're thinking..."It's a lot of information to take in." That is just a very quick run-through of what you are about to learn. Don't worry as I will break them down carefully for you in the coming chapters.

Importance of Early Intervention

When patients come to me, most of them feel they are alone in dealing with their kidney condition. They become so caught up in this belief that when you tell them how they can take action to manage their condition, it somehow reinforces that idea even more... And I understand that...

Because in the beginning, when the news was given to you, you likely found yourself in a state of shock.

Many kidney patients find it hard to believe that what the doctor is saying is true. It feels so unlikely, too overwhelming. It becomes difficult to comprehend what chronic kidney damage is, because not a lot of people talk about it like they do with diabetes or heart attack.

"No, it is not true, it will not be that bad", says your mind. This is a very normal defense mechanism: denial. But, the most important thing for you to know - in this moment - **is that taking proactive steps now may slow down your kidney disease.** Which is one of the reasons why you picked up this book, right? And as long as you're here, I'll show you the ropes little by little so that in due time, you'll be able **to learn how to do it yourself**

Studies have shown that **patients** who are actively engaged in their health and care experience better health outcomes. You can start with your lab test results. Which reminds me, have you had your lab tests done recently? Because if you have, you can use your new found knowledge to get a better picture of your overall health.

Your test results are a way **to assess the progression of your kidney condition**. For example, by keeping track of your serum creatinine or eGFR, you'll have a clearer idea of the state of your kidneys.

Now that makes it sound a bit intimidating, but trust me, it isn't hard to do once you know what to keep track of. And self-monitoring is one way to achieve that.

Okay, okay, what exactly is self-monitoring?

Self-monitoring emphasizes how YOU are part of your own healthcare team. In terms of your kidney health, self-monitoring means noting down two important categories:

1. **Your test results**, and,
2. **Your lifestyle**, which includes your diet and exercise habits, among others (we'll be talking more about these soon in the coming chapters!)

It's a simple solution, but it works. And the experts know it:

- Researchers agree that self-monitoring (or self-management) is associated with positive patient outcomes, and that fostering this behavior can **have long-term positive effects.**
- Patients in a self-monitoring program enjoyed more health benefits than those who didn't. This includes **fewer hospitalizations, feeling healthier, and being more active, among others.**
- Guidelines by psychologists include encouraging self-monitoring among chronic kidney disease patients, **to better help them accept and deal with their condition.**

Importance of Age-Based Diet

Age and Metabolism

While anybody can benefit from this book, I did mention that CKD management is diversified by many factors, and I have particularly paid close attention to the 50+ patients who I have had most experience with over the years.

Now, since diet has a direct relationship with your metabolism, let's talk about it for a while as it relates to age as well. Metabolism refers to all the physical and chemical processes in the body that convert or use energy, such as breathing, circulating blood, controlling body temperature, cell growth, brain and nerve function, and contraction

of muscles. The rate at which these processes occur is known as metabolic rate.

There is a connection between age and metabolism. Here are some key points:

1. **Basal Metabolic Rate (BMR)**: Your BMR is the number of calories your body needs to perform basic functions, like breathing and digestion. As we age, our BMR generally decreases. This decrease is typically due to loss of lean body mass (muscle), which is metabolically active.
2. **Muscle Mass Decline**: As we age, we naturally lose muscle mass, a process known as sarcopenia. This process generally starts in our 30s and continues as we age, accelerating particularly after age 50. Because muscle tissue burns more calories than fat tissue, our metabolism slows as our muscle mass decreases.
3. **Physical Activity**: In general, physical activity decreases as people age. This decrease in activity contributes to a lower metabolic rate and can lead to weight gain if calorie intake isn't adjusted to match the lower energy expenditure.
4. **Hormonal Changes**: As we age, our bodies undergo various hormonal changes. In women, menopause causes significant hormonal changes that can slow metabolism. In men, testosterone levels slowly decrease, which can lead to a decrease in muscle mass and a slower metabolism.
5. **Cellular Aging**: At the cellular level, aging is associated with a decrease in the number of mitochondria, which are the "powerhouses" of cells where metabolic processes occur. This decrease can also contribute to a slower metabolism.

In short, as we age, our metabolism tends to slow down due to factors like loss of muscle mass, decreased physical activity, hormonal changes, and cellular aging. However, lifestyle interventions such as regular physical exercise and maintaining a healthy diet can help counter the effects of aging on metabolism. Add a Chronic Kidney Disease diagnosis in the mix, you would all the more want your metabolism to be at its best, to get the optimum results on the dietary interventions that we will be putting into practice for your kidney health.

Nutritional Needs of the 50+ Age Group

Furthermore, our bodies also undergo various physiological changes that influence our nutritional needs. While calorie needs may decrease due to a slower metabolism and less physical activity, the need for certain nutrients may increase. Here is a guide to some of the nutritional needs for individuals aged 50 and above:

1. **Protein**: During aging, there's often a loss of muscle mass. To help counteract this, older adults might need more protein than their younger counterparts. The recommended dietary allowance (RDA) for protein is 46 grams per day for women and 56 grams per day for men.
2. **Fiber**: Fiber can help reduce the risk of heart disease and type 2 diabetes, which are more common in older adults. It can also help prevent constipation, a common problem in older people. Men over 50 should aim for 30 grams of fiber per day, and women should aim for 21 grams.

3. **Vitamins and Minerals:**
   - Vitamin B12: With aging, some people lose the ability to absorb vitamin B12 from food. This vitamin is important for creating red blood cells and maintaining nerve function. People over 50 should get most of their vitamin B12 from fortified foods or dietary supplements.
   - Calcium and Vitamin D: These are crucial for bone health. With age, the skin becomes less efficient at synthesizing vitamin D, and the kidneys are less able to convert it to its active form.

Thus, older adults may need to get more of these nutrients through diet or supplements.
- Potassium: Increasing potassium intake along with reducing sodium (salt) may lower blood pressure and reduce the risk of developing kidney stones and bone loss.

4. **Hydration:** As we age, our sense of thirst may not be as sharp. This can lead to dehydration. It's important for older adults to drink water regularly, even if they don't feel thirsty.
5. **Healthy Fats**: Heart health becomes increasingly important as we age. Opting for healthy fats, such as those found in avocados, nuts, seeds, and fish, can help maintain heart health.
6. **Limited Sodium**: To help control blood pressure, it's recommended that adults over 50 limit their sodium intake to 2,300 mg per day.

That was quite a foretaste of the rich journey on CKD dieting that we will be embarking in the chapters of this book. See you in the next chapter as we begin to talk about the connection between CKD and food.

Chapter 1:

The CKD-Diet Connection

Chronic kidney disease (CKD) is a major public health burden, with a global prevalence of ~ 11% in the general adult population. If left untreated, CKD slowly progresses to end-stage renal disease, which requires dialysis or kidney transplant. CKD is bidirectionally associated with cardiovascular diseases (CVD). Hypertension and type 2 diabetes mellitus (T2DM) are independent risk factors for CKD, and their global prevalences are increasing, which will likely impact CKD. Worldwide, a 31.7% increase in CKD mortality was observed over the last decade.

What Does Food Do to Your Kidneys?

As you may have known by now, our kidneys are vital organs within our body, performing a plethora of tasks that help maintain equilibrium within our body. Among their significant roles is the processing of various nutrients from the food we consume. Allow me to bore you a bit with a quick review of how the kidneys manage different types of nutrients in our body, I promise you this will be significant later on:

Water

The kidneys play a crucial role in maintaining the body's water balance. After the body utilizes the necessary water for its various metabolic processes, the excess is eliminated through the kidneys as urine. This process is regulated by a hormone called antidiuretic hormone (ADH), which increases the water reabsorption in the kidneys, and aldosterone, which conserves sodium and eliminates potassium.

Electrolytes

Kidneys balance the levels of several important electrolytes in the body, including sodium, potassium, calcium, and phosphate. Sodium and potassium levels are particularly critical. For example, aldosterone, a hormone secreted by the adrenal glands, signals the kidneys to retain sodium and water and excrete potassium, thus helping to maintain electrolyte balance.

Proteins

Typically, proteins are not excreted in the urine because they are large molecules and cannot pass through the glomerulus during filtration. However, the kidneys do play a role in metabolizing proteins. They help to extract excess amino acids and other byproducts of protein metabolism (like urea) from the blood and excrete them in urine.

Carbohydrates

After carbohydrates are broken down into glucose in the digestive system, the kidneys help reabsorb glucose back into the bloodstream. The kidneys also have a minor role in gluconeogenesis - the production of new glucose.

Fats

The kidneys do not play a major role in processing fats. However, they can be affected by a high-fat diet, which can lead to kidney disease over time.

Vitamins and Minerals

The kidneys help maintain the balance of many vitamins and minerals in the body. For example, they help regulate levels of vitamin D and calcium - the kidneys convert vitamin D from supplements or the sun to its active form in the body, which helps regulate calcium and phosphate levels.

Please remember that this is a simplified overview. The actual processes involve complex biochemical and physiological mechanisms. It's also important to note that while kidneys are very efficient at their jobs, they can be damaged by poor nutrition, high blood pressure, diabetes, and other health conditions. Therefore, maintaining a healthy diet and lifestyle is crucial for kidney health.

The Impact of Overworking Your Kidneys

Now when we err to the side of being nonchalant about taking care of our kidney health by probably taking excessive protein, high sugar consumption, poor fluid intake just to name a few, we overwork our kidneys, also known as kidney overload which now leads to several adverse health effects, which collectively or on its own progress into Severe Kidney Damage, Chronic Kidney Disease, and worst End Stage Renal Disease:

Proteinuria

When kidneys are overworked, they may allow some proteins to pass through their filters into the urine, a condition known as proteinuria. This can be an early sign of kidney damage.

High Blood Pressure

The kidneys play a crucial role in regulating blood pressure by balancing fluid levels and releasing hormones that control blood pressure. Overworking kidneys can disrupt these processes, leading to high blood pressure, which can further damage the kidneys.

Electrolyte Imbalances

Kidneys are responsible for balancing various electrolytes in the body. Overworking the kidneys can lead to imbalances in electrolytes, such as potassium, calcium, and phosphate, which can affect multiple body functions.

Kidney Stones

Overworking the kidneys, especially due to high protein diets or dehydration, can lead to the formation of kidney stones. These are hard deposits of minerals and salts that form inside your kidneys.

Kidney Infections

Overworked kidneys may not effectively remove waste and toxins from the body, potentially leading to infections.

Edema

The kidneys also remove excess fluid from the body. If they are overworked and unable to efficiently perform this task, fluid can build up leading to edema (swelling), particularly in the legs, ankles, and feet.

Foods That Put Extra Strain on Your Kidneys

While some of the causes of kidney damage are linked to certain disease conditions, even these, at the very root can be traced back to food and nutrition. Certain foods can put extra strain on the kidneys, particularly when consumed in excess. These include:

High-Sodium Foods

Too much sodium can cause the kidneys to work harder and can also lead to high blood pressure, which can damage the kidneys over time. Processed foods tend to be especially high in sodium.

High-Protein Foods

While protein is an essential part of a balanced diet, eating excessive amounts of animal protein (like red meat) can strain the kidneys. This is because metabolizing protein produces a waste product called urea that the kidneys must filter out.

High-Potassium Foods

Kidneys help balance potassium levels in the body. If your kidneys are not functioning properly, consuming foods high in potassium can cause levels to build up in your blood.

High-Phosphorus Foods

Similar to potassium, kidneys also manage the balance of phosphorus in your body. High levels of phosphorus, often found in processed foods and sodas, can be harmful to kidneys, especially for those with kidney disease.

Artificial Sweeteners

Some studies suggest that consuming large amounts of artificial sweeteners may increase the risk of kidney function decline.

Carbonated Beverages

Drinks like soda are often high in phosphorus additives and sugars, which can put additional strain on the kidneys.

How Diet Can Slow CKD Progression

We have fairly established that diet and nutrition play a very big role in causing and worsening kidney damage, however, there's also truth in the saying "Your poison can also be your medicine".

A study on The Effect of Diet on the Survival of Patients with Chronic Kidney Disease *assessed the association between four lifestyle factors (diet, physical activity, body mass index—BMI, and smoking) with all-cause mortality among CKD participants. It demonstrated that individuals in the highest quartile of the weighted healthy lifestyle score had a 53% lower risk of death compared with those in the lowest quartile.*

You **NEED** to make changes to your diet when you have Chronic Kidney Disease.

The truth is, the renal diet is not easy to understand at first glance because it is NOT intuitive. Broccoli is a "YES", but Spinach "NOT TOO MUCH"... But they're both green vegetables? You have probably started searching for information on your own and found conflicting information on what foods you can eat and avoid.

These changes may include limiting your Sodium, Potassium, Protein, and Phosphorus (also known as your SPPP) to keep them below dangerous levels. So, what should you do?

Now, how come Renal Diet is not intuitive? It's because depending on your lab test results and your nutritionist's expert recommendation, you may need to restrict ALL of SPPP or only one of those nutrients. This would then change what food you can eat and what food you should avoid. This is why it's important to start by finding out what restriction applies to you. With how much thought goes into it, you should also begin to think of your diet as part of your treatment.

What do we mean by thinking of diet as treatment?
Does that mean I shouldn't take medication from my MD?

CKD Chef Duane Sunwold shares...

"*A colleague at Spokane Community College, my friend Erin, a Registered Dietitian, asked to see my labs and challenged to take me off animal protein for 90 days. It wasn't easy, but it was the best thing I could have ever done. Within two weeks, I started feeling better. Who knew, Kevin and Karl [referring to his kidneys] like plants, and they started doing their job again.*

And in no time, I began to review my new kidney-friendly recipes healthy eating plan as the greatest culinary challenge a chef could have.

As time went by, this new plant-based cuisine brought my creatinine level from 4.99 to a 0.8. Today, I'm in complete remission. **And I'm off all medication, with the blessing of my medical team, thanks to my diet.**

Taking control by making the necessary diet and lifestyle changes recommended by your medical team is part of self-management. But, don't forget that this is meant to COMPLEMENT your medical team's recommendations, not REPLACE them."

The Connection Between Diet and Dialysis

There is a long history linked between diet and dialysis and one study even divided these periods in history as different eras.

For a time, Potassium played a role in making or breaking the deal for a dialysis patient. The focus of this adjunct therapy to dialysis is the avoidance of high-potassium foods, putting lesser emphasis on giving plant-derived proteins that caused an imbalance in another nutrient's capacity to help in slowing disease progression.

Sodium has always been on the low as it's been earlier identified, to cause excessive thirst, thereby paving the way for increased fluid intake and overload.

Then, Phosphorus followed suit in the second era, where phosphate had been almost banned from a patient's diet and had been linked to a rising mortality rate.

When things weren't adding up, and dialysis had been failing, thanks to these extreme measures in nutrition, the biggest hurdle became malnutrition. Restricting almost all nutrients was by far the worst decision that has ever been made.

These scenarios should allow you to paint a better picture of the relationship between Diet and Chronic Kidney Disease where it's not just about limiting some and increasing some, but a well-thought-off treatment plan that revolves around your diet and nutrition.

Research on Diet and CKD

A review of more than 20 prospective cohort studies by A.C. van Westing et. al. of the Division of Human Nutrition and Health, Wageningen University focused on meat, fish, dairy, vegetables, fruit, coffee, tea, soft drinks, and dietary patterns, revealed convincing evidence that following a healthy dietary pattern increases the chances of lowering risks for Chronic Kidney Disease.

The study revealed benefits from plant-based food options and beverages e.g. coffee and some dairy. The components of unhealthy dieting that add stress to the kidneys were also identified to include red meats (especially processed ones) and sugar-sweetened beverages. Some other food groups included in the studies came back with inconclusive results, such as being neutral, but should not be automatically ruled out to be beneficial as there might be not enough evidence to conclude from.

The Importance of Controlling Blood Sugar and Blood Pressure

1. Control your blood pressure

I may have mentioned that your blood pressure is determined by **what you eat** and that you have to lower your SPPP intake to manage your blood pressure. For now, **the most important one is sodium.**

A huge portion of sodium in our diets comes from packaged and processed foods. And take note that your recommended daily sodium intake should be no less than 2,000 milligrams.

Aside from high blood pressure, a high sodium diet can result in other complication including:

- Swelling in the legs, and face.
- Heart failure
- Shortness of breath: Fluid can build up in the lungs which causes breathing problems.

Since **your target blood pressure should be lower than 130/80 mmHg,** lowering your sodium intake will improve your blood pressure. An additional reason to be good about sodium? Blood pressure medication becomes more effective when sodium levels are normal.

2. Manage your blood sugar levels

To prevent or slow down kidney damage, you have to keep your blood sugar controlled. It's usually done with diet, exercise, and taking insulin *(if needed)* or hypoglycemic pills *(helps lower your blood sugar level).*

Being keen with the amount of sugar present in your food and beverages will really help make sure you don't damage your kidneys further and keep yourself at lower risk for developing diabetic kidney disease. Be deliberate in adjusting your sugar intake, may it be keeping yourself from adding more teaspoons of it in your coffee, indulging in that luscious devil's food cake, or even controlling your portions with that sweet juicy mango.

Renal Dieting may not be intuitive, but it doesn't mean it has to be impossible. Follow along in the next chapter as we explore the basics and the "what you can do" areas for CKD-Friendly Diet.

Chapter 2:

The Basics of a CKD-Friendly Diet

Scientific consensus underscores that dietary modifications can significantly affect Chronic Kidney Disease (CKD) progression.

Optimal nutrition—emphasizing a low-protein, low-sodium, and high-fiber diet—has been shown to decelerate kidney function decline. Such dietary shifts not only support kidney health, but also mitigate associated risks like hypertension and diabetes. Therefore, bridging the knowledge gap in dietary management is critical for improving CKD outcomes.

What Makes a Diet CKD-Friendly?

As a general rule, anything that does not stress the kidneys, allowing them to function to their best, and making you feel great inside and out defines something as CKD-friendly. But that sure is too broad isn't it?

This question ultimately led me down the rabbit hole, as you may already know, conflicting information may be available just about everywhere, making this more complicated than it already is. But to make sure you don't go through the same, I have validated a working definition for a "CKD-Friendly Diet" through my personal experience with patients, and through digging deep into countless evidence-based studies over the years. Here it goes:

A CKD-Friendly diet should be one that slows down the progression of the disease to kidney failure. It should show clear signs of improving toxicity in the blood test results. It must help the patient maintain a favorable and sustainable nutritional status and should decrease the risk of any possible secondary complications.

The Role of Macronutrients and Micronutrients

Macronutrients are the nutrients we need in large amounts: proteins, carbohydrates, and fats. They're the main source of energy for our bodies. Let's take a closer look at how these macronutrients influence our health and our kidneys.

Proteins

Proteins are important for repairing and building tissues, but people with chronic kidney disease (CKD) should be careful about their intake. When our bodies use protein, they produce a waste product called urea. Healthy kidneys can remove this, but in CKD, it can build up in the blood and cause symptoms like fatigue and loss of appetite. Most guidelines suggest a low to moderate protein diet for CKD patients.

Carbohydrates

These provide our bodies with energy. People with CKD should focus on complex carbs (like whole grains and fruits) instead of simple ones (like sugar). However, those on dialysis may need extra carbs to balance the energy used during treatment.

Fats

Not all fats are bad. Healthy fats (like those in olive oil, avocados, and certain fish) may help reduce inflammation and improve heart health, which is particularly important for CKD patients.

Now let's also talk about micronutrients which includes vitamins and minerals. They are needed in smaller amounts, but they're still very important. Here are some of the micronutrients that are very relevant to Chronic Kidney Disease.

Sodium

In Chronic Kidney Disease (CKD), the kidneys struggle to balance sodium levels. Consuming too much sodium can cause fluid retention, leading to higher blood pressure and further kidney damage. It might also increase proteinuria, a key marker of CKD progression. Therefore, a diet low in sodium is often recommended for those with CKD to help manage blood pressure and prevent further deterioration of kidney function.

Potassium

Our bodies need potassium for nerve and muscle cell functioning, including for the heart. But in CKD, the kidneys may not be able to remove excess potassium, leading to high levels in the blood. This can be dangerous for the heart. Hence, potassium intake often needs to be limited.

Phosphorus

Phosphorus helps build strong bones and teeth, but in CKD, the kidneys can't excrete excess phosphorus, leading to high levels in the blood. This can cause bone and heart problems.

Vitamin D

It's important for bone health and the immune system. Yet, CKD often leads to vitamin D deficiency because the kidneys play a key role in activating vitamin D. Therefore, patients often need supplements.

Remember, every person is different, and dietary needs can vary greatly among people with CKD. It's crucial to work closely with your healthcare team to create a diet plan that's right for you.

Importance of Individual Dietary Requirements

From the beginning, I cannot emphasize enough the fact that CKD care and the management of it is not generic, and that every patient's general wellbeing should be the top basis of their individualized care.

The same is true with renal diet, as we have established that it is part of your treatment plan. Now you may ask, "what is the importance of individual's dietary requirements?" That's a great question! Individual dietary requirements are important because they take into account a person's unique needs and circumstances. Here's why this matters, especially for people with chronic kidney disease (CKD).

1. Stage of CKD

Different stages of CKD require different dietary adjustments. For example, in early stages, you may only need to watch your protein intake, but in later stages, you might need to limit nutrients like potassium and phosphorus too.

2. Other Health Conditions

Many people with CKD also have other health conditions like diabetes or heart disease. These conditions often require different or additional dietary modifications.

3. Nutritional Status

People with CKD are at risk of malnutrition. They need a diet that ensures they get enough calories and nutrients to stay healthy, but doesn't overload their kidneys. This balance can be tricky and depends on factors like age, sex, weight, and physical activity level.

4. Personal Preferences and Lifestyle

A person's cultural background, personal tastes, and lifestyle also play a big role. A diet that doesn't consider these factors may be hard to stick to and could lower the quality of life.

5. Treatment Plan

People on dialysis have different dietary needs than those who aren't. For example, dialysis patients often need more protein to compensate for losses during treatment.

Because of all these factors, it's crucial to work with a dietitian or healthcare provider to create a personalized eating plan. This plan should meet your nutritional needs, be realistic for your lifestyle, and accommodate your personal preferences.

Remember, managing CKD isn't just about avoiding certain foods. It's about creating a healthy, enjoyable diet that supports your overall well-being. And that's best achieved when the diet is tailored to you!

The Role of Different Food Groups

Proteins: Animal vs. Plant-Based

Does switching to a plant-based diet help?

Protein could be tricky for Chronic Kidney Disease patients. While it may be one of the essential nutrients for a healthy, normal kidney, too much protein is bad for a malfunctioning one. A plant-based diet is **beneficial if you have early kidney disease.** Plant-based foods have fewer calories compared to their animal-based counterpart and are beneficial if you have early kidney disease.

A plant-based diet helps lower blood pressure and cholesterol thereby reducing heart-related diseases. It also improves antioxidant levels that fight against cell damage. Minimizing animal-based food lowers acid buildup in the blood, which puts less stress on the kidneys.

It is recommended to eat just small portions of protein foods that may be sourced from animals, e.g. chicken, fish, meat, eggs, and dairy, and from plants, e.g. beans, nuts, and grains.

Recommended sources of proteins for CKD patients include fish, chicken breast, low-fat soy products, and low-fat dairy products.

Be sure to talk to your dietitian to get the specific amount of protein that your body—especially your kidney—needs.

Animal-protein foods

- Meat, such as pork, beef, chicken, turkey, duck
- Eggs
- Dairy products, such as milk, yogurt, cheese
- Fish

Plant-protein foods

High protein

- Beans, peas, lentils

- Soy foods, such as soy milk, tofu
- Nuts and nut spreads, such as almond butter, peanut butter, soy nut butter
- Sunflower seeds

Low protein

- Bread, tortillas
- Oatmeal, grits, cereals
- Pasta, noodles, rice
- Rice milk (not enriched)

TINY HABIT 1. After I know my recommended protein intake, I will integrate a plant-based substitute to my kidney diet.

But what if I'm not ready to make that switch yet?

If you don't like to prepare or cook them at all, CKD Chef Duane suggested that you can fill half your plate with fruits and vegetables. Quarter the other half into starch, rice, and pasta. While the other quarter is protein.

And when you go grocery shopping, you go through and look at the meat section and pick your meal. CKD Chef Duane thinks it's such a creative way to live when he went through the produce section.

But more importantly, you need to plan your meals ahead of time. In your meal planning, you can implement things like beans, lentils, portobello mushroom, or tofu as a great protein source of your diet.

Yes, I know that most people probably don't like the texture or the taste of tofu. BUT you can get creative with some great tasting tofu recipes.

Here's another, you can take cashew nuts, soak them in hot water, and then drain them. Once you're done, you can puree them in your tofu in a food processor, which results in a thick texture. And yes, you can season it anyway you like. You can do a southwest flavor or you can use italian herbs and make them into a stuffing like zucchini boats or pasta shells.

And if you're having trouble figuring out what recipes you would like to prepare, Northwest Kidney Center has shared some of its recipes to help you.

As for timing like that souffle, plan ahead; **people who plan ahead almost always make a healthier choice than those we make because we don't have enough time.**

The Right Kind of Carbohydrates

Now, time to talk about the other nutrient factors to consider: **fat and sugar (carbohydrates).**

Earlier in this chapter, we touched the basics of macronutrients or the three (3) major nutrients found in foods: Protein, carbohydrates, and fat. Carbohydrates are a **major fuel source for your body.**

When you eat carbohydrates, your body turns them into glucose *(the energy source for the cells in the body)*. With insulin, cells are able to use that energy to perform everyday functions and help you feel your best. Besides providing energy for your body, foods that are rich in carbohydrates are good sources of vitamins, minerals, fiber, and other compounds that help protect your body. Some carbohydrate foods actually contain fiber. Fiber plays an important role in protecting your heart, blood vessels, and colon.

As I may have previously mentioned a couple of times, once you are diagnosed with Chronic Kidney Disease, you are at risk of having health complications like heart disease, which is the leading cause of death, especially in dialysis patients.

So, high fiber diets will help lower your cholesterol levels and reduce your risk for heart attack and other cardiovascular conditions. You need to ask your dietitian which high fiber foods may work in your kidney diet. But for now, I want to share with you how CKD Chef Duane did it.

Since CKD Chef Duane finds sugar addictive, the more he uses it, the more he craves it, he stopped himself from that cycle by slowly weaning himself down. **He uses and eats fresh fruits as much as possible for dessert.** A trick he learned from a clever chef in Scottsdale is that he would make smaller protein portions and give the customers larger portions of fresh fruit for dessert.

"The flavors eaten during the last course are the ones that stay on our palates the longest", he said. So, when he applied what he learned, he didn't feel deprived of the foods that he likes.

The Importance of Healthy Fats

Let's move on to fat...

For fat, it also provides energy and helps produce hormones that regulate blood pressure and other heart functions and carries fat-soluble vitamins. But it's also important to know about fat sources because eating the wrong kinds and too much of **it increases the risk of clogged vessels and heart problems.**

You should talk to a dietitian about healthy and unhealthy sources of fat since for example, there are saturated fats and trans-fatty acids like red meat, poultry, whole milk, and butter could raise blood cholesterol levels and clog blood vessels. He or she can suggest healthy ways to include fat in the diet especially if your diet needs more calories. Vegetable oils such as corn or safflower oil are healthier than animal fats such as butter or lard.

But then again, you **should speak to your dietitian** before moving forward. However, CKD Chef Duane took as much fat from recipes as he could without giving up his goal of keeping the flavor in.

How? He uses vegetable stock in place of salad oils when making salad dressings. Another gifted chef instructor at his culinary school taught him that technique.

Fluids and CKD - Hydration and Fluid Restrictions

Hydration is important for everyone, but it can be a delicate balance for people with chronic kidney disease (CKD). Here's why:

The kidneys' job is to filter waste products from the blood and regulate fluids in the body. When they're not working well, they can't remove excess fluid. This excess fluid can build up in the body, a condition called fluid overload, which can cause problems like:

- High blood pressure, where extra fluid increases the volume of blood in your veins and arteries, raising your blood pressure.
- Swelling. You might notice it in your legs, ankles, or hands. This is called edema.
- Shortness of breath. Again, fluid can accumulate in the lungs, making it hard to breathe.

Because of these risks, people with advanced CKD or those on dialysis often need to limit their fluid intake. However, the amount of fluid restriction can vary significantly from person to person. It depends on factors like the stage of CKD, urine output, whether the person is on dialysis and the type of dialysis they're receiving.

On the other hand, it's also important to avoid dehydration, which can happen if you don't drink enough water. Dehydration can cause headaches, and dizziness, and in severe cases, can further damage the kidneys.

Remember, "fluid" doesn't just refer to water. It includes anything that turns into liquid at room temperature, like ice cream, gelatin, and soup, as well as beverages like coffee, tea, and soda. And because managing fluid intake can be complex in CKD, it's essential to work closely with your healthcare team who can help you figure out the right balance for your unique situation.

Choosing the Right Beverages

Certainly, choosing the right kind of beverage when you have CKD involves a few considerations. Here are some tips to guide you:

1. **Avoid high-potassium drinks.** Some beverages, like orange juice and tomato juice, are high in potassium, which can be dangerous in CKD. A safer choice might be apple juice or cranberry juice, which are lower in potassium.
2. **Limit high-phosphorus drinks.** Dark-colored sodas often contain phosphorus additives, which can be harmful for people with

CKD. Instead, choose light-colored or clear sodas, like lemon-lime soda or ginger ale.

3. **Watch out for caffeine and alcohol**. Both can dehydrate you, so it's important to consume them in moderation. Water, herbal tea, or decaffeinated coffee can be good alternatives.
4. **Stay away from high-sodium drinks.** Some vegetable juices and canned soups can be high in sodium. Look for low-sodium versions or make your own at home.
5. **Be mindful of fluids in foods.** Remember, foods that are liquid at room temperature, like ice cream and gelatin, count towards your fluid intake.
6. **Water is always a good choice.** But remember to keep track of how much you drink, especially if you've been advised to limit your fluid intake.

Remember, these are general guidelines. The best beverage for you will depend on your individual circumstances, including your stage of CKD, any other health conditions, and your personal preferences. Always check with your healthcare team or dietitian to make sure your choices fit within your dietary plan.

Having learned of the "basics", the science, and the important foundational truths about the CKD diet, I would like to take you more into what it means to apply it to your lifestyle. I will be teaching more "TINY HABITS" that you can do in order to start incorporating changes into your diet and really get into that journey of making that positive change toward health.

Chapter 3:

The Role of Protein, Potassium, Phosphorus, and Sodium in CKD

Understanding the impact of these nutrients on chronic kidney disease (CKD) progression can be quite surprising. Here's a fact about each nutrient and its relationship to CKD:

Sodium
A study found that people with CKD who consumed high-sodium diets had twice the risk of progressing to end stage renal disease. This shows how a high-sodium diet can accelerate the progression of CKD.

Protein
Research suggests that a low-protein diet can slow the progression of CKD and reduce the symptoms. In one study, a low-protein diet reduced the risk of kidney failure by 32%.

Potassium
While it is important to avoid high potassium levels (hyperkalemia) in CKD, it's also crucial not to have too low levels (hypokalemia). A study found that both hyperkalemia and hypokalemia are associated with an increased risk of death in people with CKD.

Phosphorus
High phosphorus levels can lead to serious health problems, including heart disease, bone disease, and even death. Surprisingly, even within the "normal" range, higher phosphorus levels can be harmful. A study

found a 27% higher risk of death in CKD patients with phosphorus levels at the high end of the normal range, compared to those at the low end.

These statistics underline how important it is to manage these nutrients in your diet when you have CKD. As always, the best way to do this is by working closely with your healthcare team.

Protein and CKD

Let's start by making one thing clear: **protein is good for you.**

Without protein, your body won't function the way it's supposed to. It's needed for most bodily processes, especially for growth, maintenance, and repair. It also plays a major role in building up muscle and fighting infection.

But here's the catch— Whenever your body breaks down protein from food, a waste product called urea is produced. High levels of urea can cause fatigue and poor appetite. Too much protein in the body can also cause a buildup of creatinine, another by-product of metabolism as protein is used up. Creatinine, whether you're aware or not, is one of the key determinants of kidney damage.

Your kidneys work to remove these by-products from your system. That means, *the more protein you eat, the more work your kidneys have to do. A*nd that's basically the reason why **a low-protein diet** may be recommended by your nutritionist. Give your kidneys a lighter workload. This will help you slow down your kidney's deterioration, if not maintain the level of kidney function you still have.

Now that you understand why it's important to control your protein intake, let's explore the **how.**

We were able to discuss the importance of protein and the negative effects it can have on your kidneys, but this chapter will focus on the causes of too much protein in the urine *(proteinuria)*, what lab tests should be done, and what the next step is.

Protein is needed for most bodily processes, especially for growth, maintenance, and repair. It also plays a major role in building up muscle and fighting infection. Without protein, your body won't function the way it's supposed to. When healthy kidneys filter fluid, minerals, and wastes from the blood, they usually do not allow large amounts of serum protein to escape into the urine.

But when the kidneys are not filtering properly, protein in urine *(proteinuria)* **can occur**. For this reason, an abnormal amount of protein is then present in the urine. Having too much protein in the urine is not good for the kidneys because it's a sign of kidneys damage AND can scar the kidney because your kidneys are not able to remove all the extra waste. In most cases, proteinuria has no symptoms but if kidney damage gets worse and large amounts of protein escape from your blood through your urine, you may notice the following symptoms:

- Foamy or bubbly pee
- Swelling (edema) in your hands, feet, belly, and face
- Peeing more often
- Shortness of breath
- Fatigue
- Loss of appetite
- Upset stomach and vomiting
- Muscle cramps at night

What causes proteinuria?

There are actually a few causes to proteinuria, so be sure to take note of your other symptoms that will help your doctor **identify the underlying cause**:

1. **Dehydration** - This happens when your body loses too much fluid. Your body uses water to deliver nutrients, like proteins to the kidneys but without enough fluid, it will have difficulty doing so. In turn, the kidneys can't properly recapture proteins. It ends up in the urine instead.
2. **High Blood Pressure** - High blood pressure *(hypertension)* can weaken the blood vessels in the kidneys. This decreases their ability to reabsorb to protein, which flows into the urine.

3. **Diabetes** - With diabetes, high blood sugar forces the kidneys to over filter the blood. This can cause kidney damage, allowing protein to leak into the urine.
4. **Glomerulonephritis** - When glomeruli filter blood, they reabsorb protein. But if they're injured, protein can pass through and enter the urine.
5. **Chronic Kidney Disease** - CKD may cause proteinuria in the early stages, but it usually doesn't cause any noticeable symptoms.
6. **Autoimmune Diseases** - The immune system normally produces antibodies and immunoglobulins that fight foreign organisms. But if you have an autoimmune disease, the immune system makes antibodies and immunoglobulins that attack the body's tissues. These substances are called autoantibodies.

If the autoantibodies injure the glomeruli, inflammation can occur. This leads to kidney damage, and eventually, proteinuria.

What lab tests should be done?

The only way to diagnose proteinuria is through a **urine test,** which measures the amount of protein in your urine. The urine test takes place in a doctor's office. During the procedure, you have to urinate into a specimen cup which the doctor places a dipstick, or a small plastic stick coated with chemicals, into the urine sample.

If your urine has too much protein, **it changes color.** The rest of the urine will be sent to a lab where it will be examined under a microscope. A doctor might also use the following tests to determine what's causing your proteinuria:

- **24-hour urine collection.** In a 24-hour urine test, your urine is collected over 24 hours and sent to a lab.
- **Glomerular Filtration Rate blood test.** This test checks your kidney function.
- **Imaging tests.** You may get an ultrasound or CT Scan, which takes detailed photos of your kidneys and urinary tract.
- **Kidney biopsy.** A sample of your kidney is removed and examined for signs of kidney damage.

Can proteinuria be treated?

So treatment depends on figuring out what caused it. You might not need treatment if proteinuria is mild or lasts only a short time. But it's crucial to treat kidney disease before it leads to kidney failure. Your doctor might prescribe medication, especially if you have diabetes and/or high blood pressure. Most people will take one of two types of blood pressure medicine:

- ACE Inhibitors (angiotensin-converting enzyme inhibitors)
- ARBs (angiotensin receptor blockers)

What should I do next?

If you have temporary or mild proteinuria, you likely won't need treatment. But if you have consistent proteinuria, you'll need to treat the underlying condition. Treatment may include:

- Dietary changes
- Weight loss
- Blood pressure medication
- Diabetes medication
- Dialysis

Protein could be tricky for CKD Patients like yourself. While it may be one of the essential nutrients for a healthy, normal kidney, too much protein is bad for a malfunctioning one.

Take note that all foods contain protein, but there are two general types of sources you can choose from:

- **High-value proteins refers to protein you get from animal sources.**

    These are easier for your body to use, but can also be rich in fat and cholesterol. **They are often also high in phosphorus, so you might have to limit your intake of them.**

- **Low-value proteins refers to protein you get from plant sources**. Vegetables, cereals, beans, bread, rice, and pasta or noodles are some good examples.

To maintain a healthy diet, it's important to strike a good balance between these two.

Since they're usually high in fat, high-value protein should only make up around 70% of your total protein intake. The rest (30%) should come from low-value proteins—so don't forget your grains and vegetables!

TINY HABIT 2: After I pick a high-value protein, I will add a low-value protein to my shopping cart.

Most processed foods are meat. Animal protein produces **high amounts of acid in the blood that can be harmful to the kidneys** and cause acidosis. Acidosis is an illness where malfunctioning kidneys cannot eliminate acid from the body fast enough. Although protein may be needed for growth and repair, your kidney-friendly diet should be supplemented with fruits and vegetables.

Renal dietitians recommend that instead of animal protein from ground beef, shrimp, salmon, tuna, chicken breast, roasted chicken, or their processed versions, plant-based protein (from beans, nuts, or whole grains) or these lower-protein alternatives are preferable:

- Chili con carne
- Beef stew
- Egg substitutes
- Tofu
- Imitation crab meat

TINY HABIT 3: After I decide on a lower-protein alternative, I will apply one of the handy tips listed below.

Controlling your portions is a very handy technique in keeping your protein intake within your limits. Here are some handy tips to get you started:

FOR SANDWICHES:

- Slice your meat very thinly. This way, the flavor is spread out and the portions look larger.

- Cut your bread more thickly. This will help you feel fuller even with less meat.
- Try breads with a more distinct taste, like rye or sourdough, to add more flavor.
- Fill up your sandwich with other ingredients, like lettuce, cucumbers, parsley, alfalfa sprouts, water chestnuts, celery, or even apples, instead of protein sources.

FOR SOUPS:

- Use low protein milk substitutes when cooking cream soups. Or stay away from them altogether.
- Add relatively low protein ingredients like pasta or rice to make your soup more hearty and filling.

FOR MAIN DISHES:

- Have grains and vegetables as the main dish more often, and use high-value proteins like meat as side dishes.
- Eat more kebabs. Add more fruits and vegetables and use smaller pieces of meat.
- Adjust your casserole recipes. Use smaller amounts of protein than the recipe calls for, and increase the starch (pasta or rice) to make up for it.
- Mix protein with rice and pasta often. Pasta with ground meat and fried rice recipes are good examples.
- Chef salads are great for you. Just toss lettuce and fresh veggies with small strips of egg and meat, and you've got a quick and tasty meal.
- Use cheeses with stronger tastes, like Parmesan or Romano. That way, you'll only need a small amount to get a good flavor.
- Increase your servings of pasta, rice, and bread. Cutting down protein from your diet can cause you to eat less calories than usual. Make up for the difference by eating more of these relatively low protein foods.

I know that at this point in the book, it seems like a lot to take in but don't forget that taking this step is important to achieving your kidney health goal.

*"You don't have to see the whole staircase. Just take the **first step**."*

- Martin Luther King Jr.

Potassium's Impact on CKD

Potassium is a fairly common nutrient which can be found in almost any food. It is responsible for **keeping your nerves and muscles healthy** and **maintaining the normal rhythm of your heart beat.** The kidneys help maintain your potassium at normal level. However, if your potassium levels are too high or too low, **it is not good.**

So, *what happens if my potassium levels are too high or too low?*

When the kidneys can no longer remove excess potassium, it only builds up in the body which causes it to rise. Having too much potassium affects the way your heart and muscles work. Therefore, **your heart may beat irregularly**, which in worst cases, **can cause a heart attack.** And if your potassium level is too low *(also known as hyperkalemia),* it can cause **weakness, numbness, and may develop abnormal heart rhythms.**

To avoid these complications, it is important that you **HAVE TO** consult your kidney doctor and nutritionist and work on a plan that will help keep your potassium level in normal range based on what your lab results show.

So, what is the secret to maintaining potassium levels?

The answer: MODERATION.

According to The National Kidney Foundation, the normal amount in a typical healthy American is **3,500 to 4,500 milligrams per day.** For patients with a potassium-restricted diet, they can go as low as **2,000 mg per day.** However, it depends on what your physician or dietitian advises you to take based on your health.

You'll need a blood test to confirm whether your current potassium levels are high or not and you can use these values as a general reference:

Blood Potassium Level (mmol/L)	Description
3.5 – 5.0	your blood potassium level is **normal**
5.1 – 6.0	your blood potassium level is **elevated**
6.0 and above	your blood potassium level is **exceedingly high**

TINY HABIT 4: After I decide on a vegetable/fruit to add to my shopping list, I'll ask my doctor or dietician if it is good for my potassium level

You have to be careful with what you eat, as well as how much, is the most important point in a low-potassium diet. In general, any food that contains more than 200 mg potassium per serving is **high in potassium.** So, you'll have to start watching out for high-potassium foods such as bananas, potatoes, spinach, brussels sprouts, and avocados.

TINY HABIT 5: After I get home from shopping, I will try leaching one of my vegetables

Leaching is a process that helps reduce the potassium content of food. It means that you don't have to give up high potassium vegetables, you just need more time to prepare them. Here's how you can do it:

For beets, carrots, potatoes, sweet potatoes, rutabagas, and winter squash:

1. Peel and place vegetables in cold water (to avoid darkening)
2. Slice into 1/8 inch thick pieces
3. Briefly rinse in warm water
4. Soak in warm water for a minimum of 2 hours. Use ten times the amount of water to the amount of vegetables. For example, 10 cups of water for 1 cup of vegetables.

5. Rinse in warm water again for a few seconds
6. Cook vegetables. Use 5 times the amount of water to the amount of vegetables. For example, 5 cups of water for 1 cup of vegetables.

Now remember, although leaching is an effective process, it only **reduces potassium but DOES NOT eliminate it entirely**.

Potassium and phosphorus may be listed on a label in milligrams or percent daily value (% DV), but they are not required to be on a label. If potassium and phosphorus are not listed, it does not mean that they are not present in that food. Your needs are different from the daily value when you have CKD. If percent daily values for potassium and phosphorus are listed, you can use them to help with your diet.

	Low Potassium	Medium	High	Very high
mg per serving	<100	101-200	201-300	>300
% DV	<3	3-6	6-9	over 9

Ask your dietitian about your potassium needs. Some foods with higher levels may be on your plan if they are good sources of protein. If amounts or percent daily value for potassium are not listed on a food, you can also look at the ingredient list to identify high potassium or phosphorus ingredients. Ingredients are listed from highest to lowest quantity on a food label.

As mentioned, Potassium does not need to be declared on a food label. If it is not listed, it does NOT mean there is no potassium in your food. Your needs are different from the daily value of a person without CKD.

Aside from cooking foods that are low in potassium, you may need to completely stopped drinking fruit and vegetable juice since they can be a high source of digestible potassium. I strongly recommend that you to get a list of high and low potassium foods from your kidney doctor or dietitian.

Now, you won't be able to understand all of these in the first try, but with practice, it will become part of your routine.

Sodium and CKD

In the right amounts, sodium is actually an important part of one's diet. Our bodies need this mineral in order to:

- Keep our muscles and nerves functioning,
- Keep our cells properly hydrated, and;
- Maintain our blood volume and blood pressure, among others.

Unfortunately, since most foods naturally have some sodium in them + we love table salt, it is common for people to go overboard and have too much.

In fact, the National Kidney Foundation (NKF) estimates that on average, **Americans consume 50% more sodium than the recommended daily amount.**

Normally, the kidneys are responsible for removing excess sodium. But when they aren't functioning at full capacity, a buildup is inevitable. This can cause a lot of problems, such as:

- Puffiness and swelling, mostly in the legs and ankles,
- Fluid retention around the heart and lungs,
- Shortness of breath,
- High blood pressure, and;
- Decreased kidney function, due to damaged blood vessels in the kidneys.

To avoid these complications, the USDA advises those with kidney conditions to limit themselves to **1500 mg of sodium per day,** in accordance with the USDA's Dietary Guidelines for Americans 2010.

So, what are TINY habits you can do NOW to control your sodium intake?

TINY HABIT 6: After I pick something from the grocery shelf, I will compare it with 2 other brands to choose the one with the lowest sodium

Reading food labels is a step in the right direction. Look at the *Nutrition Facts* section of the food item you bought and see how much **sodium** is in it. You can use this screenshot as a guide:

% Daily Value	Amount of sodium per serving	What it means...
Less than 5%	Less than 125 mg	Good choice – a low sodium product that you can have often
5 – 10%	Less than 250 mg	Good choice – a low sodium product that fits your low sodium diet easily
10 – 20%	Between 250 – 500 mg	Be cautious – this can still fit into a low sodium diet, but you'll have to observe caution
More than 20%	More than 500 mg	Beware – this is a high sodium product that should not be eaten in a low sodium diet

*Adapted from information by The Kidney Foundation of Canada

What you can do next time, is make a simple swap. For example, if you decide to buy chicken stock...

...pick up the brand you usually get and look at the sodium per 100g

...pick up a 2nd brand and look at the sodium per 100g

...pick up a 3rd brand and look at the sodium per 100g

...choose the one with the **lowest sodium per 100g**

Do this for **one** grocery item every time you shop. Don't try to replace everything in one go, we're creating easy, tiny habits that you can do every time!

TINY HABIT 7: After I go through my shopping list, I will add one fresh ingredient to my shopping cart

According to data from the Centers for Disease Control and Prevention (CDC), **more than 75% of the sodium Americans consume** comes from processed food, pre-packaged meals, and restaurant food. So, a significant way to cut down on your sodium intake is to choose fresh ingredients when cooking.

TINY HABIT 8: After I pass by the salt aisle, I will get an additional non-salt spice to try

One more surefire way of reducing your sodium intake is to switch up your cooking methods. **Instead of using salt on your recipes, use other herbs and spices to add flavor to your dishes.** Some very good examples of these are the following:

Spice	Food its Best Paired With
Allspice	beef, eggs, fish, fruits, vegetables, beverages, baked products, desserts
Basil	lamb, fish, eggs, vegetables, sauces
Bay Leaf	beef, chicken, veal, fish
Cinnamon	chicken, pork, fruits, baked products, beverages, vegetables
Cloves	beef, pork, fruits
Curry (salt-free)	beef, chicken, lamb, veal, eggs
Dill	chicken, veal, fish, vegetables
Ginger	chicken, pork, fruits, vegetables, baked products, beverages
Marjoram	eggs, fish, meat, poultry

Mustard Powder	meat, poultry, fish, eggs, vegetables
Parsley	beef, chicken, fish, salads, sauces
Rosemary	beef, lamb, chicken, turkey
Sage	meat, fish, stuffing, vegetables
Savory	egg dishes, meat, poultry, stuffing, rice, vegetables
Tarragon	chicken, fish, meat, egg dishes, sauces, vegetables
Thyme	fish, meat, poultry, eggs, stuffing, vegetables

Phosphorus and Your Kidneys

Fact: Every nutrient we take into our body does serve a purpose.

For example, sodium helps the body regulate its fluids. Protein, on the other hand, mainly builds our muscles, tissues, and organs. And potassium adds to the functions of the two, helping muscle-building and fluid regulation.

For phosphorus, it is important for your bones and joints. It works with Calcium and Vitamin D in your body to keep your bones healthy and strong. When you have healthy kidneys, they help keep the right amount of phosphorus in the body. But with Chronic Kidney Disease, your kidneys cannot do that job as well as before, allowing phosphorus to build up to dangerous levels in the blood. Too much phosphorus may cause bones to lose calcium instead, making them brittle and weak. This lost calcium can pile up in blood vessels, causing them to harden, leading to even more problems down the line—**joint pain, itchy skin, and lung, eye, or heart problems**, to name a few.

Excess phosphorus in the body is usually filtered out by the kidneys and excreted. But when kidney function is compromised, it can be difficult to keep blood phosphorus levels within the healthy range.

The normal blood phosphorus level is 2.5–4.5 mg/dL (milligrams per deciliter), and your kidneys are largely responsible for maintaining that normal range. Any excess phosphorus is excreted through urine.

To avoid those health concerns, you need to keep your blood phosphorus level within the normal range. This is why as much as possible, you **should avoid processed foods**. Additionally, this will also help you limit your sodium, because that's also high in processed foods.

So what steps can I do to help limit phosphorus intake?

1. Check food labels for "phos-" ingredients.

Yes, the Nutrition Facts section of food labels don't indicate how much phosphorus is in a particular food item. But, they do indicate their phosphorus additives in their list of ingredients. All you have to do is steer clear of foods with "phos-" additives in them. Components like:

- Calcium **phos**phate
- Dicalcium **phos**phate
- Disodium **phos**phate
- Monopotassium **phos**phate
- Monosodium **phos**phate
- **Phos**phoric acid
- Pyrophosphate poly**phos**phate
- Sodium hexameta-**phos**phate
- Tetrasodium pyro**phos**phate
- Tricalcium **phos**phate
- Trisodium **phos**phate

Always remember to be extra vigilant when grocery shopping!

TINY HABIT 9. After I pick a canned ingredient, I will check food labels for "phos-" ingredients.

2. Talk to your health professional about phosphate binders.

I'm always hesitant about recommending medication. People tend to become overly dependent on drugs, and they neglect what diet and lifestyle changes can do. But if your phosphorus level is getting out of hand, then you can talk to your healthcare professionals about using **phosphate binders.**

Phosphate (or phosphorus) binders are medications that help you control phosphorus levels in your body. They absorb excess phosphorus from the food you eat and help you pass it out of your body through your stool. There are many types of this -- pills, powders, liquids, and even chewable tablets.

HOWEVER... Keep this in mind: **DO NOT take phosphate binders without the approval of a doctor or dietitian.** The assessment of a medical professional is absolutely necessary before starting this type of medication.

3. Switch to a low-phosphorus diet.

As suggested by the National Kidney Foundation (NKF), **the ideal phosphorus intake limit for people with kidney conditions is 800-1000 mg daily.** But limiting this nutrient is easier said than done. You see, most of the things that we enjoy are actually high-phosphorus food items, such as:

- Organ meat
- Dairy products
- Beans
- Lentils
- Nuts
- Cola
- Bran cereals
- Oatmeal

But you don't need to worry much about it, as there are low-phosphorus alternatives, such as these:

- Fresh fruits and vegetables
- Breads
- Pasta

- Rice
- Milk
- Corn and rice cereals
- Light color soda

TINY HABIT 10. After checking food labels for "phos-" ingredients, I will pick a low-phosphorus alternative.

I hope that this chapter has fully equipped you with the right knowledge that you need to move forward not only with this book but towards your journey to better kidney health. Flip through the next chapter and we will put what you have learned here into practical and actionable applications.

I would love to hear from you!

It's through your support and reviews that my book is able to reach other Chronic Kidney Disease patients who are still struggling to figure out how they could take a proactive approach in managing their CKD. Please take 60 seconds to kindly leave a review on Amazon. Please scan the QR code below, alternatively, you may use the link provided in your Amazon order.

Please follow these simple steps to rate/review my book:

1. Open the camera on your phone
2. Hover it over the QR code below
3. You may also type this link on your phone or browser: **https://go.renaltracker.com/bookreview**
4. Rate/Review my book

I appreciate you taking the time, your review will surely make a difference.

Thank you!

Janeth Kingston

Chapter 4:

Translating Diet into Daily Meals

"How can meal planning and portion control strategies be effectively integrated into the daily routine of a patient with CKD to manage their protein, potassium, phosphorus, and sodium intake, while also maintaining a balanced and enjoyable diet?"

Importance of Meal Planning

A kidney-friendly meal plan is essential for people with Chronic Kidney Disease. The nutritional needs of people with CKD differ and change as their disease progresses. Which is why it's important to talk to a registered dietitian to find a kidney-friendly meal plan that works best for you since following a healthy diet plan can also possibly slow down CKD progression.

The National Kidney Foundation defines a well-balanced diet as a meal plan that "gives you the right amounts of protein, calories, vitamins, and minerals each day. Eating a healthy diet, staying physically active, and taking all your medicines as prescribed are all important parts to keeping you healthy and feeling well." To know which nutrient to personally restrict and the right amounts you will need, you have to ask your renal dietitian (who would consult closely with your nephrologist).

CKD Chef Duane, as you have already known, gave a talk at the American Society of Nephrology Kidney Week, the world-leading congress on kidney science, and said this:

"Because I have kidneys on crutches, I got to explore a whole new world of cooking. Creating kidney-friendly diets is one of the most interesting culinary challenges I have ever had to face in my professional cooking career."

CKD Chef Duane agreed that salt is the most boring flavor there is. Salt masks taste. Unfortunately, humans are programmed to crave salt. It was scarce for our ancestors. However, once you learn to cook with less salt, you will find that you will start to hate salt. Importantly, when you start replacing salt, you will discover a whole new range of tasty food that is healthier for your kidneys too!

Sticking to a healthy diet plan can be challenging. However, you can see this as an opportunity to feel and eat better, have a greater quality of life and do more of what you enjoy.

What can you do?

Here are 5 actionable ways to Kickstarting Kidney-friendly meal plan:

Kickstarting Kidney-friendly Meals 1: <u>Consult a Registered Dietitian</u>

According to an article in the Journal of the Academy of Nutrition and Dietetics, 90 percent of non-dialysis kidney disease patients never meet with a dietitian. The authors added that adults with CKD are poorly informed on how diet influences disease management and progression.

Working with a registered dietitian is crucial in managing your CKD. Your dietitian will track your nutritional health and recommend customized meal plans and food substitutes that are nutritious as they are enjoyable. Dietitians will also check your blood results to suggest adjustments to balance your nutrition.

Kickstarting Kidney-friendly Meals 2: <u>Think forward</u>

Tweaking your lifestyle is necessary for healthy kidneys. However, you don't have to make such drastic changes immediately otherwise, you'd fall short on your goals. A very concrete and useful way to bring about the change you want is learning to plan. Take small, important steps towards making these changes. Consider the following:

- Food has natural sodium in them. Try to limit your sodium intake from 3 teaspoons to 1 or limit sodium intake at 20% to

40% to avoid making your food taste bland. You may not even notice the reduced sodium content.
- Plan out your daily or weekly meals.
- Write down a shopping list and follow it (this will save you a great deal of money, too).
- Design how you will prepare the food and what to put in it.
- Decide on where you will eat—home, restaurant, at the picnic with loved ones, or someone else's home, etc.

TRIVIA:

A 2017 study among French adults published in the International Journal of Behavioral Nutrition and Physical Activity revealed that meal planning encouraged home meal preparation which is linked to improved diet quality.

It will seem usual and effortless to keep up with your new diet once you get into the practice of planning meals. A small venture of time and effort, they say, brings a great return.

Kickstarting Kidney-friendly Meals 3: Keep a food journal

Keeping a nutrition journal will help you keep track of how you feel, based on what you eat, how much you weigh, what questions you have, and what you will learn. You can use it to write down:

- Daily or weekly food and beverage intake. Include portion sizes and how the foods are prepared.
- Your notes about exercise, meal plans, what you've learned from your research, readings, and experience on CKD and nutrition, etc.
- Stuff you want to mention to your doctor and/or dietitian, e.g. food choices and preference, preparation, etc.

The US Department of Health and Human Services-National Institute of Diabetes and Digestive and Kidney Diseases gives an informative guideline on the intake of the crucial nutrients such as calories, protein, fat, sodium, potassium, and phosphorus.

With good nutrition—eating the right foods and drinking the right beverages— a CKD patient may avoid or postpone some health problems since nutritional needs can vary as CKD progresses

Kickstarting Kidney-friendly Meals 4: Learn to read nutrition labels

Food labels are helpful in understanding the nutrients that food has. It guides you in choosing the right food for your CKD. Food labels have percent daily values based on the Food and Drug Administration (FDA) recommended a 2000 calorie diet.

Consult with your dietitian to learn reading nutrition labels as well as your diet restrictions.

Kickstarting Kidney-friendly Meals 5: Eyes on the Prize: Stay healthy!

The National Kidney Foundation lists down reasons good nutrition is important for people with CKD:

- It provides energy for daily tasks
- It prevents infection
- It helps you avoid muscle-mass loss
- It helps maintain a healthy weight
- It slows down the progression of the kidney disease

TRIVIA:

A 2018 study by researchers from the Harvard T.H. Chan School of Public Health showed that there are five areas of healthy living worth focusing on: healthy diet, healthy physical activity level, healthy body weight, smoking, and moderate alcohol intake.

Just one healthy habit (and it didn't matter which one) ... just one... extended life expectancy by two years in men and women. It goes on to point out that "Not surprisingly, the more healthy habits people had, the longer their lifespan."

Embracing a CKD diet plan doesn't mean self-deprivation. You don't have to entirely give up the flavor as well as your favorite food to stick to a healthier lifestyle. Talk to your registered dietitian to find healthy alternatives to your favorite food. Having great support and the right perspective can help you stick to a healthy CKD meal plan.

Meal Planning Tips for Success

Let's get to the benefits of a specific kind of self-monitoring: food logging or the practice of writing down what you ate so you can get feedback on it.

The reason why you should monitor your meals is perfectly simple...

Whatever your ultimate kidney health goal is—improve kidney functions, lose weight, or simply eat healthier for your kidneys. Keeping food logs can help you do it.

With a diet that's as full of possible restrictions as a kidney diet (sodium, potassium, protein, and more...) food logs are among the best ways to get feedback from your dietitian. It's a simple solution that will help you achieve your goals.

Here are a couple of reasons why:

1. It holds you accountable.

By keeping track of your food, you are also keeping track of the choices you make about your diet. For many people, that's all the inspiration it takes to make better decisions about what to eat.

The majority of people will think twice about "cheating" on their renal diet, if they know they'll have to record what they actually ate.

What about omitting entries entirely? Sure, nothing can stop you from doing that. But if that's what you plan to do, then you might as well save yourself the trouble:

There's no point in simply PRETENDING to change. Only genuine effort will yield results.

2. It motivates you.

Food logging helps you remember and celebrate those small quotas. It's motivating to see your progress in a concrete form, even if it is just one small step at a time.

Your meal log is not only a record of what you ate—it's a list of your achievements, a catalog of all the good choices you make.

3. It helps you evaluate.

Sometimes, despite your best efforts, you don't always get the results you expect. When that happens, you need to take a step back and evaluate what you've been doing so far. But how can you do that if you don't have a record in the first place? And that's where your food logs come in.

With actual records to look over, you have a better chance of finding out what's wrong and figuring out how to correct it. And with those three reasons, we hope that you can see now why it's important to:

"Keep track of what you eat."

Creating a CKD-Friendly Meal Plan

This entire book may be a trove of valuable information on how to personalize your diet as a PERSONALIZED treatment and that can take you some time going back and forths and accomplishing a lot of things for you to finally master it.

But we can already start small!

What you need is a solution, a tool, that will help keep track of your diet: something that can help you track your progress and will give you insights as to what works and what doesn't work in helping your kidneys improve over time...and it's called a food journal.

If you are new to kidney dieting, having a food journal will help you stick to your diet plan. Hence, it can improve your kidney functions and prevent further kidney damage.

Most patients own a food journal to help them be more cautious and be more aware of their daily intake and to make sure that they are taking in the right amount of nutrients that boost your kidney health.

In totality, a food journal/diary looks like this:

Wk 9 Monday Food Plan		TOTAL DAILY INTAKE			
		Calories	Protein (g)	Carbs (g)	Fat (g)
		1159	190	79	78
Breakfast 7.00am	3 egg whites	48	11	0	0
	30g WPI (Biofumace)	112	26	1	0
	30g raw rolled oats (complex carb)	113	3	17	3
Supplements: 1x Swisse Woman's Ultivite, 3x Fish oil 1500mg, 2 x Super Greens, 2 x Vitamin C 1000mg & 1 CLA					
Morning Snack	25g almonds	150	5	1	14
	1 Atkins Caram/Nut Chew Protein Bar	144	5	3	8
Pre Training 11.30am	130g Tuna in oil drained	277	31	0	17
	120g Salad Leaves with Beetroot	34	5	3	0
	1/2 cup brown rice	122	2	25	1
	10g Creatin (Biocharge)	42	7	0	0
Supplements: 4 x Super Greens, 1 CLA, 2 x Vitamin C 1000mg					
Weights 12.30pm	Back/Biceps/Abs (50 min)	-250			
	Treadmill inclined 4kmph (30min)	-150			
Post Training 2.00pm	30g WPI (Biofumace)	112	26	1	0
	100g mixed berries	57	1	10	1
	1 cup skim milk	85	9	12	0
Dinner 5.30pm	150g Chicken Breast	248	47	0	5
	Green vegetables (1/2 cup broccoli, 50g beans, 6xasparagus)	64	8	3	1
	1/2 tbs olive oil + vinegar	80	0	0	9
Cardio 7.00pm	Zumba (60 min)	-350			
Before Bed 9.00pm	1 egg	71	6	0	5
	25g almonds	150	5	1	14
Supplements: 3 x Fish oil 1500mg, 4 x Super Greens, 2 x Vitamin C 1000mg & 1 CLA					

https://healthiestlife4me.wordpress.com/2012/03/25/week-9-food-diary-sample

Important note: The image shown above is for illustration purposes only and differs from the food journal template provided on the annex section of this book.

You have to diligently write down everything you eat and drink for every meal. By doing so, your dietitian can help you record specific details like calories, proteins, carbs, and fats that each food and beverage contains. The most important thing is that you have to be completely honest with yourself and your healthcare team as this can help you with your process and progress.

According to LiveStrong, an organization that has been supporting millions of people in pursuit of living healthy, keeping a food journal not only carries benefits such as keeping track of one's diet, but can also help you focus on your diet, and can help you attain and maintain your goals.

How do you keep a food journal?

Here are 5 steps on how to get started with food journaling:

STEP #1: SET UP YOUR JOURNAL

You will need to keep track of the following: date, time, place, item eaten, quantity consumed, and extra notes.

STEP #2: RECORD WHAT YOU EAT AND DRINK

Try to take note of everything that goes into your mouth. Be sure to include all meals, drinks, snacks, and even the small bites of food you eat while you cook.

Here are some important guidelines I teach my patients when starting kidney diet journaling:

- Be very specific when you record and break down complicated foods by ingredient. This will help you remember what the total amount of each nutrient is.
- All beverages should be recorded as well, especially the total water intake of the day. By doing so, this will give you an idea of whether or not you need to consume more water to help you stay hydrated.

STEP #3: WRITE DOWN ACCURATE AMOUNTS

Since you need to keep track of how much nutrients you need to consume in a day for your kidney condition, you have to write down the accurate quantities as this is important data.

I suggest you purchase a food scale or measuring cups to help confirm that the amounts are correct.

CKD Chef Duane TIP:

Take your favorite glass, bowl, or plate, and measure how much drink/food is in it!

That way, every time you use your favorite glass, you immediately know that it's 8 oz. of whatever you're drinking.

If you eat at a restaurant, you can check online if they have accurate quantities of the ingredients used in their serving sizes.

STEP #4: WRITE THE DATE, TIME, AND PLACE

By writing down the date, time, and place, you can find patterns in your eating habits. If you're making the necessary changes to your diet and lifestyle, this information may provide insight into why you eat specific foods at specific times. Or find out if you are dining out all too often in places that tend to go way above your salt recommendation.

STEP #5: RECORD YOUR FEELINGS AFTER EATING.

It is also important that you jot down notes on how a food or meal makes you feel. After eating, wait 10-20 minutes to assess how you feel. It takes approximately 20 minutes for the body to know that you're satisfied.

Don't forget to also include any physical symptoms or side effects after eating. For example, you may notice that you have an upset stomach after eating dairy products.

Once you have done these 5 steps, you can then analyze your data after a specific period of time.

Recording everything you eat and drink provides regulation and accountability for what you put in your mouth and it can provide valuable insight for your doctor of what you eat. With this, it can also point out if you need more variety.

For example, if you need to eat more vegetables, or more meat, and less processed food. It can also lead to decreased caloric intake and can help you lose weight at the same time, too.

In addition, it will reveal if you are eating larger portions than your daily requirement. If you continue to keep track of your daily consumption for an extended period of time, you will start to notice the changes in your food intake and you will be able to monitor the progress you have made towards reaching your goal. After all, it's not about the data that you get. It's about the actions you do with those data. Don't you agree?

Just a little assignment for you so you can begin by starting small. Using the food diary on the annex section (page 155), try starting to record your meal starting today for one full week.

Understanding Portion Sizes

One thing you need to learn, in the case of renal diet nutrition, is to portion your food. Finding the right size of food servings for you will greatly help in regulating the amount of nutrients and wastes your kidneys filter.

Which leads me to my first question: *How much should you eat?*

Controlling what you eat is a vital step in achieving great results in following a renal diet. Your kidneys will find it easier to filter off your wastes if you don't eat more than what's necessary.

Also, a balance between the calories you eat and the ones you burn is one of the secrets to keep a healthy weight. The less sedentary you go (I'll discuss this in another chapter), the more calories you offset.

Picture this: a 120-pound man who burns a lot of calories through intense physical activity several times a week may need to eat more calories, than a man of similar size but mostly inactive and goes for a short walk once a week.

Portion Distortion

A study published in 2012 found that 96% of restaurant meals exceed USDA recommendations for fat, salt, and overall calories.

That's mainly due to the fact that restaurant and fast food chains are now serving food in gigantic plates, big cups, and king-sized packages. This is also part of the reason why fast foods are part of restrictions in a renal diet.

Another study found that modern portion sizes of popular foods added *an extra 50-150 calories*. Let's take an example:

Coffee (20 years ago)

WITH WHOLE MILK AND SUGAR

8 OUNCES

45 CALORIES

Coffee (today)

MOCHA COFFEE (WITH STEAMED WHOLE MILK AND MOCHA SYRUP)

16 OUNCES

350 CALORIES

That's a difference of 305 calories!

A 130 pound person would need to walk for an hour and 20 minutes to get rid of that many calories.

Luckily, there are certain fast foods you can enjoy, with a few modifications to your order, of course.

Portion Size vs Serving Size

Basically...

SERVING SIZE - the recommended amount of food, as stated on the product's food label.

PORTION SIZE - the amount of food you choose to eat at one time, whether you're at home or in a restaurant.

Sometimes, the serving size matches the portion size, but it most often will be up to you. To help you decide for your renal diet, here's a serving size guide you can use. So, here is a food portioning hack chart to help you easily remember how to adjust food portions on your plate.

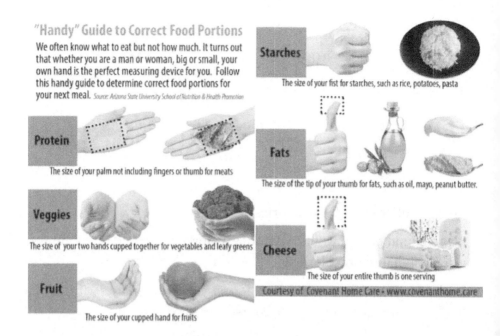

Properly portioning your food will give your body time to digest the food effectively, allowing better absorption of nutrients and reducing the amount of waste that your kidneys have to filter.

If you want to optimize your kidney functions, then I suggest you learn the charts above by heart. You can put it somewhere in your kitchen or dining area for easy reference! That way, you will be able to commit them into memory effectively. This will really help you determine if you are eating the proper amount of food. And I want you to practice this in your next meal. It may take a while for you to get it, but with practice, the habit will surely stick and the benefits you're going to get will be spectacular.

First, your body will be so used to eating small portions, that it will condition your body to become full just by eating small.

Second, most people will eventually feel better and will have more energy to do things once they have eaten moderate portions compared to how they used to eat.

Finally, if you monitor your portions properly, it can improve your digestion process. By doing so, it is more effective even when you want to lose weight.

But it sounds easier said than done, right? Don't worry, I'll help you get there with these 3 Portion Practice Tips:

1. Practice your plate control

Take a plate and divide it into 3 compartments in your mind:

- Remember that... 50% should be for vegetables
- 25% for carbohydrates *(rice, beans, and etc.)*
- 25% should be for lean protein *(chicken, fish, etc).*

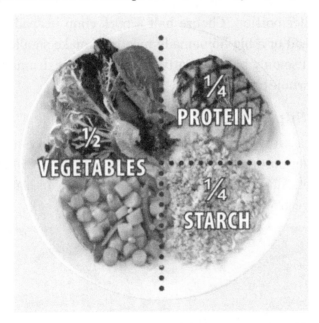

Image from: https://www.pinterest.ph/pin/298152437809682150/

For protein, if you remember from our lesson where we presented a food that's high on Protein and replaced them with ones that are lower and kidney-friendlier, the portion size of each food item was 100g.

So, how much is 100 grams? If you've never had to think about this before, that's perfectly normal. One of the most surprising things is starting to be conscious of the amount of food you are eating – especially when it comes to your favorites. The best thing to do is to actually get a kitchen weighing scale and measure the food that makes up your usual meals.

The second best thing to do is to always look at the nutrition labels because it specifies how many grams/ml there is of the food you are getting.

IF you also have to follow a protein-restricted diet, you should make it a point to calculate the protein portion in your meals. Small changes you can do to portion control:

- Eat more of things that are low-protein. Adding more of the good stuff tends to be easier than removing the bad stuff.
- If you absolutely have to have a high-protein food, then eat a smaller portion. Choose half a pork chop instead of a whole. Instead of a big homemade meatball, make smaller meatballs and use only half the portion. Take just the drumstick instead of a whole chicken leg.

2. Don't "Super Size" it

There's a reason why the Super Size Me documentary struck such a nerve – bigger portions are not always better, especially when it comes to a CKD diet. An article points out how since the 1970s, American food portions have grown as much as 138%!

Whether we are really hungry or not, the more food that is put in front of us, the more food we end up eating.

Just like the example on portion distortion earlier, you must keep in mind the calories (and sodium!) that you will be consuming. It's also a bad cycle: by eating a lot, your stomach gets used to expecting more food, so you find yourself to be hungry sooner... which urges you to eat more.

3. Take a look at labels

The Nutrition Facts Label is that friend you can count on to always tell you what you need to hear. It helps you determine what an appropriate portion should be for you. And based on the nutrients, steer you towards eating healthier and aim for more kidney-friendly foods.

Nutrition Facts	
2 servings per container	
Serving size	1 cup (140g)
Amount per serving	
Calories	**160**
	% Daily Value*
Total Fat 8g	10%
Saturated Fat 3g	15%
Trans Fat 0g	
Cholesterol 0mg	0%
Sodium 60mg	3%
Total Carbohydrate 21g	8%
Dietary Fiber 3g	11%
Total Sugars 15g	
Includes 5g Added Sugars	10%
Protein 3g	
Vitamin D 5mcg	25%
Calcium 20mg	2%
Iron 1mg	6%
Potassium 230mg	4%
*The % Daily Value tells you how much a nutrient in a serving of food contributes to a daily diet. 2000 calories a day is used for general nutrition advice.	

CKD-Friendly Recipes

As I have promised in the beginning, I cannot just keep on babbling about the basics, the fun-facts, and the truths about kidney dieting without sharing with you some recipe ideas that I have shared with my patients before.

However, though these recipes are created by a Nutritionist Dietitian for CKD patients, it is still best to consult your own dietitian in terms of the your diet restrictions and needs. I have included the macronutrient and micronutrients summary in there to make it extra easy for you.

Breakfast Ideas
Easy Stir Fry Cabbage
⏱ 15 min 🍴 4 servings   *230 Kcal / serving*   *9g Protein*   *9g Fat*   *39g Carbs*

INGREDIENTS

Vegetable broth, 100 ml (100 g)
Bell pepper, 1 (100 g)
Spring onions, 1 tbsp chopped (6 g)
Olive oil, 1 ounce (28 g)
Garlic, 2 cloves (6 g)
Cabbage, 1 head, medium (about 5-3/4" dia) (908 g)
Soy sauce, 2 tbsp (36 g)
Bell peppers, 2 (238 g)
Ground pepper, 1 tsp (2 g)
Onion, 1 medium size (150 g)
Paprika, 1/2 teaspoon (1 g)
Oyster mushroom sauce, 2 tbsp (100 g)

Instructions

1. Core and shred the cabbage into pieces, wash and dry well; set it aside.
2. Heat a wok over high heat, add the oil, and saute onion slices and minced garlic for a minute.
3. Toss in bell peppers, shredded cabbage and continue sauteing for 4 minutes stirring occasionally.
4. Add vegetable broth, soy sauce, and oyster mushroom sauce and mix well.
5. Continue tossing for another 3 minutes until the cabbage has wilted.
6. Season with smoked paprika, ground black pepper, and salt, and garnish with chopped spring onions and serve immediately. *Source: https://simplybakings.com/easy-stir-fry-cabbage*

MACRONUTRIENT SUMMARY

	TOTAL	PER 100 G	PER SERVING
Energy (kCal)	921.7	50.6	230.4
Protein (g)	34.3	1.9	8.6
Fat (g)	33.8	1.9	8.5
Carbs (g)	157	8.6	39.3
Fiber (g)	59.6	3.3	14.9

MICRONUTRIENT SUMMARY

	TOTAL	PER 100 G	PER SERVING
Sugars (g)	48.9	2.7	12.2
Fiber (g)	59.6	3.3	14.9
Calcium, Ca (mg)	910.8	50	227.7
Iron, Fe (mg)	18.7	1	4.7
Magnesium, Mg (mg)	367.4	20.2	91.9
Phosphorus, P (mg)	274	15.0	68.5
Potassium, K (mg)	2263	124	565.75
Sodium, Na (mg)	1245	68.21	311.25
Zinc, Zn (mg)	4.9	0.3	1.2
Vitamin D (ug)	0.7	0	0.2
Vitamin C (mg)	725.5	39.9	181.9
Cholesterol (mg)	0	0	0

Cauliflower Rice and Lentils

⏱ 25 min 🍽 2 servings   *155 Kcal / serving* *6g Protein* *8g Fat* *18g Carbs*

INGREDIENTS

Vegetable broth, 1/4 cup (47.1 g)
Oregano, 1 teaspoon (2 g)
Celery, 1/4 cup (21.3 g)
Carrots, 1/4 cup (30.8 g)
Olive oil, 1 servings (14 g)
Onion, 1/4 cup (38.5 g)
Lentils, 1/2 cup (99 g)
Cauliflower rice, 1/2 cup (80 g)
Garlic Powder, 1 teaspoon (3 g)
Pepper, 1/4 tsp (0.5 g)

Instructions

Heat the olive oil in a large skillet over medium heat.
Add the onion, celery, and carrots to the skillet and cook until softened, about 5 minutes.
Add the cauliflower rice and vegetable broth and cook for an additional 5 minutes.
Stir in the cooked lentils, garlic powder, oregano, and black pepper. Cook for an additional 5 minutes, stirring occasionally, until the cauliflower rice is cooked through.
Serve hot.

Comments

You can replace/ substitute lentils with preferred plant-based protein Additionally, the same goes with substitution of vegetables to other low potassium ones.

MACRONUTRIENT SUMMARY

	TOTAL	PER 100 G	PER SERVING
Energy (kCal)	309.3	92	154.7
Protein (g)	12.2	3.5	6.1
Fat (g)	14.9	4.4	7.5
Carbs (g)	35.4	10.5	17.7
Fiber (g)	12.5	3.7	6.3

MICRONUTRIENT SUMMARY

	TOTAL	PER 100 G	PER SERVING
Sugars (g)	7.1	2.1	3.6
Fiber (g)	12.5	3.7	6.3
Calcium, Ca (mg)	102	30.3	51
Iron, Fe (mg)	4.9	1.5	2.5
Magnesium, Mg (mg)	66.6	19.8	33.3
Phosphorus, P (mg)	258	75.8	129
Potassium, K (mg)	891.6	265.3	445.8
Sodium, Na (mg)	211.2	62.8	105.6
Zinc, Zn (mg)	1.8	0.5	0.9
Vitamin D (ug)	0	0	0
Vitamin C (mg)	45.6	13.6	22.8
Cholesterol (mg)	0	0	0

Stir-Fry Tofu

⏱ 25 min 🍽: *4 servings   464 Kcal / serving   15g Protein   32g Fat   36g Carbs*

INGREDIENTS

Hoisin sauce, 4 Tbsp
Shiitake mushrooms, 2 ounces (56.7 g)
Snow peas, 1 oz (113.4 g)
Sesame oil, 1 dash (2 g)
Vegetable oil, 100 grams (100 g)
Garlic, 3 cloves (9 g)
Soy sauce, 1 tsp
Extra tofu, 16 ounce (453.6 g)
Cornstarch, 2 tsp (4 g)
Brown sugar, 1 tablespoon (12 g)
Salt and pepper, to taste
Onions, 1 portion (100 g)
Pepper Flakes, 1 tsp (100 g)
Rice Vinegar, 1 tablespoon (16 g)

Instructions

1. In a medium-sized bowl, add soy sauce, rice black vinegar, brown sugar, cornstarch, red pepper flakes, and mix until combined, set aside.
2. Heat a large pan on medium heat with oil and fry the tofu until all sides are golden, then remove, transfer to a plate lined with paper towels, and set aside.
3. Add the remaining oil into the same pan and saute sliced red onions and crushed garlic cloves for about 1 minute.
4. Add slices of mushrooms and continue cooking for 3 minutes on medium-high heat.
5. Stir in the snow peas and cook for 2 minutes.
6. Add the fried tofu and the soy sauce mixture.
7. Cover and allow it to steam for 2 minutes on medium-low heat.
8. Add hoisin sauce and adjust the seasoning.
9. Turn off the heat and add a touch of sesame oil.
10. Serve with steamed Jasmin Rice.

Source: *https://simplybakings.com/tofu-stir-fry-with-snow-peas/*

MACRONUTRIENT SUMMARY

	TOTAL	PER 100 G	PER SERVING
Energy (kCal)	1854.6	169.2	463.7
Protein (g)	59.5	5.4	14.9
Fat (g)	129	11.8	32.3
Carbs (g)	144.6	13.2	36.2
Fiber (g)	44.6	4.1	11.2

MICRONUTRIENT SUMMARY

	TOTAL	PER 100 G	PER SERVING
Sugars (g)	61.3	5.6	15.3
Fiber (g)	44.6	4.1	11.2
Calcium, Ca (mg)	608.7	55.5	152.2
Iron, Fe (mg)	27.5	2.5	6.9
Magnesium, Mg (mg)	359.2	32.8	89.8
Phosphorus, P (mg)	766	69.95	191.5
Potassium, K (mg)	1694	154.70	423.50
Sodium, Na (mg)	2027	185.11	506.75
Zinc, Zn (mg)	8.6	0.8	2.2
Vitamin D (ug)	0.2	0	0.1
Vitamin C (mg)	79.3	7.2	19.8
Cholesterol (mg)	3	0.3	0.8

Lunch and Dinner Ideas

Cauliflower Crust Pizza

⏱ 45 min　　🍴 4 servings　　143 Kcal / serving 11g Protein 8g Fat 9g Carbs

INGREDIENTS

Parmesan, 1/2 cup (48.5 g)
Mozzarella, 1/4 cup (29.3 g)
Egg, 1 medium (51 g)
Dried basil, 1/2 teaspoon (0.5 g)
Oregano, 1 teaspoon (3 g)
Arugula, 2/3 cup (13.3 g)
Mushrooms, 1/2 cup (46.5 g)
Pepperoni, 5 piece (10 g)
cauliflower rice, 3 cups (480 g)
marinara sauce, 61.3 g
Cherry Tomatoes, 4 100 gram (68 g)

Instructions

Pre-heat oven to 425 F
(If youre using a pizza stone, place it in the oven now)
Place the cauliflower rice in a large microwave safe bowl and microwave on high for 3-5 minutes. Allow to cool in bowl.
When the cauliflower is cool, add the parmesan, egg and optional herbs. Mix well until a dough forms.
Line an oven tray with parchment paper and form a circle with the dough, creating a raised lip around the edges.
Bake in preheated oven for 20 minutes. Remove from oven and spread marinara sauce evenly on top of the crust.
Sprinkle with grated mozzarella followed by desired toppings.
Bake again for 10 minutes, or until the cheese melts. Slice and serve hot.

Source: https://lifemadesweeter.com/cauliflower-crust-pizza

MACRONUTRIENT SUMMARY

	TOTAL	PER 100 G	PER SERVING
Energy (kCal)	570.8	70.4	142.7
Protein (g)	44.9	5.5	11.2
Fat (g)	30.5	3.8	7.6
Carbs (g)	36.8	4.5	9.2
Fiber (g)	13.1	1.6	3.3

MICRONUTRIENT SUMMARY

	TOTAL	PER 100 G	PER SERVING
Sugars (g)	15.2	1.9	3.8
Fiber (g)	13.1	1.6	3.3
Calcium, Ca (mg)	955.9	117.8	239
Iron, Fe (mg)	6.6	0.8	1.7
Magnesium, Mg (mg)	144.5	17.8	36.1
Phosphorus, P (mg)	856.4	105.6	214.1
Potassium, K (mg)	2178	268.4	544.5
Sodium, Na (mg)	1530.2	188.6	382.6
Zinc, Zn (mg)	5	0.6	1.3
Vitamin D (ug)	1.6	0.2	0.4
Vitamin C (mg)	254.2	31.3	63.6
Cholesterol (mg)	255.5	31.5	63.9

Quick Easy Fish Stew

⏱ **30 min**　🍴 **4 servings**　*440 Kcal / serving*　*36g Protein*　*24g Fat*　*17g Carbs*

INGREDIENTS

Thyme, 1 pinch (0.1 g)
Oregano, 1 pinch (0.1 g)
Salt, 1 tsp
Canned tomatoes, 1/2 cup (116.3 g)
Onion, 1 1/2 cup (236.8 g)
Wine, 1/2 cup (113.5 g)
Clam juice, 4 ounces (226.8 g)
Pepper, 4 servings (0.4 g)
Parsley, 2/3 cup (39.2 g)
Garlic cloves, 3 (9 g)
Extra virgin olive oil, 6 tablespoon (84 g)
Tomato paste, 2 teaspoons (12 g)
Fish fillets, 1 1/2 lb (671.4 g)
Tabasco sauce, 1/8 teaspoon (0.4 g)

Instructions

1. Heat olive oil in a large thick-bottomed pot over medium-high heat.
2. Add onion and sauté 4 minutes, add the garlic and cook a minute more.
3. Add parsley and stir 2 minutes.
4. Add tomato and tomato paste, and gently cook for 10 minutes or so.
5. Add clam juice, dry white wine, and Bsh. Tring to a simmer and simmer until the Fish is cooked through and easily flakes apart, about 3 to 5 minutes.
6. Add seasoning (oregano, thyme, Tabasco).
7. Add salt and pepper to taste. Ladle into bowls and serve.
8. Great served with crusty bread for dipping in the fish stew broth.

Source: https://www.simplyrecipes.com/recipes/dads_fish_stew

MACRONUTRIENT SUMMARY

	TOTAL	PER 100 G	PER SERVING
Energy (kCal)	1758.7	116.3	439.7
Protein (g)	143.1	9.5	35.8
Fat (g)	96.9	6.4	24.2
Carbs (g)	65.9	4.4	16.5
Fiber (g)	9.3	0.6	2.3

MICRONUTRIENT SUMMARY

	TOTAL	PER 100 G	PER SERVING
Sugars (g)	24.6	1.6	6.2
Fiber (g)	9.3	0.6	2.3
Calcium, Ca (mg)	259.4	17.2	64.9
Iron, Fe (mg)	9.6	0.6	2.4
Magnesium, Mg (mg)	267.7	17.7	66.9
Phosphorus, P (mg)	1319.7	87.3	329.9
Potassium, K (mg)	3300.2	218.3	825.1
Sodium, Na (mg)	2301.3	152.2	575.3
Zinc, Zn (mg)	3.7	0.2	0.9
Vitamin D (ug)	20.8	1.4	5.2
Vitamin C (mg)	97.6	6.5	24.4
Cholesterol (mg)	335.7	22.2	83.9

Chicken Pelau

🕐 **60 min**   🍴 **4 servings**   *653 Kcal / serving*   *36g Protein*   *31g Fat*   *57g Carbs*

INGREDIENTS

boneless skinless chicken thighs, target stores, 6 serving (672 g)
Onion, Fresh, 1 medium (105.8 g)
Ginger, fresh, 1 tbsp (20 g)
Lime juice, fresh, 1/2 ounce (14.2 g)
peeled garlic cloves, 2 clove (8 g)
Coriander (cilantro) leaves, raw, 1/4 cup (4 g)
Parsley, 1 tablespoons (5 g)
Chives, 1 tsp chopped (1 g)
Spices, oregano, dried, 1 teaspoon (3 g)
Spices, thyme, dried, 1 teaspoon (2 g)
TABASCO PEPPERS PEPPER SAUCE, 1 serving (5 g)
Oil, olive, salad or cooking, 3 tbsp (42 g)
Sugars, brown, 3 tbsp (3k g)
Pigeon peas (red gram), mature seeds, cooked, boiled, without salt, 1 cup (168 g)
Carrots, raw, 1 portion (61.6 g)
Peppers, sweet, red, raw, 1 medium (k3 g)
Celery, raw, 1 stalk (44 g)
Tomato, Fresh, 1 small (k5 g)
Worcestershire sauce, 1 tsp (5 g)
coconut cream, thai agri foods co., ltd., 1 serving (k0 g)
Rice, white, long-grain, parboiled, unenriched, cooked, 2 cup (316 g)
Table salt, 1 teaspoon (5 g)
Black Pepper, 1/2 tsp, ground (1.2 g)
Water, 3 portion(s) (630 g)

Instructions

1. Marinate the chicken pieces with the seasoning/marinade above for a few hours or overnight.
2. When ready to cook, heat a large pot on high heat and add oil. When the oil is hot, add the brown sugar. Don't stir yet. Let it melt and start to get dark brown around the dome of the edges. Don't let it burn.
3. Start adding the seasoned chicken, a few pieces at a time, stirring to ensure all the pieces get coated evenly with the caramelized/burnt sugar. Don't add the seasoning from the bowl yet. You will add that later.
4. After adding all the chicken pieces, cover the pot and allow to cook on medium heat for about 10 minutes. Stir up a few times to

get all the pieces well covered. This will create some liquid from the chicken.

5. Then open he pot lid, turn up the heat for about 3-5 minutes to allow the chicken to get a nice brown color.
6. Add the drained cooked pigeon peas. Stir. Cover pot with lid for about a couple more minutes.
7. Now you can add any seasoning that was left over the marinated chicken bowl
8. Add onion, hot pepper and/or pimiento, carrot and/or pumpkin, bell peppers, and tomato.
9. Add about ¼ cup of water if needed and cover the pot to help them cook a little – maybe 3 – 4 minutes.
10. Add the ketchup, Worcestershire sauce, salt and pepper.
11. Then add the 3 cups of water and mix all together.
12. Add the soaked and drained rice and stir well. Turn the heat to high to bring to a boil.
13 Then run the heat to very low, cover the pot and simmer for about 30 to 35 minutes, checking periodically to ensure it's not sticking to the bottom of the pot. Taste and adjust seasoning as needed.
14. After you turn the heat off, add some fresh parsley if you want and mix it in with you pelau. Finely chopped celery leaves also works well.

MACRONUTRIENT SUMMARY

	TOTAL	PER 100 G	PER SERVING
Energy (kCal)	2611.8	101.7	653
Protein (g)	143.2	5.6	35.8
Fat (g)	125.3	4.9	31.3
Carbs (g)	226.1	8.8	56.5
Fiber (g)	25.3	1	6.3

MICRONUTRIENT SUMMARY

	TOTAL	PER 100 G	PER SERVING
Sugars (g)	83.9	3.3	21
Fiber (g)	25.3	1	6.3
Calcium, Ca (mg)	365.7	14.2	91.4
Iron, Fe (mg)	15.3	0.6	3.8
Magnesium, Mg (mg)	200.7	7.8	50.2
Phosphorus, P (mg)	944	36.68	236
Potassium, K (mg)	2838	110.29	709.50
Sodium, Na (mg)	2665	103.57	666.25
Zinc, Zn (mg)	4	0.2	1
Vitamin D (ug)	0	0	0
Vitamin C (mg)	163.6	6.4	40.9
Cholesterol (mg)	631.7	24.6	157.9

Double Tomato Pesto Spaghetti with Zucchini Noodles

⏱ 30 min   🍽 4 servings   454 *Kcal / serving*   *13g Protein*   *22g Fat*   *55g Carbs*

INGREDIENTS

Basil leaves, 1/2 cup (12 g)
Lemon zest, 1/2 tsp (1 g)
Lemon juice, 1 tablespoons (15 g)
Salt, 1/4 teaspoon (1.8 g)
Olive oil, 2 servings (28 g)
Zucchini, 1 large (324 g)
Garlic cloves, 2 clove (6 g)
Walnuts, 2/3 cup (76.7 g)
Oil packed sun dried tomatoes, 1/4 cup (28.8 g)
bell pepper, 4 medium (298 g)
nutritional yeast, 1 teaspoons (4 g)
red pepper flakes, 1/4 teaspoon (0.5 g)
spaghetti, 1/2 lb (226.8 g)

Instructions

1. Bring a large pot of salted water to boil for the spaghetti. Cook the pasta until al dente, according to package directions. Drain and transfer to a large serving bowl.
2. Spiralize the zucchini with a spiralizer, or turn the zucchini into noodles with a julienne peeler, or grate the zucchini the long way on a large box grater.
3. Toast the walnuts: In a medium skillet over medium heat, cook the walnuts, stirring occasionally, until they smell nice and fragrant, about 7 minutes. Set aside to cool.
4. Cook the cherry tomatoes: In a large saucepan over medium-high heat, combine the cherry tomatoes, olive oil and a pinch of salt. Cover the pot and cook, stirring occasionally, until the tomatoes have burst open and they are cooking in their own juices, about 7 to 8 minutes. Set aside.
5. In a food processor, combine the walnuts, half of the cooked tomatoes, sun-dried tomatoes, garlic, lemon zest, 1 tablespoon lemon juice, red pepper flakes, teaspoon salt and several twists of freshly ground black pepper. Blend until the mixture is pretty smooth, then season to taste with additional lemon
6. juice, salt and/or pepper until the flavors really sing. Blend again.
7. Pour the pesto over the spaghetti and toss to combine. If you'll be consuming this dish in one sitting, go ahead and toss in all of the zucchini noodles now,
8. too. (If you plan on having leftovers, store the zucchini noodles separately from the rest, as they leach water when they're exposed to salt. I just pile the noodles on top of my individual bowls and wait to stir them in when I'm ready to eat). Pour the rest of the cherry tomatoes on top of

the dish, and sprinkle the basil over them. Toss gently, and divide the mixture into bowls. Top individual bowls with Parmesan or nutritional yeast, if you'd like, and a light drizzle of olive oil. Serve immediately.

MACRONUTRIENT SUMMARY

	TOTAL	PER 100 G	PER SERVING
Energy (kCal)	1816	177.5	454
Protein (g)	52.5	5.1	13.1
Fat (g)	87.8	8.6	22
Carbs (g)	220	21.15	55
Fiber (g)	25.2	2.5	6.3

MICRONUTRIENT SUMMARY

	TOTAL	PER 100 G	PER SERVING
Sugars (g)	29.2	2.9	7.3
Fiber (g)	25.2	2.5	6.3
Calcium, Ca (mg)	245.7	24	61.4
Iron, Fe (mg)	9.4	0.9	2.4
Magnesium, Mg (mg)	369.7	36.2	92.4
Phosphorus, P (mg)	953.2	93.2	238.3
Potassium, K (mg)	2934.9	287	733.7
Sodium, Na (mg)	818.2	80	204.6
Zinc, Zn (mg)	7.8	0.8	2
Vitamin D (ug)	0	0	0
Vitamin C (mg)	480.8	47	120.2
Cholesterol (mg)	0	0	0

Curried Butternut Squash Soup

⏱ 30 min   🍴 4 servings   541 *Kcal / serving*   *16g Protein*   *27g Fat*   *72g Carbs*

INGREDIENTS

Vegetable broth, 100 ml (100 g)
Shallots), 2 (50 g)
Garlic, 2 (6 g)
Curry powder, 1 jar (100 g)
Butternut squash , 1 portion(s) (100 g)
Avocado oil, 1 tbsp (14 g)
Full-fat coconut milk, 1 ml (1 g)
Pumpkin seeds, 1 portion(s) (100 g)
Sea salt, 1 serving (100 g)
Ground cinnamon, 1 tsp (0.7 g)
Maple syrup), 1 tbsp (100 g)
Chili garlic paste, 1 teaspoon (100 g)
Coconut milk, 14 ounce (396.9 g)

Instructions

1. Heat a large pot over medium heat.
2. Once hot, add oil, shallots, and garlic. Sauté for 2 minutes, stirring frequently.
3. Add butternut squash and season with salt, pepper, curry powder, and ground cinnamon. Stir to coat. Then cover and cook for 4 minutes, stirring occasionally.
4. Add coconut milk, vegetable broth, maple syrup or coconut sugar, and chili garlic paste (optional - for heat).
5. Bring to a low boil over medium heat and then reduce heat to low, cover, and simmer for 15 minutes or until butternut squash is fork tender.
6. Use an immersion blender, or transfer soup to a blender, and purée on high until creamy and smooth. If using a blender, return soup back to pot.
7. Taste and adjust seasonings, adding more curry powder, salt, or sweetener as needed. Continue cooking for a few more minutes over medium heat.
8. Serve as is or with garnishes of choice (options above). Store leftovers covered in the refrigerator for 3-4 days or in the freezer up to 1 month. Best when fresh.

Comments

You can upgrade nutritionally by adding greens, such as, chopped spinach, moringa leaves, boiled/ chopped broccoli
Source: https://minimalistbaker.com/curried-butternut-squash-soup/

MACRONUTRIENT SUMMARY

	TOTAL	PER 100 G	PER SERVING
Energy (kCal)	2164	185.2	541
Protein (g)	64.2	5.5	16.1
Fat (g)	107.7	9.2	26.9
Carbs (g)	287.4	24.6	71.9
Fiber (g)	90.7	7.8	22.7

MICRONUTRIENT SUMMARY

	TOTAL	PER 100 G	PER SERVING
Sugars (g)	77.8	6.7	19.5
Fiber (g)	90.7	7.8	22.7
Calcium, Ca (mg)	1282.1	109.7	320.5
Iron, Fe (mg)	40.9	3.5	10.2
Magnesium, Mg (mg)	1090.9	93.4	272.7
Phosphorus, P (mg)	1987.6	170.1	496.9
Potassium, K (mg)	4277.1	366	1069.3
Sodium, Na (mg)	936.9	80.2	234.2
Zinc, Zn (mg)	15.3	1.3	3.8
Vitamin D (ug)	0	0	0
Vitamin C (mg)	61.1	5.2	15.3
Cholesterol (mg)	0	0	0

Cauliflower Risotto with Brie and Almonds

⏱ 45 min   🍽 4 servings   596 *Kcal / serving*   17g *Protein*   27g *Fat*   69g *Carbs*

INGREDIENTS

Thyme sprigs, 3 handful (6 g)
Unsalted butter, 1 tablespoon (14 g)
Vegetable broth, 4 cups (784 g)
Brie, 5 ounces (145 g)
Cauliflower, 1/2 head (276.5 g)
Olive oil, 2 servings (28 g)
Almonds, 1/3 cup (49.7 g)
Water, 2 1/2 cup (587.5 g)
Dry White Wine, 1/3 cup (83.3 g)
arborio rice, 1 cups (300 g)

Instructions

1. Bring broth, water, and thyme sprigs to a bare simmer in a medium saucepan.
2. Meanwhile, heat butter and 1 tablespoon oil in a 4-quart heavy saucepan over medium-high heat until foam subsides, then sauté cauliflower with ¼ teaspoon salt until crisp-tender and golden brown, about 6 minutes.
3. Add thyme leaves and sauté 1 minute.
4. Transfer to a bowl. Add remaining tablespoon oil to pan, then add rice
5. and cook, stirring constantly, 1 minute.
6. Add wine and simmer briskly, stirring, until wine has been absorbed,
7. about 1 minute.
   Add 1/2 cup hot broth and briskly simmer, stirring, until broth has been absorbed. Continue simmering and adding hot broth, about 1/2 cup at a time, stirring constantly and waiting until each addition has been absorbed before adding the next, until rice is just tender and looks creamy, 18 to 22 minutes. (There will be leftover broth.)
8. Stir in cauliflower, Brie, and salt and pepper to taste.
9. Thin with some of remaining broth if desired. Serve topped with almonds.

   Source: https://www.epicurious.com/recipes/food/views/cauliflower-risotto-with-Brie-and-Almonds-350559

MACRONUTRIENT SUMMARY

	TOTAL	PER 100 G	PER SERVING
Energy (kCal)	2384.3	104.9	596.1
Protein (g)	67.7	3	16.9
Fat (g)	107.3	4.7	26.8
Carbs (g)	274.2	12.1	68.6
Fiber (g)	21	0.9	5.3

MICRONUTRIENT SUMMARY

	TOTAL	PER 100 G	PER SERVING
Sugars (g)	13.4	0.6	3.4
Fiber (g)	21	0.9	5.3
Calcium, Ca (mg)	546.8	24	136.7
Iron, Fe (mg)	18.5	0.8	4.6
Magnesium, Mg (mg)	305.5	13.4	76.4
Phosphorus, P (mg)	819	49.69	204.75
Potassium, K (mg)	1373	83.3	343.25
Sodium, Na (mg)	2402	145.75	600.5
Zinc, Zn (mg)	9.6	0.4	2.4
Vitamin D (ug)	0.7	0	0.2
Vitamin C (mg)	146	6.4	36.5
Cholesterol (mg)	175.1	7.7	43.8

Snack Ideas and Healthy Desserts

Almond Berry Smoothie

⏱ 10 min   🍽 1 servings   305 *Kcal / serving* 6g *Protein*   11g *Fat*   52g *Carbs*

INGREDIENTS

Banana, 1 medium (7" to 7-7/8" long) (118 g)
Blueberries, 1 cup (148 g)
Water, 1 serving (236.6 g)
Almond butter, 1 tbsp (16 g)
Almond milk, 1/2 cup (125 g)

Instructions

1. Combine blueberries, banana, almond milk, and almond butter in a blender; blend until smooth, adding water for a thinner smoothie.

Source: *https://www.allrecipes.com/recipe/246613/almond-berry-smoothie/*

MACRONUTRIENT SUMMARY

	TOTAL	PER 100 G	PER SERVING
Energy (kCal)	305.1	47.4	305.1
Protein (g)	6.4	1	6.4
Fat (g)	11.3	1.8	11.3
Carbs (g)	51.9	8.1	51.9
Fiber (g)	8.6	1.3	8.6

MICRONUTRIENT SUMMARY

	TOTAL	PER 100 G	PER SERVING
Sugars (g)	30	4.7	30
Fiber (g)	8.6	1.3	8.6
Calcium, Ca (mg)	227.4	35.3	227.4
Iron, Fe (mg)	1.3	0.2	1.3
Magnesium, Mg (mg)	87.7	13.6	87.7
Phosphorus, P (mg)	125	19.4	125
Potassium, K (mg)	656.1	101.9	656.1
Sodium, Na (mg)	178.1	27.7	178.1
Zinc, Zn (mg)	1	0.2	1
Vitamin D (ug)	0	0	0
Vitamin C (mg)	24.6	3.8	24.6
Cholesterol (mg)	0	0	0

Oatmeal Cookies

🕐 41 min   ℃ 24 servings   12*Kcal / serving* 1*g Protein*   0*g Fat*   3*g Carbs*

INGREDIENTS

Vanilla extract, 1 tsp (5 g)
Applesauce (Mott's LLP), 1 serving (123 g)
Salt, table, 1 teaspoon (5 g)
Oat bran, raw, 1 cup (94 g)

Instructions

1. Preheat oven to 200F
2. Mix all ingredients in a bowl
3. Scoop out 1 tablespoon dough and shape into balls
4. Prepare baking sheets lined with parchment paper and press cookie balls on the baking sheet to flatten a bit
5. Bake in the oven for 10 to 15 minutes or until cookies look golden.
6. Cool in a cooling rack for at least 10 minutes before eating.

MACRONUTRIENT SUMMARY

	TOTAL	PER 100 G	PER SERVING
Energy (kCal)	296.1	130.4	12.3
Protein (g)	16.3	7.2	0.7
Fat (g)	6.6	2.9	0.3
Carbs (g)	76.9	33.9	3.2
Fiber (g)	15.5	6.8	0.6

MICRONUTRIENT SUMMARY

	TOTAL	PER 100 G	PER SERVING
Sugars (g)	14	6.2	0.6
Fiber (g)	15.5	6.8	0.6
Calcium, Ca (mg)	56.3	24.8	2.3
Iron, Fe (mg)	5.1	2.2	0.2
Magnesium, Mg (mg)	221.16	97.6	9.2
Phosphorus, P (mg)	690.3	304.1	28.8
Potassium, K (mg)	629.6	277.4	26.2
Sodium, Na (mg)	1942.1	855.6	80.9
Zinc, Zn (mg)	2.9	1.3	0.1
Vitamin D (ug)	0	0	0
Vitamin C (mg)	12.1	5.3	0.5
Cholesterol (mg)	0	0	0

While managing Chronic Kidney Disease (CKD) through a carefully monitored diet is crucial, it's only one piece of a larger, intricate puzzle. A balanced, low-sodium diet with controlled protein intake is essential, but it's not all-encompassing. A more holistic approach to CKD management exists, one that integrates not just dietary changes, but also lifestyle modifications.

Consider the impact of regular physical activity, adequate hydration, stress management, and quality sleep to overall wellbeing. How could these elements be intertwined with a CKD-friendly diet to create a comprehensive healthcare strategy? The answer lies in a broader perspective, one that values the interconnectedness of our daily habits. But what does this really mean for a patient with CKD? How does each aspect influence kidney health?

As we delve deeper into CKD management beyond dietary changes, you'll discover that there's more to this story than meets the eye...

Chapter 5:

Adapting Your Diet to Your Lifestyle

"Personalized nutrition is not just a trend, but a fundamental shift in how we approach health and wellness. Recognizing that each person has unique dietary needs is the cornerstone of effective nutritional therapy. It's about more than just the food on your plate; it's about how it interacts with your unique biochemistry."

Working with a Dietitian

I cannot stress enough and have repeatedly encouraged you and mentioned to you about "ask your dietitian this", "tell your dietitian about this", "let your dietitian confirm this" and so on.

At this point I don't think you need more convincing that a dietitian plays a crucial role in the management of Chronic Kidney Disease (CKD) and has the key responsibilities in your treatment process. But allow me to talk about some of these key roles so we can keep reminding ourselves how important they are for our overall wellness:

Nutritional Assessment

A dietitian conducts a comprehensive nutritional assessment to identify any nutritional deficiencies or excesses. They also evaluate a patient's dietary habits, preferences, and adherence to dietary recommendations.

Diet Planning

Based on the assessment, the dietitian creates an individualized diet plan. The dietitian takes into account the patient's CKD stage, other health conditions (like diabetes or hypertension), and dietary preferences.

Education

A dietitian educates the patient about the importance of nutrition in managing CKD. This includes explaining why certain foods should be limited (like those high in sodium, potassium, phosphorus) and others should be included.

Monitoring and Adjusting the Diet

The dietitian continually monitors the patient's health status, lab results, and adherence to the diet plan. They adjust the diet as necessary to account for changes in the patient's health.

Interdisciplinary Collaboration

The dietitian collaboratively works with the rest of the healthcare team, sharing their expertise on dietary issues to provide the best possible care for the patient.

Research and Advocacy

Dietitians stay informed about the latest research on CKD and nutrition. They also advocate for the nutritional needs of their patients.

Maximizing Your Dietician Appointments

With all those in mind, just like your doctors' visits, you may want to maximize your dietitian appointments which makes it crucial in managing Chronic Kidney Disease (CKD). Here are some strategies to make the most out of your time with your dietitian:

1. Preparation: Before your appointment, write down any questions or concerns you have. This could include queries about specific foods, how to manage your diet in social situations, or how to cope with dietary restrictions.
2. Honesty: Be honest with your dietitian about your eating habits, even if they're not always in line with dietary recommendations. Your dietitian is there to help, not judge. The more accurate

information they have, the better they can tailor the dietary plan to your needs.

3. Open-Mindedness: Be open to trying new foods and recipes suggested by your dietitian. Diversifying your diet can make it more enjoyable and ensure you're getting a range of nutrients.
4. Record Keeping: Keep a food diary to track what and when you eat, as well as any symptoms you experience. This can provide valuable insights for your dietitian and may clarify areas where changes can be made.
5. Active Learning: Make an effort to understand the rationale behind dietary recommendations. This can help you make good dietary decisions in different situations.
6. Regular Feedback: Regularly communicate with your dietitian about what's working and what's not. This will help them adjust your diet plan as necessary.
7. Consistent Follow-Up: Regular appointments allow your dietitian to monitor your progress and make adjustments to your diet plan as needed. Don't skip these unless absolutely necessary.
8. Integration of Advice: Try to integrate the advice given by your dietitian into your daily life. This might require planning and prepping meals in advance or making conscious choices when dining out.
9. Involve Your Support System: If you're comfortable doing so, consider involving family members or close friends in your dietary management. They can provide support and help maintain the dietary changes you are making.

Remember, managing CKD is a team effort. Your dietitian is an important teammate in this journey, and maximizing your appointments with them can contribute significantly to your overall health and well-being. Finding one and being able to work consistently and openly would be one of the considerably major decisions and modifications you'll make in the course of your treatment plan.

Diet Adjustments for Common Comorbidities

Adjusting for Diabetes

Whether you have them or not, I would also like to take a little step further in including adjustments that you have to make for two of the most common chronic illnesses that may be due to or may have developed prior to CKD: Diabetes and Hypertension.

What's the relationship between Diabetes and Chronic Kidney Damage?

Diabetes is actually one of the risk factors and **leading cause to kidney failure.**

High blood glucose *(blood sugar)* can damage the blood vessels in your kidneys. When the blood vessels are damaged, your kidneys cannot clean your blood properly.

In turn, your body will retain more water and salt than it should, which can result in weight gain and ankle swelling.

Other health results include high blood pressure and having protein in your urine.

Since diabetes can damage the nerves in your body, it can cause a difficulty in emptying your bladder. With the pressure, it will result from your full bladder can back up and **injure the kidneys.**

What does that mean?

It means that if the urine stays in your bladder for a long period of time, you can develop an infection from the rapid growth of bacteria in urine that has a high sugar level.

So...what are the symptoms of diabetic kidney disease?

Most people with diabetic kidney disease *(diabetic nephropathy)* do not have symptoms because the only way to know if you have diabetic kidney disease is to **get your kidneys checked.** However, for some, there are early signs such as:

- Increased excretion of protein in urine

- Weight gain
- Leg or ankle swelling/cramps
- Increased need to urinate *(especially at night)*
- High blood pressure

Before we continue...I want to discuss the differences between diabetic kidney disease with type 1 & 2 diabetes.

Diabetic kidney disease is kidney damage that results from having diabetes. Because diabetes can cause high blood sugar, it can damage the part that filters the blood. For this reason, the damaged filter becomes leaky and then lets protein into your urine.

With *diabetic nephropathy*, it can progress to kidney failure compared to that of type 1 & 2 diabetes.

People with type 1 diabetes do not produce insulin, while type 2 diabetes do not respond to insulin. They both do not develop kidney disease that eventually progresses to kidney failure.

Now, moving on...

What lab tests do I need do to know that I have diabetic kidney disease?

First, take note of the signs or symptoms that you experienced since that will be the first thing that your doctor will ask you. Then, he or she will conduct a physical exam which afterwards, they will ask about your medical history. Once that's done, they will then refer you to a nephrologist or a diabetes specialist *(endocrinologist)*.

To really determine if you have diabetic kidney disease, you may be advised to do these tests and procedures:

- **Blood tests.** If you have diabetes, you will need blood tests to monitor your condition and determine how well your kidneys are working.
- **Urine tests.** Urine samples provide information about your kidney function and whether you have too much protein in the urine. High levels of a protein called microalbumin may indicate your kidneys are being affected by the disease.

- **Imaging tests.** Your doctor may use X-rays and ultrasound to assess your kidneys' structure and size. You may also undergo CT scanning and magnetic resonance imaging (MRI) to determine how well blood is circulating within your kidneys. Other imaging tests may be used in some cases.
- **Renal function testing.** Your doctor can assess your kidneys' filtering capacity using renal analysis testing.
- **Kidney biopsy.** Your doctor may recommend a kidney biopsy to remove a sample of kidney tissue. You'll be given a numbing medication (local anesthetic). Then your doctor will use a thin needle to remove small pieces of kidney tissue for examination under a microscope.

Okay....how about medication?

In the early stages of the disease, your treatment plan may include various medications that will help:

- **Control high blood pressure.** Medications called angiotensin-converting enzyme (ACE) inhibitors and angiotensin II receptor blockers (ARBs) are used to treat high blood pressure. Using both of these together isn't advised because of increased side effects. Studies support the goal of a blood pressure reading below 140/90 millimeters of mercury (mm Hg) depending on your age and overall risk of cardiovascular disease.
- **Manage high blood sugar.** Several medications have been shown to help control high blood sugar in people with diabetic nephropathy. Studies support the goal of an average hemoglobin A1C of less than 7%.
- **Lower high cholesterol.** Cholesterol-lowering drugs called statins are used to treat high cholesterol and reduce protein in the urine.
- **Foster bone health.** Medications that help manage your calcium phosphate balance are important in maintaining healthy bones.

- **Control protein in urine.** Medications can often reduce the level of the protein albumin in the urine and improve kidney function.

Along the way, your doctor may recommend follow-up testing at regular intervals to see whether your kidney disease remains stable or progresses.

Can diabetic kidney disease be treated?

Treatment for diabetic kidney disease include:

- Controlling and managing blood sugar levels
- Controlling high blood pressure
- Reducing dietary protein intake
- Avoiding medications that may damage kidneys
- Treat urinary tract infections
- Exercise/Lose weight *(under the supervision of a physician)*

If I have diabetic kidney disease and CKD, how should I balance both diets?

It's true that the **right diet** helps your body function properly. However, figuring out what to eat especially if you have both diabetes and Chronic Kidney Disease can be a major challenge because when one meal plan may be good for you, it may not be good for the other. Which is why, **you need to consult a registered nutritionist dietitian** who is trained in both diabetes and Chronic Kidney Disease nutrition for this one. Together you will create a diet plan that will help keep your blood sugar levels steady and reduce the waste and fluid your kidneys have to handle. He or she will give nutritional guidelines to you on how much nutrients *(SPPP)* you can have each day and limit or avoid them while planning your meals.

Remember that portion is also important to do. If you remember from our previous lesson, I taught you how to do so below:

But if you want, you could talk to your nutritionist regarding tips to accurately measure a serving size because what may be measured as one serving size on a regular diet may count as three times more on a kidney diet.

The meal planning also includes eating meals and snacks that have the same size and calorie/carbohydrate content at certain times of the day in order to keep your blood glucose at an even level. Again, it's important to check your blood glucose levels often and share the results with your doctor.

Believe it or not, diabetes and Chronic Kidney Disease share a lot of the same food BUT of course, there are some important differences.

So, what can I eat then?

What I will list down below are examples of food choices that are usually recommended on a typical renal diabetic diet since this list will be based on sodium, potassium, phosphorus, protein, and high sugar content of foods.

CARBOHYDRATE FOODS
Milk and non dairy products

- Skim/Fat-free milk
- Non-dairy creamer
- Sugar-free yogurt

- Sugar-free ice cream
- Sugar-free non dairy frozen desserts

BREADS AND STARCHES

- Whole wheat
- Whole grain
- Unsalted crackers
- White/Whole Wheat Pasta
- Grits

FRUITS AND JUICES

- Apples/Applesauce/apple juice
- Raspberries
- Blueberries
- Low-sugar cranberry juice
- Grape/grape juice
- Grapefruit

STARCHY VEGETABLES

- Corn
- Peas
- Potatoes *(soaked in order to reduce potassium)*

NON-STARCHY VEGETABLES

- Asparagus
- Beets
- Broccoli
- Brussels sprouts
- Cauliflower
- Cabbage
- Cucumber

HIGH-PROTEIN FOODS

Meats, cheeses, and eggs

- Lean cuts of meat

- Eggs
- Poultry
- Low-cholesterol egg substitute

HIGHER-FAT FOODS

Seasonings and calories

- Sour cream
- Low-fat mayonnaise
- Low-fat cream cheese

Again, these are all just recommendations on a typical renal diabetic diet. You need to ask your nutritionist if you can have any of these listed foods and make sure that you ask your recommended servings size as well. I want to share four (4) tips on how to keep your kidneys healthy with diabetic kidney disease.

The best way to slow it down or prevent it from progressing is to try to reach your blood glucose and blood pressure goals. Healthy lifestyle habits and taking in your prescribed medications can help you achieve those goals and at the same time, improve your overall health.

1. Reach your blood glucose goals

A healthcare professional will need to test your A1C. This is a blood test that will show your average blood glucose level over the past three months, which is different from the blood glucose checks that you may do yourself at home.

The higher your A1C number, the higher your blood glucose levels have been during the past three months. The goal for many people with diabetes is **below 7 percent.** However, you may ask your health care team what your goal should be since reaching it will help protect your kidneys. After which, you will use those results to discuss with your healthcare team that will help decide on food, physical activity, and medicines.

One more thing to ask your healthcare team is how often you should check your blood glucose level.

2. Control and manage your blood pressure

High blood pressure *(hypertension)* happens when the pressure of your blood against the walls of your blood vessels increases. If left uncontrolled, it could cause stroke, heart attack, and Chronic Kidney Disease.

For this reason, ask your health care team to help you set and reach your blood pressure goal. The blood pressure goal for most people with diabetes is below 140/90mmHg.

Taking in prescribed medication that can help lower blood pressure and slow down kidney damage is also important.

3. Develop or maintain healthy lifestyle habits

Forming healthy lifestyle habits can help you reach your blood glucose and blood pressure goals. Following these steps below will help you keep your kidneys healthy:

- Stop smoking
- Work with a nutritionist dietitian to develop a diabetes meal plan and limit salt and sodium
- Get physical! Make it part of your routine *(with the supervision of a physician)*
- Stay at or get to a healthy weight
- Get enough sleep. Be sure to aim for 7-8 hours of sleep each night.

4. Take prescribed medications

Taking in medications may be an important part of your treatment plan as your health care professional will prescribe them based on your specific needs and can help meet your blood glucose and blood pressure goals.

High Blood Pressure and CKD

I know it's been briefly discussed almost althroughout this book and even when talking about diabetic nephropathy, but I want us to take a closer look at high blood pressure's (hypertension) relationship with

Chronic Kidney Disease, the negative effects of high blood pressure, and how to manage it.

So, are you ready? If you are, let's start with what it means...

Blood pressure refers to the force of blood against the walls of your blood vessels as your heart pumps blood around your body. If it becomes too high, you can be diagnosed with high blood pressure or hypertension. Simply put, it's the pressure that prevails in the blood vessels.

Did you know that your blood pressure results are written with two values?

- The upper pressure *(systolic pressure)* is the pressure you have at the moment your heart contracts and pushes the blood through all blood vessels.
- The bottom number *(diastolic pressure)* indicates the pressure you have when your heart relaxes between the contractions. The heart functions as a pump.

Normal Blood Pressure

It is important for everyone to maintain normal blood pressure, appropriate to age, especially for patients with CKD.

Your blood pressure should be lower than 130/80 mmHg. If it's higher than 130/80 mmHg, it puts extra strain on your heart and blood vessels. This increases your risk of developing cardiovascular disease. The blood vessels can get thicker walls, the heart is negatively affected, just like the eyes. In short, the higher the blood pressure over a longer period of time, the greater the risk of a heart attack, or stroke.

High blood pressure is one of the causes of CKD, making it more serious. But, it also works the other way around. CKD sooner or later causes blood pressure to rise. This is partly because the kidneys can no longer properly regulate blood pressure. In other words: High blood pressure and CKD reinforce each other in a negative way. So, how can you determine if your blood pressure is too high?

The only way is to measure it with a blood pressure monitoring device. To make things worse, high blood pressure may not reveal obvious symptoms. That's why it has been called a "silent killer". A single reading of high blood pressure doesn't confirm that you have it. It is confirmed through follow-up visits to your doctor or clinic. Symptoms of severely elevated blood pressure include:

- Headache
- Confusion
- Blurry or double vision
- Bloody (pink colored) urine
- Nose bleed

When visiting your doctor, make sure to have your blood pressure measured. During this visit, they may focus on lowering and managing your blood pressure – one of the most important goals of treatment to improve and maintain your kidney functions.

Treatment Plan

Well, a treatment plan is necessary especially when it should be based on your CKD stage. In some cases, your doctor may recommend you to see a specialist in high blood pressure or CKD. The goals of the treatment are:

- To lower your blood pressure,
- To keep kidney disease from getting worse, and
- To lower your chances of getting heart disease.

To help reach these goals, you will need a combination of lifestyle changes, such as switching to a kidney-healthy diet, exercise, and taking medications especially prescribed for your condition.

To Do's to Lower Your Blood Pressure

But for now, we would like to focus more on the first goal which is to lower your blood pressure because it can have a positive ripple effect. Here are 6 ways you can do that:

☑ To Do 1: Exercise

- Exercise is important for heart health.
- Set a goal to exercise for 30 minutes a day, 5 days per week.
- Try walking or dancing.

☑ To Do 2: Maintain a healthy weight

Being overweight normally increases blood pressure, while reduced weight can lower blood pressure.

☑ To Do 3: Quit smoking

Nicotine causes the smallest blood vessels to constrict and thereby increases blood pressure.

☑ To Do 4: Limit sodium intake

Stop adding salt to your meals. Try to prepare the meal with as little salt as possible. Salt ensures that you retain moisture and that again causes the blood pressure to rise. If you use less salt you will quickly get used to the taste and feel better.

☑ To Do 5: Take prescribed medications

It is very important that you take the blood pressure medication that the doctor prescribed and that you do exactly as he has advised. You can get one or two different blood pressure medications prescribed which all have a slightly different effect and together ensure that your high blood pressure will decrease.

☑ To Do 6: Reduce stress

Stress is normal. And yes, stress can be detrimental, but ONLY IF YOU LET IT. Properly dealing with stress not only helps you manage it, but it will also serve to strengthen you and make you more resilient.

Constant and excessive stress does take a toll on your health. This is why stress management is very important, especially for people with a chronic kidney condition.

So, how does stress affect the kidneys? Usually, the body's response to stress and anxiety are the following:

- Increase in breathing and heart rate
- Blood pressure spikes
- Pupil dilation
- Muscle tension
- Increase in fat and sugar levels in the blood

These responses are normal and can actually help you when dealing with crises and immediate danger.

However, constantly experiencing these bodily reactions because of high stress levels for long periods takes a toll on your health.

I hope that I was able to shed light, or add important bits of information in the management of comorbidities that may have come along with CKD, or help you prevent them from sabotaging your goals for health. Now that that's out of the way, how about we take care of other serious business? Like planning your lunch out next weekend?

"Am I even allowed to do that?"...

Sure you are, and I might have just the thing to help you out!

Chapter 6:

Handling Special Occasions and Dining Out

*I*n the heart of Foodville lived a kidney patient, Kevin, with a mighty appetite. Dining out was his hobby, but health was his priority.

When "Salty Spud" opened, renowned for its potato delights, Kevin's face lit up. However, he knew the drill: no excess salt, no potassium overload.

As the waiter recommended the "Spud Supreme," Kevin's mouth watered. But he ordered the "Low-Sodium Salad" instead. The waiter blinked, surprised. "Are you sure, sir? It's rather...bland."

"Absolutely," replied Kevin, with a twinkle in his eye.

The salad arrived, plain as plain can be. Then, Kevin unveiled his secret weapon - a small bottle of homemade, kidney-friendly seasoning. A sprinkle here, a dash there, and the salad was transformed!

That night, Kevin left the restaurant, belly full, spirits high. Health restrictions couldn't dampen his dining adventures. Kevin, the ever-ready foodie, had once again found joy in the culinary battlefield.

Navigating Different Eating Situations

That was a little too playful, wasn't it? But let me ask you, have you ever been tempted to break your diet when you're eating at home or at a restaurant? Well, the reality is, **we've all been there.**

Whether it is with friends or with family, it can be quite stressful to stay on-track with your needs to make healthy choices and be mindful of what you are eating, especially if they're not going through the same journey as you. This anxiety can lead to poor food decisions and hinder you from achieving a healthier lifestyle. Growing up, our parents are our first role models and teachers, so we tend to mirror our behavior after what we have been shown or taught. If we have always experienced an unhealthy lifestyle, we are more likely to make poor dietary choices — even as an adult.

Therefore, it can be difficult to overcome that kind of eating style, especially if we are dining with our family or friends. Such situations can be a trigger and may push us back into our old eating habits.

Dining out with friends can be just as stressful because you are not conforming to the "norm" of the social circle. Most of us, *I know I do*, want to feel included, so we tend to give into "peer pressure" especially in a social setting that involves eating. Most of the time, this leads to guilt or shame because you abandoned everything that you have been working hard for.

However, in making small changes in our thoughts and behaviors, we can better handle some of the situations mentioned above that can help keep us on track and positively impact those we care about. Every step that you take to improve your overall health and well-being is a positive step in **the right direction.**

Eating alone at home

When you are at home you can of course think about what you will eat. You can plan food so that it contains exactly the amount of protein you are allowed to have. Certainly if you cook yourself. Do not add salt to the food.

Eating with family at home

When more people in the family eat together, things get a bit more complicated. Not everyone in the family will appreciate the protein-restricted meals. There are at least two ways to work around this problem:

- One way is to prepare different dishes; for those who have chronic kidney damage and for the rest of the family. For example: for the kidney patient, instead a bowl of yogurt or

custard for dessert or no cheese sauce over the vegetables. And vegetables, potatoes and meat without salt for the kidney patient and with salt for the rest of the family.
- The other way is that you prepare food that most of the family likes without thinking about the kidney patient. Then it is up to you to determine what you eat or not eat (or less) of. For example: you take more potatoes, more vegetables and less meat (and preferably an extra cube of diet-margarine through the food). Do not add salt to the food. The family members can add salt to their own dish if necessary.

In most families, it will be some sort of mix of these two ways. Sometimes you can prepare something for the kidney patient. But usually everyone eats the same and the difference is in the quantities. Of course, you are the one having CKD and therefore you should be able to assess what you can and cannot eat. You are the one in control of the grams of protein you eat.

Eating at work

When you bring your food from home to work, you decide what you eat - food and drinks appropriate for someone with CKD. If you eat in the staff restaurant it would be nice if you can choose different dishes. Again, as a kidney patient you must have enough knowledge to make a responsible choice - for instance, choose something of which you roughly know how much protein it contains, and of which you can take the right amounts.

Dining out

The best thing is of course if you can choose your restaurant yourself. For someone with chronic kidney disease, a "steakhouse" where mainly large steaks are served is not the best option. It is best to go to a restaurant with a wide and varied range of dishes, where you have more "kidney-friendly" dishes. Ask if they can prepare the food without any added salt.

The important thing is that you have so much knowledge of the amount of protein in the various

foods that you know which dishes to avoid, of which you can take bits and from which you can take somewhat larger portions. You can have that knowledge by plunging into the tables a little further in the book.

*For Chef Duane, one of his **AHA! Moments** where he felt normal again was when he ordered side dishes at a Mexican restaurant and felt normal. Not only that, he could also eat rice, beans, guacamole with "no salt added" chips, and learned to make spinach and mushroom enchiladas. Because of this, he doesn't miss the beef tacos or the chicken taquitos.*

*If you're trying to limit animal protein like him, here's his advice: **Read the entire menu.** Read it like it's a grocery list. Yes, a grocery list. But you have to look at the side dishes with every entree on the menu.*

What he does is he'd take all the side dishes and request a plate be made into a meal. But he cautions you that with this kind of creativity, it can cause some surprises when the bill comes at the end of the meal.

Eat with family or friends

All good hosts and hostesses ask themselves: what can I prepare for a person with chronic kidney disease, what can he have? That is quite thoughtful and nice.

An answer to the question can be: "In principle I eat everything, so prepare something you want". And then you adjust how much you eat, that is, a little bit of what contains a lot of protein and more of other things. But ask if they don't add salt to it.

Another answer can of course be that you indicate more precisely what you like and that you explain something about the protein-restricted diet and about cooking without salt. Most people who invite someone with chronic kidney damage would like to make an effort to offer something suitable, that is after all the reason they ask.

The most important thing is that you stick to the number of grams of protein per day that are recommended. So if you take a little more protein with lunch then you need one take a little less when eating at night - and vice versa. It is about the average dividend amount per day. And all this of course with the note that you are well.

Eat if you go by plane

Eating on board of a plane can become a minor problem, as there usually is little to choose. You usually have to take what is there and then you have to determine what and how much you can eat from what is available.

Another way is to prepare, for example, a vegetarian and sodium meal that is likely to have less protein (and no salt) than the normal meat and fish dishes. Watch out for soy dishes, which are high in protein. With some airlines you can even eat protein-restricted and sodium-restricted foods, if you order this well in advance.

Strategies on Staying On-Track

When the time comes where you will feel pressured to eat something that you shouldn't, here are **four (4) tips to help yourself stay in control and on track with your health:**

1. Visualize yourself making good choices

Scientific research shows that if you visualize yourself doing something that has a successful outcome, you are able to reinforce the neural pathways in your brain and **increase your chances for success**.

For example, if you're afraid to go to a party because you know the host will expect you to eat the meals they have prepared, visualize yourself enjoying the party, and calmly explaining to the host that you're practicing health-consciousness.

Imagine yourself feeling calm, relaxed, happy, and satisfied. You'll notice that when you mentally prepare yourself in this manner beforehand, you'll experience much more success at being able to avoid certain foods.

2. Eat a healthy meal beforehand

If you're getting ready to attend an event that you know will offer unhealthy foods, make plans to eat before you go so you won't be hungry, tempted, or forced to eat anything at the event.

For example, eat a large green salad followed by a chicken breast and some steamed veggies to give yourself the nourishment and energy you need to sustain yourself throughout the course of the event.

These types of foods will also provide you with a lasting feeling of fullness that will help prevent you from being hungry and experiencing cravings later on.

3. Bring your own healthy dish

If you're attending a party or event where bringing food is allowed, make your own healthy meals or side dishes at home and bring them with you to the party.

In most cases, the host will be thankful that you contributed to the party. Bring homemade salad and dressing, or crackers made with healthy ingredients and hummus dip.

4. Assess your options before digging in

If the event you're attending is offering catered food, or food laid out in buffet style, take a moment to walk through and assess your options before loading up your plate.

Look for salads, vegetables, drumsticks, and other whole foods that aren't processed or made with artificial ingredients. Start off with a large plate of salad, then go back for various other whole foods that won't harm your kidneys.

As far as drinks go, stick to water and avoid drinking sugary fruit juice or punch. If alcohol is being served, limit yourself to one or two glasses of wine or consume small amounts of liquor without adding mixers. This too will depend on your healthcare team's advice on alcohol consumption. If you are unsure, let's stick with water!

And that's it! As mentioned, taking the first step is the most difficult to make. But once you take it, everything will fall into place.

You will become more invested in your journey to a healthier lifestyle. Who knows, along the way, you may even inspire those around you to eat healthier. You will feel better about yourself and the choices that you are making.

Every step in the right direction will get you one step closer to achieving your goals of creating the healthy lifestyle you desire.

While social pressure can be quite stressful, **it can be managed.** Remember that **YOU ARE IN CONTROL.** Just don't forget to take the first step because your body and mind will thank you in the future.

Chapter 7:

Exercise and CKD Management

As Dr. Patel explained the importance of exercise in managing Chronic Kidney Disease, Alex felt a pang of guilt. Those unused running shoes gathered dust in the corner, a stark reminder of abandoned resolutions. "Start slow, Alex," Dr. Patel advised, "your kidneys will thank you." The next morning, lacing up those shoes, Alex stepped outside, heart pounding. Nervous energy filled the air. The jog was tougher than expected, but it had begun. Just as Alex was finding rhythm, a sharp pain shot through his side. Doubled over, he saw a figure approach. "Are you okay?" the stranger asked.

Alex grimaced, clutching his side. His breaths becoming short and fast. "Just...a cramp," he panted, trying to wave the stranger away. But the stranger, a woman with kind eyes and a runner's physique, didn't budge.

"Try slow, deep breaths," she suggested, her tone laced with concern. Alex followed her advice, the pain slowly subsiding. As he straightened up, he noticed her runner's bib. 'Marathoner', it read.

"You new to running?" she asked, handing him a water bottle. Alex nodded, explaining about his CKD and the doctor's advice. A smile of understanding crossed her face. "It's tough at first, but it gets better," she said, "Want some company on your journey?"

How about you? Yes, you! Do you want some company in this journey?

While I can't technically be physically with you, let me help you with the following:

- Understand the role of exercise in improving your kidney health,
- Learn how to sketch out your own exercise plan and overcome common objections and excuses,
- Learn exercise tips and tricks that you can follow and take inspiration from, and
- Learn how to combine both diet and exercise.

Before we begin, I'd like to share this piece of advice with you:

"How we spend our days is, of course, how we spend our lives." - Annie Dillard

Now, it may seem like we're stating the obvious. But the truth is, not everyone grasps the gravity of those words.

Few of us are consciously aware that everything we do—down to the tiniest, most seemingly inconsequential action—defines the quality of the life we live. But what does that have to do with today's discussion? Or with your kidneys for that matter?

Well, we brought it up because today, we're going to talk about a particular action that a lot of people with kidney conditions have questions about: **exercise!**

Normally, exercise is a vital part of a healthy daily routine. But considering you have CKD, you might be wondering what effect working out will have on your kidneys and your life. *Should you still do it, or should you take it easy because of your condition?* If you're not sure of the answer, worry not; that's the first question we'll answer today.

A few years back, the answer would have been a resounding "no".

Doctors used to think that kidney disease patients shouldn't exercise—vigorous physical activity was too much for them to handle and would do more harm than good. But things have changed a lot since then. Now we know different things. The newest research shows that:

Kidney disease patients who exercise enjoy a lot of health benefits.

However, there is a **bit of a catch.** As someone with a kidney condition, your exercise routine should be tailored to fit your condition. We'll talk about how you can do that later on. For now, let's go into more detail on those "health benefits" we just mentioned.

The Benefits of Exercise

Here's a list of the major advantages you can get by engaging in proper exercise:

1. Lower blood pressure

This can have a direct effect on your renal health, since high blood pressure is one of those conditions that **can cause kidney function to decline.** Keeping it in check is crucial.

2. Reduced risk of diabetes or better glucose control

Diabetes is another condition that has a direct effect on kidney function. If you don't have it, do everything in your power to keep it that way. If you already have diabetes, exercise is still beneficial, since it helps your body control your glucose level better.

3. Improved muscle strength and function

Weakness and fatigue is a common complaint for those with kidney conditions. Exercise can alleviate that by developing your muscles which leaves you feeling stronger and more able to move around.

4. Helps you lose excess weight or maintain your current weight

Being overweight really isn't a problem you want to have on top of dealing with kidney disease—you'll be at risk of developing even more health complications. A healthy weight is vital.

5. Lower levels of blood fats (like triglycerides and cholesterol)

At high levels, triglycerides and cholesterol can damage your blood vessels. Kidney function depends a lot on the condition of your kidneys' blood vessels, so make sure to keep them damage-free.

6. Better sleep

Few things are as relaxing as a good night's sleep, right? Sleep is when our bodies rest and regenerate, and studies show that catching enough Z's can do wonders for your health.

7. Reduces anxiety and depression

Your emotions and outlook can have a surprisingly large impact on your physical condition. Exercising encourages the release of *"happy hormones"*, combating depression, or simply giving your mood a lift.

And there you have it! Those are some great benefits, right? All that through the simple act of proper exercise.h

But before you start working out, there are some things you should take into consideration, especially because you have a kidney condition... To find out what those are, read on!

Personalizing Your Exercise Plan

You'll notice that I mentioned the words *"proper exercise"* more than once.

The reason for that is because we want to emphasize the importance not just of exercising, but of **exercising the right way.**

And that means personalizing your workout — taking into account your strengths and weaknesses, as well as any health conditions that may hinder you. But planning the right exercise program can be a bit tricky, so it's best to have the opinion of a health professional who is familiar with your condition.

Together, you can decide on the specifics, like:

- **Type:** What type of exercise should you do?

- **Frequency:** How often should you do it?
- **Duration:** How long should you do it each time?
- **Intensity:** How hard should you push yourself?

Those are basic questions you need to answer before you begin any exercise plan. Personalize your exercise plan by choosing the right type, frequency, duration, and intensity of exercise.

Too Busy For Exercise?

Sometimes, it doesn't matter whether there's an exercise plan in place or not, because we often get in our own way when it's time to work out.

You can come up with a thousand reasons why you're "too busy" to exercise right now, but here's the truth:

You should never be too busy to prioritize your own health.

Putting your health first sounds like common sense, but unfortunately, it's not something that comes easy for many of us.

So to help you put all your objections behind, here's the University of Houston's list of the most common excuses we make to avoid exercise, and counterpoints for each of them:

EXCUSE	COUNTERPOINT
"I'm too busy, I only have 20 minutes"	Not only is that enough time, **it's far better than doing nothing**.
"I'm too tired"	Exercise will give you energy. You'll feel better when you're done.
"My husband or wife won't join me"	**Set a good example** that may inspire your partner to join you.
"I'm on vacation"	What better time to exercise than when you have so much free time? Walking is a great travel pastime.

| "I can come up with more reasons **not to exercise**" | That still doesn't mean you can't. |

We hope that with the examples in this list, you can identify the excuses you use to avoid exercising and come up with your own counterpoints.

Exercise doesn't have to be boring. Tying it into your hobbies, like dancing or hiking, can make it a bit easier to deal with. Even chores, like walking the dog or tending the garden, can be considered exercise as well.

Which is why we'll be showing you some actual exercise routines through easy-to-follow videos. But before I do, here's what Lee Haney, a fitness expert and champion bodybuilder once said:

*"Exercise to **stimulate** not to **annihilate**; The world wasn't formed in a day and neither were we. **Set small gals and build upon them**." – Lee Haney*

Don't exercise with the goal of eliminating your health issues as quickly as possible, because honestly, **nothing will change overnight. Be patient with yourself.** Remember to set goals that are **achievable and realistic**. Work on achieving those goals, one step at a time, and eventually, you'll notice a big change!

Types of Exercises That Should Be In Your Plan

Since we talked about the four aspects of exercise: ***type, frequency, duration, and intensity,*** we'll focus on the **type** first. There are three major types of exercise that should always be part of any workout plan:

1. Flexibility Exercises

Stretching activities fall under this category. They're usually used as warm-ups for exercise routines. Here are some sample routines: *(scan the code with your phone camera to watch the exercise videos)*

- **Desk Stretches** - A series of flexibility exercises you can perform anytime, even on your desk. *(https://youtu.be/DKnJh2wJvHE)*

- **Hamstring Stretch** - A stretch you can do with a simple tool, like a belt. *(https://youtu.be/2-plTieJyFs)*

2. Aerobic Exercises

Aerobic exercises improve your endurance. It involves moving large muscle groups in a continuous way. These are also used as **warm up and cooling down exercises** when done lightly for a short period. But when done for longer and with a higher intensity, they can be the main focus of your exercise routine.

Good examples include **walking, running, swimming, dancing, and cycling**—whether outdoors, or indoors on a stationary bike, as you will see in the next slide. Here are some sample routines:

- **Seated Bike** - A good example of aerobic exercise which requires equipment. You can also use a regular bike instead and go outdoors. *(https://youtu.be/X7NYGzDMzYo)*

- **High Knees** - One of many aerobic exercises you can do that are easy and don't require equipment. *(https://youtu.be/SC_Y1Ri_S6I)*

- **Jumping Jacks** *(optional)* - A familiar exercise that can be a warm up when done in a short period, but can also be high intensity when done longer. *(https://youtu.be/CV_BOYUA63c)*

3. Resistance Exercises

The focus of this type of exercise is to improve your strength. That's why they are also called **strength training exercises.** They are typically the main part of routines, which means they are done **after warming up and before cooling down.**

Examples include weight lifting, and activities that involve lifting your own weight like **jumps, squats, lifts, lunges, push-ups (and its modified forms), and even climbing stairs.**

Important Note: Overall, resistance exercises are beneficial, but since you have a kidney condition, avoid routines that require heavy lifting. If you want to push yourself harder, do more repetitions instead of using heavier weights. Here's another set of sample routines:

- Forward Stepping Lunge - A resistance exercise you can do with or without additional weights.
  (https://youtu.be/LuqNTCGIqUo)

- Bicep Curl - A very simple weightlifting exercise. You can gradually increase the difficulty level by doing more repetitions. *(https://youtu.be/S-jAVi4NFVs)*

Duration, Frequency, and Intensity: Tips and Tricks

Now that we're done with the types of exercise, let's talk about the other three aspects: duration, frequency, and intensity.

Let's go through them one at a time:

1. Frequency. This refers to how often you should exercise. As you might expect, this varies from case to case, but generally, most people should exercise **at least 3 days a week.** Quick Tips:

- **Do not exercise on consecutive days.** Leave a "rest day" in between your workout sessions. This prevents muscle damage and fatigue.
- **Alternate between aerobic and resistance exercises for the main parts of your routines.** Different types of exercise have different effects on your body, so make sure to strike a balance between the two for maximum benefit.

2. Duration. This refers to how long your exercises should be. Ideally, you should aim for at least 30 minutes for each session.

- **Don't worry if you think 30 minutes is too long for you.** For now, just go with the duration you're most comfortable with and gradually increase the time until you reach 30 minutes. For example, you can start at 15 minutes, and then increase each session 1 minute at a time.

- **Spend around 5-10 minutes on warming up.** Do this so that your body isn't "shocked" by sudden activity. You can start with light aerobic exercise, and then move on to stretching.
- **Cool down before stopping.** Gradually end each session with exercises that are similar to your warm up. Stopping your routine all of a sudden (without a cool down) can cause negative effects, like dizziness or nausea.

3. Intensity. This refers to how hard you should push yourself while exercising.

We've told you before that exercise should be personalized, and this is especially important when determining the intensity of your workout. Here are some quick tips to check for the right intensity:

- **Your breathing shouldn't be so hard that you can't talk while exercising.** You can check this by talking to yourself (or someone else if possible) once in a while during your workout.
- **You should feel completely normal an hour after ending your session.** If you don't, you're probably pushing yourself too hard. Slow down and cut back on the number of exercises or repetitions you're doing.
- **Your muscles shouldn't be sore enough that you can't exercise for the next session.** Consistency is important. Don't set a pace you can't keep up with.
- **Aim for a comfortable push.** Exerting yourself is part of working out, so you should feel like you're pushing yourself – just not too much.

Remember, starting slowly and progressing gradually over time is the best way to exercise.

Don't forget Mr. Lee Haney's quote at the beginning of this chapter – exercises to stimulate, not to annihilate. Give your body enough time to adapt to your increasing physical activity.

Making Sense of the Whole Package: Integrating Nutrition, Diet and Exercise

Diet and exercise go hand in hand. If your goal is to achieve better overall health—and that includes your kidney health, of course—then you can't have one without the other.

Both are also vital for weight management. This is especially important, since for someone with a kidney condition, any problems with weight (or fat) will likely have more consequences down the line...

To sum it up simply, it's like this:

Diet controls weight, while exercise controls body composition.

Basically, **what you eat** determines how fast you lose or gain weight, and **physical activity** determines if you're losing or gaining fat or muscle. I know that might be just a bit confusing, so let me clarify with a few examples:

1. If you want to lose weight...

Losing weight depends mainly on your diet. If you're eating too many calories, you won't lose weight no matter how much exercise you put in.

On the flip side, if you eat too little calories, you're starving yourself. Your body responds to that by trying to save as much energy as possible, which means less weight loss for you. **Aim for a daily calorie intake that's around 300-500 calories below your daily recommendation.** This is just enough to prevent your body from going into *"starvation mode"*.

Exercise contributes by controlling your body composition as your weight goes down. **If you don't exercise, your body will burn off muscle instead of fat during weight loss.** This will leave you feeling weak and fatigued.

But when you do exercise, you keep (or maybe increase) your muscle mass while dropping off the pounds in fat. This is the healthy type of weight loss that you should aim for—it should leave you feeling stronger and more energetic, and not the other way around.

2. If you want to maintain your weight (and lose fat while gaining muscle)...

If you're currently at your ideal weight—and want it to stay that way—then your focus should be on exercise. Still, you shouldn't disregard your diet altogether.

A healthy balanced diet is vital for keeping up your energy level, repairing and replenishing your muscles, and promoting the growth of new muscle.

3. If you want to gain weight (by adding muscle, not fat)...

You have to eat more!

Of course, it goes without saying you should eat healthy food—trying to gain weight is not an excuse to eat anything you want. To gain weight the healthy way, a balanced diet is vital. You just need to increase your portion sizes.

Trying to gain weight is also not an excuse to slack in the exercise department.

You want to add muscle mass to your body, not fat, so exercise is an absolute must. Just make sure that your diet makes up for the calories you burn during exercise.

Your Diet and Activity Plan

> "A goal without a plan is just a wish." -
> Antoine de Saint-Exupery

In order for a goal to become reality, you need a plan to make it happen!

Right now, your goal is to maintain your kidney health. To do that, you need a diet and activity plan. It doesn't have to be ultra-detailed, just clear enough to help you stay on track and not lose focus.

To get started, here are a few questions you should be able to answer:

1. What are your bad health habits? What nutrients should you be limiting? (For example, sodium or phosphorus, maybe?)

2. How many calories do you consume per day? Is it more than what you need, less, or just enough?
3. How much exercise do you get right now? Is it enough?
4. What healthy foods and recipes do you like? What physical activities do you enjoy?
5. What challenges and roadblocks have you encountered in the past?

You can use your answers to those questions to come up with a diet and exercise plan that addresses your personal needs.

The first three of those questions are all about self-assessment. Before you can come up with a plan, you need to get a good idea of where you are at the moment—and where you want to be.

The 4th question is the key to creating a plan that's enjoyable for you—or at least, one that won't make you miserable! Use the answers you have to create a plan that's tailored to your preferences.

The last question identifies the things that have stopped you from being healthy in the past, so you can avoid them in the present. Don't make the same mistakes twice!

You have all you need to create a great diet and exercise plan... and you're good to go!

Chapter 8:

Stress, Mental Health, and CKD

The mental health aspect of managing Chronic Kidney Disease (CKD) is frequently overlooked, yet it is a crucial component of comprehensive patient care. Living with CKD is not just a physical challenge; it is an emotional and psychological battle as well. The diagnosis often brings a profound life change, triggering feelings of fear, stress, and uncertainty.

Additionally, the ongoing management of the disease - the strict dietary restrictions, the regular medical appointments, and the necessary lifestyle alterations - can cause significant psychological distress. It is paramount that healthcare providers recognize this and integrate mental health care into the treatment plans. Psychological support, including counselling and therapy, should be readily available to patients, helping them navigate their feelings and cope more effectively with their condition. The interplay between physical health and mental well-being is undeniable; addressing both is key for improving the overall quality of life for CKD patients.

Understanding the Mental Impact of CKD

A 2019 study on neuropharmacology states that "neuropsychiatric conditions including depression, anxiety disorders, and cognitive impairment are prevalent in patients with chronic kidney disease (CKD)". And often, these conditions can further prevent patients' progress.

Because of such, it's crucial for us to learn about the role of your mental health too. This includes your thoughts, feelings, and behaviors related to improving your condition.

So remember: don't stick to your health's physical aspect alone. Your health care team can provide you with all the information about your condition and even hand you over all the medications you need to improve your health.

However, being a mere recipient of your health care is sometimes not enough. You should play an active role in your own health. Because if you lacked the will to improve or recover, what use are all the medicines in the world?

Now think about our physical and mental structures having their own natural 'defense mechanisms', a 'first line of defense', or 'guards and protectors'. A simple example would be our skin as it acts as a protective barrier between invaders (pathogens) and our bodies.

Our 'psyche' (our mind) is also protected from things that prevent us from fully realizing our wills or motivations. But sometimes, our mental health isn't strong enough to combat these struggles which can make us unable to cope up with our condition properly.

And this is why we're here to talk about how you can strengthen your mental health: so that you can confront and break down the barriers that impede your recovery and improvement.

In the very beginning of this book, we talked about the different goal setting barriers you face when adjusting your diet. To overcome them, we laid down a few examples of SMART (Specific, Measurable, Action-Oriented, Realistic, and Time-framed) goals and encouraged you to use it in every goal you set.

Now, we will tackle another barrier related to healthy eating that is common among CKD patients---your motivational barriers relevant to your attitude and beliefs.

Motivational Barriers and How to Overcome Them

A qualitative study conducted in 2019 lists 4 barriers that interfere with people's motivation to improve their diet or accustom themselves to healthy eating. we've renamed them to "Bogus Barriers" because they're exactly that - untrue.

😦 Bogus Barrier 1: "Eating healthy food is undesirable"

Some people often consider healthy eating as undesirable because they have a general perception that healthy foods don't taste good. They also consider eating healthy as unsatisfying in comparison to junk food. And they feel like they are forced to eat as an obligation more than an enjoyable diet or lifestyle.

Better Belief: these perceptions usually only occur at the beginning of your shift to a healthier diet. CKD Chef Duane says, "You probably already eat some healthy foods, let's identify those and build a healthier meal plan around them!"

By being patient and giving it time, your palate or taste will adjust. Soon enough, you'll find them delicious and rewarding.

☹ Bogus Barrier 2: Lack of Knowledge

People are not motivated to adapt to a healthy diet because they don't know anything about the food they are eating. This is often caused by a lack of 'nutritional knowledge' or 'nutrition misinformation'.

Better Belief: by taking this book and still reading until this chapter, you are already getting more knowledgeable about kidney-friendly nutrition than when you started!

If you want to change your mindset or perception about healthy food, you should research well on the food's nutritional aspect. You can also seek help from your doctor or health care team and ask how exactly does a healthy diet improve your condition.

☹ Bogus Barrier 3: Prioritization

People lose motivation to eat healthily because they can't find time to start and they have other priorities like work or other personal interests.

Better Belief: We often forget how important our health is too. How can we earn a living if we're unhealthy or sick? How can we carry out the things we're passionate about if our health hinders us from doing so?

I'm pretty sure you know the answers to these. So make sure that your health is among your priorities!

☹ Bogus Barrier 4: Thriftiness

In relation to prioritization as a barrier, thriftiness is also one of the reasons why people find healthy eating extra challenging. The funny thing is, CKD Chef Duane will be the first to tell you that...

..."healthy eating has to be expensive" is a MYTH.

Better Belief: sure, you will have to be more conscious about your food choices and expenses. But by doing so, you can actually discover healthier, cheaper options. For example, when comparing price per ounce at Kroger's: Beef Shaved Steak is $0.43 but a healthier substitute like White Mushroom is only $0.24, which is almost half-priced. Beans and rice are less expensive than purchasing meat, too. And guess what, fresh fruit for your sweet fix is not only healthier, they are less expensive than buying pre-made dessert!

On a more basic level, you also need to realize that it's an investment in how you're going to spend the rest of your life. The more resources and care you put in deciding what to eat, the healthier you'll be in the long run and the less you'll end up spending for hospitalizations and healthcare.

Mental Health Journey of a CKD Patient

Linda, a vibrant woman in her fifties, had always treated life as a grand adventure until she was diagnosed with Chronic Kidney Disease (CKD). Her world seemed to shrink, and she grappled with a rush of unwelcome emotions.

She felt shocked and scared at first, the word "chronic" echoing in her mind. But Linda had always been a fighter, so she gathered her strength and embarked on this new, unexpected journey.

Dealing with CKD was challenging. Sometimes, the fatigue was overwhelming, and her radiant smile would waver. But she found solace in her beloved garden, tending to her roses and marigolds, finding peace in their blooms.

On days when the physical discomfort mounted, she turned to her close-knit book club members. Their laughter, shared stories, and words of encouragement were her balm, a sweet reminder that she was not alone.

Linda also sought professional help, speaking to a psychologist who specialized in chronic illnesses. Her therapist taught her coping mechanisms and ways to reframe her thoughts, which played an effective role in managing her anxiety.

She also joined a support group for CKD patients. Sharing experiences, fears, and small victories with those who truly understood what she was going through was profoundly comforting.

Through the highs and lows of her CKD journey, Linda realized that it's okay to be vulnerable and seek help. She learned to listen to her body and mind, to take one day at a time, and to cherish the love and support that surrounded her. She acknowledged the struggle, but refused to let it define her. And in her resilience, she found a new strength she never knew she had.

Strategies for Managing Stress

Techniques for Stress Reduction

Managing stress with chronic illness can be challenging, but there are multiple techniques that can help. Here are some recommendations:

1. **Mindfulness and Meditation**: Mindfulness is about staying present and focusing on the moment. It helps to reduce stress by preventing overthinking about past or future worries. Meditation is one way to practice mindfulness.
2. **Exercise**: Regular physical activity can boost your mood, help you sleep better, and decrease tension. It's important to consult with your doctor about suitable exercises for your condition.
3. **Social Support**: Staying connected with friends and family, joining support groups, or speaking with a mental health professional can provide emotional relief.
4. **Healthy Eating:** Certain foods can influence the body's stress response. Maintain a balanced diet with plenty of fruits, vegetables, lean proteins, and whole grains.
5. **Relaxation Techniques**: Techniques like deep breathing, progressive muscle relaxation, and yoga can reduce stress.
6. **Cognitive Behavioral Therapy (CBT)**: CBT can help you manage stress by changing negative thought patterns and developing coping strategies.

Implementing a Daily Stress-Management Routine

Implementing a daily stress-management routine is a key step in handling stress effectively. Here are some strategies you can use:

Start Your Day With Mindfulness

Spend a few minutes each morning practicing mindfulness or meditation. This can be as simple as focusing on your breath, savoring your morning coffee, or doing a guided meditation using an app like Headspace (https://www.headspace.com/) or Calm (https://www.calm.com/).

Regular Exercise

Incorporate physical activity into your daily routine. This could be a morning walk, yoga, swimming, or any exercise you enjoy. Remember to consult with a healthcare professional about what's suitable for you.

Balanced Diet

I cannot stress enough that you should ensure your meals are nutritious and balanced. Poor nutrition can exacerbate feelings of stress, while a healthy diet can boost your mood and energy levels.

Take Regular Breaks

Breaks, especially ones where you move around, can help regain focus and reduce stress during the day.

Practice Deep Breathing or Progressive Muscle Relaxation

These exercises can be done almost anywhere to help reduce immediate feelings of stress.

Connect with Others

Spend time each day connecting with loved ones, either in person, over the phone, or through video calls.

Prioritize Sleep

Good sleep hygiene is crucial for stress management. Try to have a consistent sleep schedule, and make your sleep environment as comfortable as possible.

End Your Day with Reflection

Journaling or quiet reflection can help process the events of the day, fostering gratitude and helping identify stressors.

Professional Support

If stress becomes overwhelming, consider seeking help from a mental health professional. They can provide strategies tailored to your specific needs.

Remember, different strategies work better for different people, so it's important to experiment and find what works best for you.

Chapter 9:

The Importance of Sleep in CKD Management

Understanding a your sleep patterns can provide valuable insights into your overall wellbeing and the management of Chronic Kidney Disease. I'd like you to do a quick assessment of your own sleep patterns by answering the following questions before proceeding in this chapter:

1. What time do you usually go to bed and wake up?
   _____
   This can help establish your natural sleep-wake cycle.

2. How long does it take you to fall asleep once you're in bed?
   _____

   Difficulty falling asleep can be a sign of insomnia.

3. Do you wake up during the night?
   _____

4. If so, how often and for how long?
   _____

   Frequent awakenings could indicate a sleep disorder.

5. Do you feel refreshed upon waking up in the morning?
   _____

   Feeling tired even after a full night's rest could indicate poor sleep quality.

6. Do you snore or has anyone ever told you that you stop breathing during sleep? _____
   These might be signs of sleep apnea, which is common in CKD patients.

7. Do you experience restless legs or any other discomfort that prevents you from falling asleep?
   _____

   Restless legs syndrome is also common in CKD patients.

8. Do you nap during the day?
   _____

9. How often and for how long?
   _____

   Daytime sleepiness can disrupt the sleep-wake cycle.

10. Do you consume caffeine or alcohol, and when?
    _____

    These substances can interfere with sleep.

11. Do you use any electronic devices (e.g., smartphones, laptops) in bed? _____

> *The light emitted from these devices can interfere with circadian rhythms.*

12. What is your bedtime routine?
    _____

13. _____
    _____

> *A consistent routine can help signal the body that it's time to sleep.*

Remember, these questions are a starting point. It would also be helpful to share these answers with your healthcare team, especially if you are experiencing some discomfort and abnormalities in your sleep.

Understanding Sleep and CKD

The Role of Sleep in Health

Sleep disorders are common in patients with CKD, including sleep apnea, insomnia, restless leg syndrome, and others. These disorders can increase the risk of high blood pressure, cardiovascular disease, and exacerbate kidney damage, all of which can further compromise kidney function.

In a study published in 2019, it was found that poor sleep quality was associated with faster CKD progression. The researchers suggested that sleep disturbances could be an overlooked factor contributing to the progression of kidney disease in these patients.

Additionally, a review article from 2020 discussed the complex relationship between CKD and sleep disorders. The authors suggested that effectively managing sleep problems could help slow the progression of kidney disease, reduce symptoms, and improve the overall quality of life for these patients.

Therefore, proper sleep management should be integrated into your comprehensive care plan as an individual with CKD. This can include lifestyle modifications, cognitive-behavioral therapy for insomnia, and treatment for specific sleep disorders.

However, it's important to note that the relationship between sleep and CKD is complex and multifactorial. Future research is needed to further understand this relationship, and to develop specific sleep interventions that can help slow the progression of CKD.

Sleep-Friendly Environment

While understanding the relationship between sleep and CKD could still be considered somewhat controversial, creating a sleep-friendly environment can be beneficial for a Chronic Kidney Disease (CKD) patient as good quality sleep can help manage stress levels and overall health. Here are some tips:

Maintain a Comfortable Sleep Environment.

Your bedroom should be quiet, dark, and cool for optimal sleep. Consider using earplugs, eye shades, or white noise machines if necessary.

Invest in a Good Quality Mattress and Pillows

These should support your body well and help prevent aches and pains that could disrupt your sleep.

Limit Light Exposure

Exposure to light stimulates alertness. Consider using heavy curtains or an eye mask to block out light. Limit screen time before bed as the blue light from screens can interfere with your body's natural sleep-wake cycle.

Regulate Your Room Temperature

A cooler room often promotes better sleep. The recommended temperature is usually around 65 degrees Fahrenheit (18.3 degrees Celsius), but it can vary per individual.

Manage Noise Levels

If you can't control the noise level outside your room, consider using a fan or a white noise machine to drown out disturbing sounds.

Keep Your Room Clean

A clean, decluttered room can help create a calm environment conducive to sleep.

Limit Bedroom Activities

Reserve your bed for sleep and intimacy only. This strengthens the mental association between your bedroom and sleep.

Consider Aromatherapy

Some people find scents like lavender and chamomile soothing and conducive to sleep. However, be sure to check that you are not allergic to these scents.

When to Seek Help for Sleep Problems

However, when these sleep problems are already causing a myriad of other inconveniences, not to mention hastening the progression of your CKD, you should consider seeking professional help for sleep problems in the following situations:

Persistent Insomnia

If you consistently have trouble falling asleep, staying asleep, or if you wake up too early and cannot get back to sleep.

Excessive Daytime Sleepiness

If you often feel excessively tired or sleepy during the day, even after a full night's sleep.

Snoring or Breathing Pauses During Sleep

Loud snoring that is followed by periods of silence and gasping could indicate sleep apnea, a condition common in CKD patients.

Restless Legs Syndrome (RLS)

If you often have an irresistible urge to move your legs while resting, particularly in the evenings.

Unrefreshing Sleep

If you regularly wake up feeling unrefreshed, even after sleeping for a sufficient number of hours.

Difficulty Adapting to a Dialysis Schedule

If you're on dialysis and are having trouble adjusting your sleep schedule.

Impact on Quality of Life

If sleep problems are causing significant distress or are interfering with your daily life.

Remember, sleep problems can be a symptom of underlying issues, some of which may be related to CKD or its treatments. Therefore, it's crucial to discuss any sleep issues with your healthcare provider so they can guide you on the best course of action.

Results of Improved Sleep Patterns

Though sometimes regarded with little attention, I have decided to really dedicate a chapter on this topic on quality sleep. I personally believe that it plays a significant role in the overall management of Chronic Kidney Disease (CKD) and contributes to a better quality of life. My belief springs from these facts and I genuinely believe that each patient should benefit from them:

1. **Improved Physical Health**. Adequate sleep allows the body to rest and repair. It supports the functioning of the immune system and helps manage CKD-related symptoms such as fatigue and weakness.
2. **Better Mental Health**. Good sleep can enhance mood and emotional regulation, reducing the risk of depression and anxiety, which are often prevalent in CKD patients.
3. **Enhanced Cognitive Function**. Quality sleep contributes to better cognition, including improved memory, attention, and problem-solving skills. This can help patients manage their treatment plans more effectively.
4. **Chronic Disease Management**. Sleep disorders are common in CKD patients and can worsen the disease's progression. Managing these sleep disorders, such as sleep apnea and insomnia, can therefore aid in CKD management.

5. **Improved Quality of Life.** Overall, getting a good night's sleep can enhance a patient's well-being and quality of life, making it easier for them to cope with the challenges of managing a chronic illness like CKD.

With your self-assesment at the beginning of this chapter, and with some introspection on the roles and significance of sleep for your CKD, I would need you to include this in your next discussions with your healthcare provider who can guide you on the best strategies or treatments to improve your sleep quality and thereby affecting your overall health.

Chapter 10:

Medication and Dietary Supplements

Managing Chronic Kidney Disease (CKD) with medication and diet is akin to steering a ship through stormy seas. Medication is the compass, providing precise direction and control, actively correcting course when the waves of disease symptoms grow too wild. A well-balanced diet, on the other hand, is the anchor, offering stability and resistance against the storm. It reinforces the ship's structure, preventing further deterioration from the relentless waves. Both are pivotal in the journey. The compass alone cannot prevent the ship from taking on water, while the anchor alone cannot guide the ship to calm seas. Only together, with medication and diet, can they navigate successfully through the storm of CKD, ensuring a safe and stable voyage.

Understanding the Importance of Medication

I am really hesitant to include this chapter on medications, not because I don't believe in them, but because I would really want this discussed to you by your doctor. However, I am also compelled to talk about the importance of medication for Chronic Kidney Disease to truly provide you with a holistic knowledge of your condition. The goal at the end of this chapter is for you to be able to identify and list down all the medications that you are taking for your kidney condition so that we will know if you are aware of what you're taking.

So before we continue, a word of warning. Doctors and pharmacists have spent a long time studying to learn when to prescribe what medications. When you have a kidney disease and are taking multiple different medications, there is a risk of side effects. This is why you should always consult with your doctor before you stop, start, or change the dosage of your medication.

If you have CKD, diabetes, or high blood pressure, you should take certain steps to protect your kidneys from harm. Your doctors can prescribe medications to help slow down the worsening of your kidneys, and prevent the complications that come from it, such as stroke or heart attack.

There are 3 factors that could help decide whether to reduce your blood pressure levels especially when you're diagnosed with CKD:

- How high your blood pressure is, especially if left untreated,
- If you have diabetes, and
- How much protein is in your urine *(albumin level)*.

A person with a normal blood pressure who doesn't have any other problems like diabetes or protein in the urine can get by without using any blood pressure medications. However, if you have those factors listed above, you are most likely to be advised to have treatment with Angiotensin-Converting Enzyme Inhibitor (ACE Inhibitor) or Angiotensin Receptor Blockers (ARBs, also known as sartans).

Let's find out which ones you have been prescribed...

ACE Inhibitors have names that end in -pril such as:

- Captopril (Capoten)
- Enalapril (Vasotec)
- Fosinopril (Monopril)
- Lisinopril (Prinivil, Zestril)
- and Ramipril (Altace)

And ARBs have names that end in -sartan such as:

- Azilsartan (Edarbi)
- Eprosartan (Teveten)
- Irbesartan (Avapro)
- Losartan (Cozaar)
- Olmesartan (Benicar)
- Valsartan (Diovan)

These are two types of blood pressure medications that are often prescribed to kidney patients to help slow down the loss of kidney function, delay kidney failure, and lower the amount of protein in your urine.

The Institute for Quality and Efficiency in Health Care posts that in a review of 119 studies involving over 64,000 participants with advanced kidney disease, ACE Inhibitors and ARBs offer several advantages compared with other blood-pressure-lowering medications (like beta blockers).

ACE inhibitors or ARBs were more effective at reducing the risk of complete kidney failure. They also reduce the risk of cardiovascular diseases such as heart attacks or strokes. There are other medications that can help prevent Stage 5 Kidney Disease, such as antihypertensive agents, diuretics (water tablets), and statins (cholesterol-lowering medication).

However, a person with CKD should avoid Motrin/Ibuprofen because it can cause Tubulointerstitial Nephritis – a disorder in which part of the kidneys become swollen, causing problems with the way your kidneys work.

Practical Things About Prescriptions

If the blood pressure medications will help my kidneys, why do I have to be extra careful?

Yes, taking blood pressure medicines will help protect your kidneys. But there are certain situations, such as when you're dehydrated from diarrhea or the flu when you need to pay attention to your blood pressure. Dehydration can lower OR raise your blood pressure! In either scenario, your kidneys might not be able to properly filter.

The best person to give you advice is your nephrologist. Make sure to ask them a list of symptoms or warning signs you need to be aware of for your specific medical situation.

But how about supplements? Will they help?

It's still highly questionable whether over-the-counter dietary, herbal and other natural supplements can help people diagnosed with CKD. Muscle-building supplements such as whey protein powders or creatinine supplements can also affect your lab results for kidney health numbers. If possible, avoid most herbal supplements unless approved by your nephrologist and dietitian.

It's important that you mention taking any supplements or alternative medicine.

What should I do at the pharmacy?

The next time you pick up your prescription or buy an over-the-counter medicine or supplement, ask your pharmacist how the product may affect your kidneys and how it will react with the other medicines that you're taking.

Fill your prescriptions at only one pharmacy or at least a pharmacy chain so that your pharmacist can carefully monitor your medicines and supplements. It can be helpful to bring a print-out with a list of all your prescriptions, you can ask for one at your doctor's office.

What should I do at my doctor's or dietitian's office?

Be sure to keep an up-to-date list of your prescribed medicines and supplements with you for your appointment. If possible, you can bring all your medicine bottles with you as well.

When CKD Chef Duane was still on medications, he always carried his list with him. If he ever had an emergency or questions about medications, his list was always in his wallet.

What should I remember about Over-The-Counter (OTC) medicines?

If you take over-the-counter medicines for headaches, pain, fever, or even colds, you may be taking non-steroidal anti-inflammatory drugs (NSAIDs), such as ibuprofen and motrin. As mentioned above, these drugs may be dangerous to your kidneys.

Here is a short list of the most common OTC medicines to be careful of:

PROBLEM	MEDICATION	BRAND NAMES
Pain	Ibuprofen	Advil, Motrin
Pain/Swelling	Naproxen	Naprosyn, Aleve
Constipation	Sodium Phosphorous solutions	Fleets enemas
Constipation	Magnesium citrate	MagCitrate

Here are OTC medicines you MAY take (unless advised by your physician):

PROBLEM	MEDICATION	BRAND NAMES
Cough	Dextromethorphan	Delsym
	Guaifenesin	Robitussin
Congestion (Sedating)	Diphenhydramine	Benadryl
	Chlorpheniramine	Chlor-Trimeton
Heartburn	Famotidine	Pepcid
Nausea/Motion Sickness (Sedating)	Dimenhydrinate	Dramamine
Gas and Bloating	Simethicone	Gas-X
	Alpha-D-Galactosidase	Beano
Diarrhea	Loperamide	Imodium
Constipation	Docusate Sodium	Colace
	Lactulose	Enulose
Insomnia	Diphenhydramine	Benadryl
	Acetaminophen PM	Tylenol PM

Reference: BIDMC Welcome Booklet for CKD Patients

Again, be sure to ask your doctors if the OTC medicines you are taking are safe to use with your current prescribed CKD medicines.

What is self-medication? Is that something I need to worry about?

Self-medication is when you take medicine because you or another person (who is not a doctor) think it can help with your condition. It is normal for some people. It is just something they prefer to do rather than going to the doctor which can be time-consuming and expensive. However, what they don't realize is that opting for self-medication makes us prone to allergies or even drug dependence. Or it can have the opposite effect, such as in the case of medical cannabis where kidneys become worse *faster*.

Also, remember it is your doctor's job to make sure that you get the right medical treatment. Every doctor would prefer that you call them with a question about your medication, than that you make a mistake that damages your kidneys.

Unfortunately, there is very little or almost no awareness about the disadvantages of self-medication. Taking pills may get us instant relief but it does not mean we are free from the side effects. Oftentimes, a patient may be under-prescribed medication for a different health issue, and self-medicating may lead to unfortunate reactions.

Why? Because one drug may react differently when consumed with another prescribed drug. In rare cases, this can even lead to death. Which is why <u>consulting a doctor is very important</u>.

Which leads me to my next question...

Do you keep track of your prescribed medications?

If yes, I want you to list them all down, especially if you have been prescribed a blood pressure drug. Once you've got that list ready, I need you to send them over along with the hurdles you experience when taking them to your doctor and dietitian.

Chapter 11:

Staying Motivated and Dealing with Setbacks

We are finally at the end of the book, and I can't express enough how proud I am of you for devoting your time and putting effort into having the best possible health while battling with CKD.

After reading this book is the time when you actually will start the real journey. And let me tell you, it's not always going to be easy. You will deal with some minor or even major setbacks, and them some more along the way.

But I trust that we were able to build a solid foundation and that in going through this journey, you have the right tools to break through each barrier that comes along your way. When the tools don't work anymore, all you need to do is sharpen your tools by going back and flipping through the pages of this book.

And I don't want to close this by not leaving one more secret weapon that will help you to be always on guard and ready for the battle that's ahead.

Ask For Help: Let's Overcome Those Support Setbacks

Now the question is: what are the different Support Setbacks that most patients face when trying to ask for help? More importantly, what can you do to overcome them? Let's find out!

⃠ Support Setback 1: Stigma

Did you ever feel like you were embarrassed about your condition? And this made it harder for you to tell people, especially your doctor, about it?

Stigma is common among patients with chronic diseases. Recent studies show that the representations of illness associated with CKD gave rise to social stigma among some diagnosed patients. This is particularly true with patients who are also experiencing depression upon knowing they are diagnosed with CKD.

And we understand that. Anyone could feel the same. It takes a lot of heart and courage to deal with the mental health challenges that come along with CKD. If you've come this far, then you're doing great and we're here to support you all the way through.

But if you have been struggling with opening up, don't worry, we're here to help and guide you.

So to overcome this barrier, you simply need to open up slowly. Don't rush it. Start sharing your thoughts and feelings with your closest circle like your family and friends first.

Once you do that, you'll be able to create your first line of support. This is important because if you establish your support system with people you're comfortable with, everything that comes next will be a lot easier.

Most of the time, they would also encourage you to open up more to someone else. Eventually, you'll feel better and more confident talking to your doctor if you have your family right beside you.

Always remember that you're not alone and you don't need to do this all by yourself.

⊘ Support Setback 2: Lack of Trust

You probably had some doubts about your doctor which made it harder for you to talk to him or her about your condition. And since we're talking about your health here, it's definitely understandable and even normal to be skeptical at first.

But the problem comes if this persists for way too long. The only way your healthcare team can help you is if you meet them halfway.

According to Dr. Carlos A. Pellegrini, the Chief Medical Officer for University of Washington Medicine and a Professor in the Department of Surgery,

> **"Trust is the keystone of the physician-patient relationship."**

Without trust, reaching out will be too difficult. So if you're struggling with trusting your healthcare team, what should you do?

Again, you need to take things slowly. Build a relationship with them. For starters, don't stop at being a care recipient. Play an active role in your own health by asking them about your condition. Ask them about your medications. And maybe from time to time, ask them about their day too. Let yourself be educated by them.

After some time, you won't even notice it but you're already going with the flow. Just like good friendships, you'll eventually trust them enough to help you out on your road to recovery – or even let them be a significant part of your life.

⊘ Support Setback 3: Hopelessness

"What's the point of asking for help when it's hopeless?"

"It's too late. No one can help me."

"There's just no way out of this."

A lot of patients also struggle to seek help because of feelings of hopelessness. You've probably had moments like these too, without a doubt. And for you to be able to seek help properly, you need to overcome these feelings.

One way to overcome hopelessness is to look for motivations. Ask yourself.

What wakes you up in the morning?

What makes you happy?

What makes you want to live?

Sometimes, looking for a single but strong motivation is all it takes to keep you hopeful and going on again.

You can also look forward to something new every day---whether that's a new hobby, a new skill or talent, or doing something you've never done before.

And it may be a cliche, but it will always stand true: don't ever stop hoping for a better tomorrow.

Once you have that motivation back, asking for help will be so much easier. And you'll be surprised by how much it will change your overall lifestyle!

So remember, to overcome these barriers: take it slow, build relationships, be educated, be motivated, and look forward to a great future just ahead of you.

3 Motivation Movers

It's one thing to be motivated, but it's another thing to keep yourself motivated. So let's lay down a few things you can do to keep the momentum for healthy eating up and running.

🏆 Motivation Mover 1: Start with your WHYs

If you find yourself lost while looking for an ounce of motivation, just ask your whys:

"Why should I lessen my sodium intake?"

"Why should I strive to do better?"

"Why did I do my best to make it this far in my health goals?"

Asking yourself these questions and finding out the reasons behind everything you do will help you direct yourself to your health goals. This will help you establish what you really want to do and accomplish.

And more often than not, directions can help you in reaching or achieving the outcomes you want.

🏆 Motivation Mover 2: Make it enjoyable

In everything that you do to change or improve your lifestyle, in this particular case, your diet or food/nutrient intake, always find a way to make it enjoyable.

You can do this in a lot of ways too! You can look for healthy and creative recipes online that can suit your health needs or you can try to learn something new every day---whether that's a new recipe or new information about your health by reading scientific articles or asking help from your doctor.

As long as you find your lifestyle enjoyable, you'll have less worrying to do in keeping yourself motivated.

🏆 Motivation Mover 3: Never hesitate to ask for help or support

Slip-ups will occur occasionally along the way and it's fine. Sometimes, it might get lonely as well – it's as if you're carrying everything on your own. But this is simply not true. You have your doctor, healthcare team, friends, and family to help you every step of the way.

Surround yourself with people you care about and you don't have to do things alone.

If you ever find yourself losing motivation and you feel like you can't pull yourself together on your own, remember that you have people around you who will never think twice before helping you. It's always more motivational and encouraging to keep going on if you know that you will always have company around no matter what.

Remember, your mental health is just as important as your physical health. For you to improve your overall health, these two aspects should work together.

While what we've discussed are just a few of the things you can do to strengthen your motivation, and consequently your mental health, they're a great way to start. So as long as you keep your mental health in check, your will and motivation to make changes in your lifestyle and to do better will never burn out.

Now, all throughout this book, we've established the undeniable fact that making changes to your lifestyle (and ultimately adapting to them) can require a tremendous amount of work and effort from your end. This can make your nutritional or diet adaptation (along with your overall behavior and habits relevant to your health) quite challenging and overwhelming.

But we've also established that this takes time and a few slip-ups along the way are to be expected – and these are all fine!

Eventually, though, you'll get the hang of it. Especially when you know that making even the littlest changes to your diet, your workout, and your overall daily routines, as a significant part of managing your own health, could go a long way in the future. In fact, you probably are now too! And you're definitely taking big steps towards your recovery.

At some point, however, if we were to look through a long-term prospect, you might start to realize and ask yourself the question: *how will you know if the self-management practices you've been carrying out are actually working?*

Of course, one way to check your progress is to consult your healthcare team. This is more particularly applicable to your health's biophysical aspect.

Through a series of medical tests, your doctor can make an assessment and conclude whether or not the changes and adaptations you're making in your lifestyle have significantly contributed to your health improvement.

But since self-management is taking charge of your own health, it's important for you to monitor your condition along with the progress you're making along the way as well.

Strategies to Overcome Setbacks

Ultimately, we all want to have more control over our health. That's what we've always been aiming for since day one – laying out the cards in the table that can help you win in the end. But we also want to go beyond that. It's one thing to change your lifestyle and recover; keeping up with it, however, is another.

And so we want to bring about a significant effect on your health that doesn't stop at your recovery. We'll do this by presenting you two simple self-assessment measures you can use that can determine if you're taking the right steps towards adapting, managing your own health, and improving your overall lifestyle.

Being able to motivate yourself

Reinforcement theories under social psychology suggest that people can devise reinforcements (rewards or things that can encourage them to carry out or maintain good habits) to help them achieve their desired outcomes.

Children, for example, are given treats or toys if they do a good job at something (let's say, winning a quiz bee or acing an exam). While this seems to be a usual thing we see in every pre-school environment we've been to, it can motivate kids to always do their best and it can carry on such a habit until they grow up.

Positive reinforcements, however, don't only work among kids. In low-key but also profound ways, it affects us too! Doing a great job at work can give us recognition from our workmates and even a promotion which can inspire us to do better. A hearty and healthy meal with good company after finishing a project can drive us to continue the hard work. And simply hearing words of encouragement from our loved ones can keep us going.

As you can see, a lot of positive reinforcements are rooted in socially based drives – we want companionship, we want to be accepted, and well, who doesn't want to be loved?

It's not that bad to look for motivation from other people too. But there will be times when you need to work on it on your own, especially in cases where others just can't seem to give you the motivation or support you need. It's part of taking charge of your own health.

You need to have your own set of personal-based motivations. You need to have control over what keeps you going. It's through this that you can truly drive yourself to always do your best.

This won't be easy the first time too because a lot of us usually rely on the support of others. But once you gain such strong control over this dynamic in your life, I'm confident that you will always be able to manage your health and maintain a healthy lifestyle under any circumstances.

Dealing with failures appropriately (Stress Management)

Sometimes, people may find themselves in more difficult situations than others when dealing with failures. Of course, feeling down for the first few missteps is normal. The problem arises, however, if you stop dealing with them maturely or realistically and just let your defeat consume you.

This is more especially common among patients who were just diagnosed with a chronic condition thinking that they need to immediately adjust their lifestyle in order to cope with it.

I'm sure that the pressure you've been feeling back then might be relatively tenser than the stress you've dealt with after a few weeks or months of your adjustments. Upon knowing about your condition, you surely had your thoughts rushing in all together. And you've probably only thought about your recovery and how to get there as fast as you can.

Most people never really give so much thought about failing, because who would want to fail in the first place? We just want to skip that part and then take the shorter route---the route without barriers. The thing though, is that it's by accepting the inevitable fact that you will certainly face a few failures, missteps, and slip-ups that can you truly deal with them. If you fed yourself with the idea that everything will be perfect in your self-improvement progress, you will only end up discouraged once you stumble upon one and fail to solve it.

You need to keep in mind that failures are part of our growth and more often than not, they have shaped some of our good qualities as individuals.

Again, to feel a bit down from a failure is normal. What matters, however, are the things that you do to overcome them. Don't let it drown you.

You'll find it easier to adapt to any lifestyle change if you learn how to appropriately deal with failures.

Now, these are just two self-assessment measures you can use to evaluate your self-improvement. But they could tell significant information about your overall progress.

Sometimes, self-perception could get tricky as well because your self-evaluation greatly rests on your own judgment. You might get to a point where you want to drop your progress even though you've barely made compelling changes and adjustments to your lifestyle because it's just simply draining and overwhelming. You might think you've failed. But as we've said earlier, it's only by recognizing the failures you'll inevitably come across somewhere along the way (coupled with your own will to compensate for your shortcomings) that can you genuinely address and win your struggles.

So just remember to try and try. Rest for a while but always pick up where you left off and continue again. And be as objective as you can when assessing yourself.

I would love to hear from you!

It's through your support and reviews that my book is able to reach other Chronic Kidney Disease patients who are still struggling to figure out how they could take a proactive approach in managing their CKD. Please take 60 seconds to kindly leave a review on Amazon. Please scan the QR code below, alternatively, you may use the link provided in your Amazon order.

Please follow these simple steps to rate/review my book:

1. Open the camera on your phone
2. Hover it over the QR code below
3. You may also type this link on your phone or browser: **https://go.renaltracker.com/bookreview**
4. Rate/Review my book

I appreciate you taking the time, your review will surely make a difference.

Thank you!

Janeth Kingston

Conclusion

As we navigate the journey of life, living with Chronic Kidney Disease (CKD) presents its own unique challenges. Over the years I've spent as a kidney nurse, I have been committed to guiding and supporting you through this journey. This book has been a part of that commitment, emphasizing the crucial role of diet and nutrition in managing CKD.

Food is not just for enjoyment; it's a primary source of fuel for our bodies. It helps build our cells, powers our activities and strengthens our immune systems. In the context of CKD, proper nutrition can help control symptoms, slow the progression of the disease, and significantly improve the quality of life. It's not a cure, but it's a powerful strategy that you have control over every day.

It's important to remember that dietary needs for CKD vary greatly from person to person. Each individual's situation is unique, influenced by disease stage, other health conditions, and personal preferences. That's why it's essential to consult with your doctor and work with a nutritionist or dietitian. Their expertise can help you tailor a diet plan that aligns with your health needs and accommodates your lifestyle and tastes.

These professionals are knowledgeable guides who can help you navigate the sometimes complex world of nutrition. They can break down the latest research, debunk common myths, and provide practical and personalized advice. They can help you understand why certain foods need to be limited, why others should be encouraged, and how to strike a balance between maintaining a healthy diet and enjoying your meals.

As we conclude this book, please know that this is not the end of our journey together. Through my other books focused on CKD, I will continue to provide you with the latest and most relevant information. Living with CKD can be challenging, but with the right guidance, a well-balanced diet, and an openness to learning, you can lead a fulfilling life.

Remember, CKD is a part of your life, but it doesn't define who you are. You have the ability to make choices, ask questions, and seek support. Your engagement is as important as the guidance you receive.

So, let's not view this as a goodbye, but rather a pause in our ongoing conversation. I look forward to our continued dialogue and shared learning. Until we meet again in the pages of another book, take care, stay curious, and continue to prioritize your health and nutrition.

Annex

DAILY FOOD JOURNAL

Date:_____ Mon   Tue   Wed   Thu   Fri   Sat   Sun
(circle)

			Calories	Protein (g)	Carbs (g)	Fat (g)		
Qty	Measure	Food	Calories	Protein (g)	Carbs (g)	Fat (g)	Mood Before	Mood After

BREAKFAST   Time of Day:

		Totals						

LUNCH   Time of Day:

		Totals						

DINNER   Time of Day:

		Totals						

SNACKS   Time of Day:

		Totals						

Check 8 Ounce Glasses of Water

Day in Review

_____
_____
_____

_____

How Did I Do Today?

Excellent   Great   OK   Not Good   Very Bad (circle)

References

Stirring the Pot: Can Dietary Modification Alleviate the Burden of CKD? Snelson et. al. https://www.mdpi.com/2072-6643/9/3/265

Importance of Age and Metabolism in CKD Dieting

- National Institute on Aging - Sarcopenia with Aging - https://www.nia.nih.gov/health/sarcopenia-loss-muscle-mass-strength-and-function-aging

Nutritional Needs of the 50+ Age Group

National Institute on Aging - Choosing Healthy Meals As You Get Older

Harvard Health Publishing - Special Nutrient Needs of Older Adults

Mayo Clinic - Dietary fiber: Essential for a healthy diet

Oregon State University - Micronutrient Information Center: Vitamin B12

National Institutes of Health Office of Dietary Supplements - Vitamin D

National Institutes of Health Office of Dietary Supplements - Potassium

American Heart Association - Shaking the Salt Habit to Lower High Blood Pressure

CDC - Nutrition for Older Adults

Impact of Food on your Kidneys

- [National Kidney Foundation: 6 Harmful Things for your Kidneys] (https://www.kidney.org/atoz/content/sixstepshealthprimer)
- [American Kidney Fund: Kidney-friendly diet for CKD] (https://www.kidneyfund.org/kidney-disease/chronic-kidney-disease-ckd/kidney-friendly-diet-for-ckd.html)
- [Mayo Clinic: Chronic kidney disease] (https://www.mayoclinic.org/diseases-conditions/chronic-kidney-disease/symptoms-causes/syc-20354521)

The Diet and Haemodialysis Dyad: Three Eras, Four Open Questions and Four Paradoxes. A Narrative Review, Towards a Personalized, Patient-Centered Approach

- https://www.mdpi.com/2072-6643/9/4/372

Vegetarian Diet in Chronic Kidney Disease—A Friend or Foe

- https://www.mdpi.com/2072-6643/9/4/374

ROLE OF MACRONUTRIENT AND MICRONUTRIENT IN CKD

- [National Kidney Foundation: Protein and Chronic Kidney Disease](https://www.kidney.org/atoz/content/protein)
- [National Kidney Foundation: Carbohydrates and Chronic Kidney Disease](https://www.kidney.org/atoz/content/carbs)
- [National Kidney Foundation: Fats and Chronic Kidney Disease](https://www.kidney.org/atoz/content/fats)
- [National Kidney Foundation: Potassium and Chronic Kidney Disease](https://www.kidney.org/atoz/content/potassium)
- [National Kidney Foundation: Phosphorus and Your CKD Diet](https://www.kidney.org/atoz/content/phosphorus)
- [National Kidney Foundation: Vitamin D and Chronic Kidney Disease](https://www.kidney.org/atoz/content/vitaminD)

IMPORTANCE OF INDIVIDUAL DIETARY REQUIREMENTS

[National Kidney Foundation: Nutrition and Chronic Kidney Disease] (https://www.kidney.org/atoz/content/nutrichronic)

IMPORTANCE OF HYDRATION AND FLUID RESTRICTION IN CKD

- [National Kidney Foundation: High Blood Pressure and Chronic Kidney Disease] (https://www.kidney.org/atoz/content/highblood)
- [National Kidney Foundation: Swelling and Chronic Kidney Disease] (https://www.kidney.org/atoz/content/swelling)
- [National Kidney Foundation: Shortness of Breath and Chronic Kidney Disease] (https://www.kidney.org/atoz/content/shortness-breath-and-chronic-kidney-disease)
- [National Kidney Foundation: Dehydration and Kidney Disease] (https://www.kidney.org/newsletter/can-dehydration-affect-your-kidneys)
- [National Kidney Foundation: What Do You Mean I Can't Have a Fresca?] (https://www.kidney.org/blog/kidney-diet-tips/kidney-diet-tips-what-do-you-mean-I-cant-have-fresca)

CHOOSING THE RIGHT BEVERAGE IN CKD

- [National Kidney Foundation: Potassium and Your CKD Diet] (https://www.kidney.org/atoz/content/potassium)

- [National Kidney Foundation: Phosphorus and Your CKD Diet] (https://www.kidney.org/atoz/content/phosphorus)
- [National Kidney Foundation: Alcohol and Chronic Kidney Disease] (https://www.kidney.org/atoz/content/alcohol)
- [National Kidney Foundation: Sodium and Your CKD Diet] (https://www.kidney.org/atoz/content/sodiumckd)

STATISTICS ON PPPS

- [American Journal of Physiology-Renal Physiology: High salt intake and chronic kidney disease] (https://journals.physiology.org/doi/full/10.1152/ajprenal.00025.2015)
- [Cochrane Database of Systematic Reviews: Low protein diets for chronic kidney disease in non diabetic adults] (https://www.cochranelibrary.com/cdsr/doi/10.1002/14651858.CD001892.pub3/full)
- [American Journal of Kidney Diseases: Serum Potassium Levels and Mortality in Chronic Kidney Disease] (https://www.ajkd.org/article/S0272-6386(10)01156-3/fulltext)
- [Journal of the American Society of Nephrology: Serum Phosphorus and Risk of Cardiovascular Disease, All-Cause Mortality, or Graft Failure in Kidney Transplant Recipients: An Ancillary Study of the FAVORIT Trial Cohort] (https://jasn.asnjournals.org/content/28/9/2756)
- http://i.imgur.com/DWeLkhA.png

Food Journal Guide/Sample

- https://healthiestlife4me.wordpress.com/2012/03/25/week-9-food-diary-sample/

Food Label Sample

- https://esha.com/blog/potassium-rounding-rules-on-the-2016-nutrition-facts-panel/

Food Portioning Guide

- https://www.pinterest.ph/pin/298152437809682150/

WORKING WITH A DIETITIAN

- The Academy of Nutrition and Dietetics (www.eatright.org), The National Kidney Foundation (www.kidney.org),

STRATEGIES FOR MANAGING STRESS

- [Mindful] (https://www.mindful.org/) and [Headspace] (https://www.headspace.com/meditation-101/what-is-meditation).
- The [Mayo Clinic]
- (https://www.mayoclinic.org/healthy-lifestyle/stress-management/in-depth/exercise-and-stress/art-20044469)
- [American Psychological Association] (http://www.apa.org/helpcenter/emotional-support).
- [Harvard Medical School]
- (https://www.health.harvard.edu/blog/nutritional-strategies-to-ease-anxiety-201604139441) website.
- [Mayo Clinic]
- (https://www.mayoclinic.org/healthy-lifestyle/stress-management/in-depth/relaxation-technique/art-20045368).
- American Psychological Association (https://www.apa.org/ptsd-guideline/patients-and-families/cognitive-behavioral).

UNDERSTANDING SLEEP AND CKD

- Masood, M., et al. (2018). Sleep Disorders and Chronic Kidney Disease. World Journal of Nephrology.
- Molnar, MZ., et al. (2019). Association of Quality of Sleep with Cognitive Decline and Risk of Incident Dementia: Reasons for Geographic and Racial Differences. Sleep.
- Roumelioti, ME., et al. (2020). Sleep Disorders and Chronic Kidney Disease. World Journal of Nephrology.
- Mayo Clinic (https://www.mayoclinic.org/diseases-conditions/insomnia/symptoms-causes/syc-20355167).
- National Kidney Foundation (https://www.kidney.org/atoz/content/sleep).
- National Kidney Foundation (https://www.kidney.org/news/ekidney/june10/SleepProblems_june10) and [American Journal of Kidney Diseases](https://www.ajkd.org/article/S0272-6386(16)30523-8/fulltext) for more information.

UNDERSTANDING MEDICATIONS

- https://www.ncbi.nlm.nih.gov/books/NBK492989

- https://www.ncbi.nlm.nih.gov/pmc/articles/PMC4421632/#:~:text=There%20is%20less%20concern%20today,should%20avoid%20using%20this%20supplement.
- https://www.sciencedirect.com/topics/medicine-and-dentistry/self-medication
- https://www.kidneyfund.org/kidney-today/a-caution-about-self-medication-for-kidney-patients.html

The
KIDNEY DIET
Food List Guide

FOR RENAL DISEASE

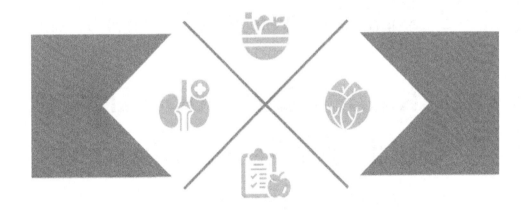

Effectively Manage CKD with Detailed
Food Lists and Meal Planning Tips

JANETH KINGSTON, BS RN

The Comprehensive Reference for Kidney Disease Food Items

Kidney Diet Food List Guide for Renal Disease

Effectively Manage CKD with Detailed Food Lists and Meal Planning Tips

By JANETH KINGSTON, BSN RN

2nd Edition

Introduction

About This Book

Purpose and Scope

Navigating the complexities of kidney disease can be daunting, especially when it comes to dietary management. This book is designed to empower you with comprehensive guidance on managing kidney disease through nutrition. Our aim is to explore a wide array of dietary options suitable for various stages of chronic kidney disease (CKD), ensuring that the information provided is both evidence-based and practical for your everyday life.

The food items featured in this guide have been meticulously selected from trusted food databases and reputable scientific sources. This rigorous selection process guarantees that all dietary recommendations are anchored in the latest nutritional research and clinical guidelines tailored for optimal kidney health.

How to Use This Book

This user-friendly guide is crafted for anyone seeking to manage kidney disease through diet, whether you're newly diagnosed or looking to refine your dietary choices. Each section is thoughtfully organized to help you easily locate the information you need. Whether you're searching for specific foods to embrace or avoid, meal planning strategies, or detailed recipes, you'll find it all here.

To simplify your journey, we have categorized foods so you can quickly identify kidney-friendly options. The comprehensive food lists are rooted in scientific research, crafted by our dedicated team of dietitians and nephrology nurses—not generated by AI. This ensures a reliable resource for making informed dietary choices that support your kidney health.

In addition to the food lists, you will discover practical meal plans and delicious recipes tailored to different stages of kidney disease. These resources are designed to help you maintain a balanced diet that meets your unique nutritional requirements.

To enhance your experience, use the detailed index on PAGE 337 to swiftly locate specific topics or foods of interest. The glossary will clarify any unfamiliar terms and additional resources to further support your dietary management journey.

Together, we can navigate the path to better kidney health, armed with the knowledge and tools necessary to thrive.

Part I: Understanding Kidney Disease and Nutrition

Chapter 1: Understanding Kidney Disease

In my previous book, *Avoid Dialysis Diet Plan for Kidney Disease*, I extensively discussed the crucial role of diet in both the progression and management of kidney disease. However, before diving into the specifics of this guide, let's take a moment to recap what we're dealing with, how we reached this point, and the primary reason you are reading this book. (If you feel confident in your understanding of CKD basics, you are welcome to skip ahead to the next chapter!)

So, What is Kidney Disease?

Kidney disease occurs when the kidneys become damaged and can no longer filter blood effectively. This damage can lead to the accumulation of waste products in the body and may trigger other health complications that jeopardize your overall well-being.

For many individuals, kidney damage develops gradually over several years, often as a result of diabetes or high blood pressure. This condition is known as chronic kidney disease (CKD). Conversely, when kidney function declines suddenly due to illness, injury, or certain medications, it is referred to as acute kidney injury. This condition can affect individuals with previously normal kidney function or those with existing kidney issues, and it may be reversible.

The Growing Concern of Kidney Disease

Kidney disease is an escalating public health concern. More than 37 million Americans may be living with kidney disease, and countless others are at risk. Anyone, regardless of age or ethnicity, can develop kidney disease. The primary risk factors include:

- Diabetes
- High blood pressure
- Cardiovascular disease (affecting the heart and blood vessels)
- A family history of kidney failure
- Unhealthy lifestyle and dietary choices

Diagnosis and Symptoms: What Causes Kidney Disease?

Diabetes and high blood pressure are the leading causes of kidney disease in the United States, as these conditions can slowly harm the kidneys over time.

Additional causes may include autoimmune diseases that lead to gradual damage to kidney tissue, such as lupus nephritis. In some cases, the underlying cause of kidney disease remains unclear, prompting your nephrologist to recommend a kidney biopsy for further investigation.

Early Stages: A Silent Threat

Kidney disease often progresses without noticeable signs or symptoms:

- You may not feel any different until the disease reaches an advanced stage.
- Blood and urine tests are essential for determining whether you have kidney disease.
- A blood test measures your glomerular filtration rate (GFR), indicating how well your kidneys are filtering blood.
- A urine test checks for protein levels in your urine.

The Importance of Early Detection

Detecting kidney disease early can lead to effective treatment or management strategies:

- The sooner you identify kidney disease, the sooner you can initiate treatment to delay or prevent kidney failure.

- Treatments may include medications like ACE inhibitors or ARBs to manage high blood pressure, ultimately helping to preserve kidney function.

- Managing kidney disease can also reduce the risk of developing heart disease.

Long-Term Outlook

While kidney disease typically does not resolve, it can worsen over time and potentially lead to kidney failure. In such cases, treatment options include dialysis or kidney transplantation. Moreover, kidney disease can contribute to various other health conditions, including heart disease, increasing the likelihood of stroke or heart attack.

Monitoring Your Kidney Health

Many individuals with kidney disease remain asymptomatic until significant damage has occurred. Regular blood and urine tests are crucial for monitoring kidney health. These tests assess your GFR and check for albumin levels in your urine, which are fundamental in tracking the progression of kidney disease.

Key Tests to Monitor Kidney Health Include:

- Blood Pressure: Keeping your blood pressure at or below the target set by your healthcare provider is the most effective way to slow the progression of kidney disease and prevent kidney failure.

- GFR: The GFR indicates how well your kidneys filter blood. While you cannot increase your GFR, your goal should be to prevent it from declining.

- Urine Albumin: Albumin is a protein that may leak into urine when the kidneys are damaged. Although kidney damage cannot be undone, you may be able to reduce the amount of albumin in your urine through effective treatment.

- A1C: For those with diabetes, the A1C test reflects average blood glucose levels over the past three months. Lowering your A1C can significantly improve your health.

Here's a quick glance of your GFR in comparison to your Kidney Function:

STAGES OF CHRONIC KIDNEY DISEASE		GFR*	% OF KIDNEY FUNCTION
Stage 1	Kidney damage with **normal** kidney function	90 or higher	90-100%
Stage 2	Kidney damage with **mild loss** of kidney function	89 to 60	60-89%
Stage 3a	**Mild to moderate** loss of kidney function	59 to 45	45-59%
Stage 3b	**Moderate to severe** loss of kidney function	44 to 30	30-44%
Stage 4	**Severe** loss of kidney function	29 to 15	15-29%
Stage 5	Kidney **failure**	less than 15	<15%

* Your GFR number tells you how much kidney function you have left. As the kidney disease progresses, the GFR number goes down so does your kidney function.

The Role of Diet in Managing Kidney Disease

I cannot emphasize enough the critical role that renal diet foods play in managing kidney disease. Scientific consensus highlights that dietary modifications can profoundly influence the progression of Chronic Kidney Disease (CKD). Optimal nutrition—focused on a low-protein, low-sodium, and high-fiber diet—has been shown to slow the decline of kidney function. Such dietary changes not only support kidney health but also mitigate associated risks, including hypertension and diabetes. Therefore, bridging the knowledge gap in dietary management is essential for improving outcomes in CKD.

Chapter 2: The Basics of a Kidney-Friendly Diet

Key Nutrients to Monitor: Potassium, Phosphorus, Sodium, and Protein

You've probably heard it countless times, yet navigating the vast sea of dietary information can be overwhelming. If only there were a shortcut to understanding what to eat for managing chronic kidney disease (CKD)! In this chapter, I've distilled essential information into bite-sized, actionable nuggets to help you effectively manage your CKD diet.

What Should You Eat for Your CKD?

Adhering to a healthy diet is crucial for maintaining good nutritional status and slowing the progression of kidney disease. Here are key steps to follow, with a particular focus on the four essential nutrients that impact your kidney health:

1. Follow a Low-Sodium Diet and Read Labels

- Aim for a Blood Pressure Below 130/80 mmHg: Keeping your blood pressure in check is vital for kidney health.

- Limit Daily Sodium Intake: Aim for less than 2000–2300 mg of sodium per day.

- Choose Fresh and Low-Sodium Foods: Opt for fresh produce and low-sodium frozen options.

- Use Herbs for Flavor: Replace regular seasonings with herbs to enhance flavor without added sodium.

- Read Nutrition Labels: Look for sodium-free, salt-free, very low sodium, light, or reduced-sodium items instead of regular options.

2. Consume an Appropriate Amount of Protein

- Portion Control: Keep protein portions small, focusing on meat, poultry, fish, eggs, dairy, and beans.
- Consult Your Dietitian: Ask your dietitian about your specific protein needs.
- Avoid Fad Diets: Steer clear of commercial weight-loss plans like South Beach or low-carb diets.

Animal Protein Sources	Plant Protein Sources
Chicken, fish, beef, pork, lamb, eggs, dairy	Beans, nuts, lentils, tofu, grains

3. Use Healthy Cooking Methods

- Opt for Healthier Preparation: Grill, broil, bake, roast, or stir-fry instead of deep-frying.
- Trim Fat: Remove excess fat from meat and skin from poultry.
- Choose Healthy Fats: Use non-stick margarine or oils instead of butter, and select low-fat products.

Heart-Healthy Foods: Lean cuts of meat (loin or round), skinless poultry, fish, beans, vegetables, fruits, and low-fat dairy products.

4. Choose Foods with Adequate Potassium

- Monitor Potassium Intake: You may need to limit potassium as CKD progresses, especially if prescribed medications like ACE inhibitors or ARBs (Lisinopril, Avapro).
- Limit High-Potassium Foods: Avoid foods that are high in potassium.
- Skip Lite Salt: Be cautious with "lite salt" as it contains potassium instead of sodium.
- Avoid Canned Fruit/Vegetable Liquids: Don't use the liquid from canned fruits or vegetables.
- Watch Portion Sizes!

High Potassium Foods	Low Potassium Foods
Potatoes (white and sweet), tomatoes, bananas, orange juice, beans, nuts, prunes, milk, peanut butter	Apples, peaches, green beans, cauliflower, onions, celery, white bread, pasta, rice, corn flakes, rice cereal, rice milk

5. Choose Foods with Adequate Phosphorus

- Limit Phosphorus Intake: As kidney function declines, a low-phosphorus diet may be necessary to protect your bones and blood vessels.

- Watch for Phosphorus Additives: Limit dairy products, beans, lentils, nuts, organ meats, and dark colas.

- Read Ingredient Lists: Look out for "PHOS" on labels, as many packaged foods contain added phosphorus.

- Avoid Processed Meats: Choose fresh meats over deli meats that often contain phosphorus.

High Phosphorus Foods	Low Phosphorus Foods
Organ meats, dairy, beans, lentils, nuts, cola, bran cereals, oatmeal	Fresh fruits and vegetables, bread, pasta, rice milk, corn and rice cereals, light-colored soda

Hydration and Fluid Management

Chronic Kidney Disease (CKD) is classified into five stages, ranging from mild (Stage 1) to severe (Stage 5), which may require dialysis or a kidney transplant. It's crucial to note that fluid intake recommendations vary widely based on individual circumstances, including body size, activity level, climate, and other health conditions. Therefore, consider these general guidelines, but always consult your healthcare provider for personalized advice.

General Fluid Guidelines Based on CKD Stages:

- Stage 1 (GFR ≥90 mL/min): Fluid intake may not require specific restrictions unless other health conditions dictate otherwise. Typically, healthy adults should aim for around 2 to 2.5 liters (8-10 glasses) of water per day, avoiding overconsumption.

- Stage 2 (GFR 60-89 mL/min): Similar to Stage 1, there may not be specific fluid restrictions unless necessary due to other health issues. Maintaining adequate hydration remains important.

- Stage 3 (GFR 30-59 mL/min): As kidney function declines, patients may experience fluid retention, leading to swelling and increased blood pressure. In this case, your healthcare provider may recommend limiting fluid intake.

- Stage 4 (GFR 15-29 mL/min): Significant loss of kidney filtering capacity occurs at this stage, making fluid restrictions more likely to prevent fluid overload.

- Stage 5 (GFR <15 mL/min or on dialysis): Fluid intake is usually closely monitored, especially for dialysis patients. Fluid allowances often depend on urine output and the amount of fluid removed during dialysis. It's common for hemodialysis patients to limit fluid intake to 1-1.5 liters per day.

Final Thoughts

These guidelines serve as a foundation for managing your kidney health through diet. However, individual recommendations can vary widely, so it's essential to collaborate closely with your healthcare provider to determine the appropriate dietary choices and fluid intake for your specific needs.

Chapter 3: The Renal Diet Food List

Welcome to the heart of this book! As previously mentioned, the data contained in this food list has been meticulously curated by a dedicated team of dietitians and nephrology nurses. They have invested countless hours gathering scientific data from reputable sources, including the USDA Food Data Central, ensuring that this information is accurate and reliable for your chronic kidney disease (CKD) diet management as prescribed by your physician and dietitian. For your convenience, you can also find an index in Appendix C (page 337) to quickly locate specific foods.

How to Use the Charts

Navigating the food list is simple! Here's a step-by-step guide to help you utilize the charts effectively:

1. Categorization: The charts are organized into general food groups:
    - Carbohydrates
    - Fats (oils, nuts, and seeds)
    - Milk
    - Fruits & Vegetables
    - Vegetable Proteins
    - Meats, Poultry, & Seafood
    - Herbs & Spices

2. Finding Specific Foods: Locate your desired food item through the categories or use the indices available in Appendix C (page 337).

3. Standardized Measurements: Each food group is further categorized by preparation styles, standardized to a measurement of 100 grams. Below this, you will find additional

measurements (slices, teaspoons, tablespoons, or cups) along with their corresponding weights in grams.

4. Nutrient Information: For each 100 grams of food, you will find the corresponding amounts of essential nutrients, including:

    - Calories
    - Carbohydrates
    - Proteins
    - Fats
    - Sodium
    - Phosphorus
    - Potassium

5. Calculating Nutrient Content: You can divide or multiply the nutrient values based on the amount of food you are preparing in your recipe.

Example 1: Actual Nutrient Content in Your Recipe

ASPARAGUS	SERVING QUANTITY	SERVING UNIT	CALORIES (kCal)	PROTEIN (g)	TOTAL CARBOHYDRATES (g)	SODIUM (mg)	POTASSIUM (mg)	PHOSPHORUS (mg)	TOTAL FAT (g)
boiled, drained	100.00	g	22	2.4	4.1	14.00	224.00	54.00	0.22
	90.00	g	20	2.2	3.7	12.60	201.60	48.60	0.20
	0.50	c							

Let's say your recipe calls for 1 cup of boiled asparagus. According to the food list chart, 90 grams of boiled asparagus is equivalent to ½ cup. Since you need a full cup, you would multiply the nutrient values by 2.

For 1 cup of asparagus, the nutrient content would be:

- Calories: 40 kCal
- Protein: 4.4 g
- Carbohydrates: 7.4 g
- Fats: 0.40 g
- Sodium: 25.2 mg
- Potassium: 403 mg
- Phosphorus: 97.2 mg

Example 2: More on Reading and Using the Chart

ASPARAGUS	SERVING QUANTITY	SERVING UNIT	CALORIES (kcal)	PROTEIN (g)	TOTAL CARBOHYDRATES (g)	SODIUM (mg)	POTASSIUM (mg)	PHOSPHORUS (mg)	TOTAL FAT (g)
boiled, drained	100.00	g	22	2.4	4.1	14.00	224.00	54.00	0.22
	90.00	g	20	2.2	3.7	12.60	201.60	48.60	0.20
	0.50	c							
frozen	100.00	g	24	3.2	4.1	8.00	253.00	64.00	0.23
	87.00	g	21	2.8	3.6	6.96	220.11	55.68	0.20
	6.00	pcs							

Consider 6 pieces of frozen asparagus, which weigh approximately 87 grams. You would reference the nutrient values based on the 87-gram line. If you wish to reduce your potassium intake, you might choose to eat only 3 pieces, which would lower the potassium content from 220.11 mg to approximately 110 mg.

Alternatively, using a kitchen scale to measure your food allows you to adjust your intake based on the 100-gram standard, tailoring your consumption to meet your daily needs and restrictions effectively.

A. Vegetable Proteins

Hey there!

Do you need to print out this Food List?

You can download a printable version of this chart by scanning the QR code below or copying the link on your computer browser.

https://go.renaltracker.com/printfoodlist

BEANS	SERVING QUANTITY	SERVING UNIT	CALORIES kcal	PROTEIN (g)	TOTAL CARBOHYDRATES (g)	SODIUM (mg)	POTASSIUM (mg)	PHOSPHORUS (mg)	TOTAL FAT (g)
Lentils/Pinto/Navy	100.00	g	131	8.6	23.9	1.67	398.91	165.76	0.49
	92.00	g	121	8.0	22.0	1.54	367.00	152.50	0.45
	0.50	c							
Lima	100.00	g	113	6.8	20.2	8.00	467.00	136.00	0.86
	78.00	g	88	5.3	15.7	6.24	364.26	106.08	0.67
	0.50	c							
Broad or Fava	100.00	g	72	5.6	11.7	50.00	250.00	95.00	0.60
	81.75	g	59	4.6	9.6	40.88	204.38	77.66	0.49
	0.75	c							
Black beans, boiled	100.00	g	132	8.9	23.7	1.00	355.00	140.00	0.54
	86.00	g	114	7.6	20.4	0.86	305.30	120.40	0.46
	0.50	c							
Mungo, boiled	100.00	g	105	7.5	18.3	7.00	231.00	156.00	0.55
	90.00	g	95	6.8	16.5	6.30	207.90	140.40	0.50
	0.50	c							
sprouts, Mung	100.00	g	30	3.0	5.9	6.00	149.00	54.00	0.18
	78.00	g	23	2.4	4.6	4.68	116.22	42.12	0.14
	0.75	c							
Kidney, boiled	100.00	g	127	8.7	22.8	1.00	405.00	138.00	0.50
	88.50	g	112	7.7	20.2	0.89	358.43	122.13	0.44
	0.50	c							
Navy, boiled	100.00	g	140	8.2	26.1	0.00	389.00	144.00	0.62
	91.00	g	127	7.5	23.7	0.00	353.99	131.04	0.56
	0.50	c							
Lupin, boiled	100.00	g	119	15.6	9.9	4.00	245.00	128.00	2.92
	83.00	g	99	12.9	8.2	3.32	203.35	106.24	2.42
	0.50	c							
Pinto, frozen	100.00	g	170	9.8	32.5	92.00	755.98	117.00	0.50
	94.49	g	161	9.3	31.0	86.93	714.34	110.55	0.47
	3.33	oz							
Pinto, boiled	100.00	g	143	9.0	26.2	1.00	436.00	147.00	0.65
	85.50	g	122	7.7	22.4	0.86	372.78	125.69	0.56
	0.50	c							
White (Cannellini), boiled no salt	100.00	g	139	9.7	25.1	6.00	561.00	113.00	0.35
	89.50	g	124	8.7	22.5	5.37	502.10	101.14	0.31
	0.50	c							

BEANS	SERVING QUANTITY	SERVING UNIT	CALORIES (kcal)	PROTEIN (g)	TOTAL CARBOHYDRATES (g)	SODIUM (mg)	POTASSIUM (mg)	PHOSPHORUS (mg)	TOTAL FAT (g)
White, small, boiled, no salt	100.00	g	142	9.0	25.8	2.00	463.00	169.00	0.64
	89.50	g	127	8.0	23.1	1.79	414.39	151.26	0.57
	0.50	c							
sprouts, Kidney	100.00	g	29	4.2	4.1	6.00	187.00	37.00	0.50
	92.00	g	27	3.9	3.8	5.52	172.04	34.04	0.46
	0.50	c							
sprouts, Navy	100.00	g	67	6.2	13.1	13.00	307.00	100.00	0.70
	78.00	g	52	4.8	10.2	10.14	239.46	78.00	0.55
	0.75	c							
sprouts, Pinto	100.00	g	62	5.3	11.6	153.0	307.00	94.00	0.90
	85.05	g	53	4.5	9.9	130.1	262.10	79.95	0.77
	3.00	oz							
French, boiled	100.00	g	129	7.1	24.0	6.00	370.00	102.00	0.76
	88.50	g	114	6.2	21.3	5.31	327.45	90.27	0.67
	0.50	c							
baked, prepared	100.00	g	155	5.5	21.6	422.0	358.00	109.00	5.15
	126.50	g	196	7.0	27.4	533.8	452.87	138.00	6.51
	0.50	c							
Refried, canned	100.00	g	90	5.0	13.6	370.0	319.00	92.00	2.01
	119.00	g	107	5.9	16.1	440.3	379.61	109.48	2.39
	0.50	c							
CHICKPEAS									
garbanzos/ bengal gram, canned	100.00	g	88	4.9	13.5	278.0	144.00	80.00	1.95
	120.00	g	106	5.9	16.2	333.6	172.80	96.00	2.34
	0.50	c							
garbanzos/ bengal gram, boiled	100.00	g	164	8.9	27.4	7.00	291.00	168.00	2.59
	82.00	g	134	7.3	22.5	5.74	238.62	137.76	2.12
	0.50	c							
garbanzos/ bengal gram, canned drained, rinsed in tap water	100.00	g	138	7.0	22.9	212.0	109.00	80.00	2.47
	152.00	g	210	10.7	34.8	322.3	165.68	121.60	3.75
	1.00	c							
garbanzos/ bengal gram, canned low sodium	100	g	88	4.9	13.5	132.0	144.00	80.00	1.95
	240	g	211	11.8	32.4	316.8	345.60	192.00	4.68
	1	c							
flour	100.00	g	387	22.4	57.8	64.00	846.00	318.00	6.69
	92.00	g	110	6.4	16.4	18.14	239.84	90.15	1.90
	1.00	c							

TOFU	SERVING QUANTITY	SERVING UNIT	CALORIES (kcal)	PROTEIN (g)	TOTAL CARBOHYDRATES (g)	SODIUM (mg)	POTASSIUM (mg)	PHOSPHORUS (mg)	TOTAL FAT (g)
soft with calcium sulfate and magnesium chloride (Nigari)	100.00	g	61	7.2	1.2	8.00	120.00	92.00	3.69
	85.05	g	52	6.1	1.0	6.80	102.06	78.25	3.14
	3.00	oz							
firm with calcium sulfate and magnesium chloride (Nigari)	100.00	g	78	9.0	2.9	12.00	148.00	121.00	4.17
	85.05	g	66	7.7	2.4	10.21	125.87	102.91	3.55
	3.00	oz							
silken tofu (Vitasoy USA)	100.00	g	43	4.8	0.6	2.00	na	na	2.40
	91.00	g	39	4.4	0.5	1.82	na	na	2.18
	0.20	package							
TEMPEH									
raw	100.00	g	192	20.3	7.6	9.00	412.0	266.0	10.80
	83.00	g	159	16.8	6.3	7.47	341.9	220.8	8.96
	0.50	c							
cooked	100.00	g	185	19.9	7.6	14.00	401.0	253.0	11.38
EDAMAME									
frozen, unprepared	100.00	g	109	11.2	7.6	6.00	482.0	161.0	4.73
	118.00	g	129	13.2	9.0	7.08	568.7	189.9	5.58
	1.00	c							
frozen, prepared	100.00	g	121	11.9	8.9	6.00	436.0	261.9	5.20
	155.00	g	188	18.5	13.8	9.30	676	169	8.06
	1.00	c							
SPIRULINA									
seaweed, fresh/raw	100.00	g	26	5.9	2.4	98.00	127	11.00	0.39
	28.35	g	7	1.7	0.7	27.78	36.00	3.12	0.11
	1.00	oz							
seaweed, dried	100.00	g	290	57.5	23.9	1,048	1363	118	7.72
	112.00	g	325	64.4	26.8	1,174	1527	133	8.65
	1.00	c							

B. Animal Protein

(Meats, Poultry, and Seafood)

Hey there!

Do you need to print out this Food List?

You can download a printable version of this chart by scanning the QR code below or copying the link on your computer browser.

https://go.renaltracker.com/printfoodlist

CHICKEN	SERVING QUANTITY	UNIT	CALORIES (kcal)	PROTEIN (g)	TOTAL CARBOHYDRATES (g)	SODIUM (mg)	POTASSIUM (mg)	PHOSPHORUS (mg)	TOTAL FAT (g)
ground, raw	100.00	g	143	17.4	0.0	60.00	522.00	178.00	8.10
meat and skin, raw	100.00	g	215	18.6	0.0	70.00	189.00	147.00	15.06
	113.40	g	244	21.1	0.0	79.38	214.33	166.70	17.08
	4.00	oz							
meat and skin, roasted	100.00	g	239	27.3	0.0	82.00	223.00	182.00	13.60
	85.05	g	203	23.2	0.0	69.74	189.66	154.79	11.57
	3.00	oz							
thigh meat only, fried	100.00	g	218	28.2	1.2	95.00	259.00	199.00	10.30
	85.05	g	185	24.0	1.0	80.80	220.28	169.25	8.76
	3.00	oz							
thigh meat only, roasted	100.00	g	179	24.8	0.0	106.00	269.00	230.00	8.15
	85.05	g	152	21.1	0.0	90.15	228.78	195.61	6.93
	3.00	oz							
wing meat only, fried	100.00	g	211	30.2	0.0	91.00	208.00	164.00	9.15
	85.05	g	179	25.6	0.0	77.39	176.90	139.48	7.78
	3.00	oz							
wing meat only, roasted	100.00	g	203	30.5	0.0	92.00	210.00	166.00	8.13
	85.05	g	173	26.0	0.0	78.25	178.60	141.18	6.91
	3.00	oz							
wing meat only, stewed	100.00	g	181	27.2	0.0	73.00	153.00	134.00	7.18
	85.05	g	154	23.1	0.0	62.09	130.12	113.97	6.11
	3.00	oz							
back meat only, fried	100.00	g	288	30.0	5.7	99.00	251.00	176.00	4.12
	85.05	g	245	25.5	4.8	84.20	213.47	149.69	3.50
	3.00	oz							
back meat only, roasted	100.00	g	239	28.2	0.0	96.00	237.00	165.00	13.16
	85.05	g	203	24.0	0.0	81.65	201.57	140.33	11.19
	3.00	oz							
back meat only, stewed	100.00	g	209	25.3	0.0	67.00	158.00	130.00	11.19
	85.05	g	178	21.5	0.0	56.98	134.38	110.56	9.52
	3.00	oz							
drumstick meat only, fried	100.00	g	195	28.6	0.0	96.00	249.00	186.00	8.08
	85.05	g	166	24.3	0.0	81.65	211.77	158.19	6.87
	3.00	oz							
drumstick meat only, roasted	100.00	g	155	24.2	0.0	128.00	256.00	200.00	5.70
	85.05	g	132	20.6	0.0	108.86	217.73	170.10	4.85
	3	oz							

CHICKEN	SERVING QUANTITY	UNIT	CALORIES (kcal)	PROTEIN (g)	TOTAL CARBOHYDRATE (g)	SODIUM (mg)	POTASSIUM (mg)	PHOSPHORUS (mg)	TOTAL FAT (g)
drumstick meat only, stewed	100.00	g	169	27.5	0.0	80.00	199.00	150.00	5.71
	85.05 3.00	g oz	144	23.4	0.0	68.04	169.25	127.57	4.86
leg meat only, fried	100.00	g	208	28.4	0.7	96.00	254.00	193.00	9.32
	85.05 3.00	g oz	177	24.1	0.6	81.65	216.02	164.14	7.93
leg meat only, roasted	100.00	g	174	24.2	0.0	99.00	269.00	205.00	7.80
	85.05 3.00	g oz	148	20.6	0.0	84.20	228.78	174.35	6.63
leg meat only, stewed	100.00	g	185	26.3	0.0	78.00	190.00	149.00	8.06
	85.05 3.00	g oz	157	22.3	0.0	66.34	161.59	126.72	6.85
pate, chicken liver, canned	100.00	g	201	13.5	6.6	386.0	95.00	175.00	13.10
	52.00 4.00	g tbsp	105	7.0	3.4	200.7	49.40	91.00	6.81
chicken tenders, fast food	100.00	g	271	19.2	17.3	769.0	373.00	282.00	13.95
	62.00 4.00	g pcs	168	11.9	10.7	476.8	231.26	174.84	8.65
chicken patty, frozen, cooked	100.00	g	287	14.9	12.8	532.0	261.00	208.00	19.58
bratwurst, chicken, cooked	100.00	g	176	19.4	0.0	72.00	211.00	160.00	10.30
	83.92 2.96	g oz	148	16.3	0.0	60.42	177.06	134.27	8.69
sausage, chicken/beef, smoked	100.00	g	295	18.5	0.0	1,020	139.00	111.00	244.00
	138.00 1.00	g c	251	15.7	0.0	867.5	118.22	94.41	20.41

TURKEY	SERVING QUANTITY	UNIT	CALORIES (kcal)	PROTEIN (g)	TOTAL CARBOHYDRATE (g)	SODIUM (mg)	POTASSIUM (mg)	PHOSPHORUS (mg)	TOTAL FAT (g)
breast, meat & skin, raw	100.00	g	144	21.6	0.1	112.00	224.00	183.00	5.64
	113.40	g	163	24.5	0.2	127.01	254.02	207.52	6.40
	4.00	oz							
breast, meat & skin, roasted	100.00	g	189	28.6	0.1	103.00	239.00	223.00	7.39
	85.05	g	161	24.3	0.1	87.60	203.27	189.66	6.29
	3.00	oz							
breast, meat only, raw	100.00	g	114	23.3	0.0	74.00	267.00	185.00	2.33
	85.05	g	97	19.9	0.0	62.94	227.08	157.34	1.98
	3.00	oz							
breast, meat only, roasted	100.00	g	136	29.5	0.0	114.00	297.00	253.00	1.97
	85.05	g	116	25.1	0.0	96.96	252.60	215.17	1.68
	3.00	oz							
ground, raw	100.00	g	148	20.0	0.0	58.00	237.00	200.00	7.66
	113.40	g	168	22.3	0.0	65.77	268.76	226.80	8.69
	4.00	oz							
ground, cooked	100.00	g	203	27.4	0.0	78.00	294.00	254.00	10.40
	85.05	g	173	23.3	0.0	66.34	250.04	216.02	8.85
	3.00	oz							
white rotisserie, deli cut	100.00	g	112	13.5	7.7	1,200	349.00	158.00	3.00
	56.70	g	64	7.7	4.4	680.40	197.88	89.59	1.70
	2.00	oz							
ham, extra lean, sliced	100.00	g	134	19.6	0.9	1,038	299.00	304.00	5.80
	20.00	g	27	3.9	0.2	207.60	59.80	60.80	1.16
	1.00	pc							
pastrami, sliced	100.00	g	139	16.3	3.3	1,123	345.00	200.00	6.21
	56.70	g	79	9.2	1.9	636.74	195.62	113.40	3.52
	2.00	slices							
bologna	100.00	g	209	11.4	4.7	1,071	135.00	114.00	16.05
	56.70	g	119	6.5	2.7	607.26	76.55	64.64	9.10
	2.00	slices							
salami	100.00	g	172	19.2	1.6	1,107	216.00	266.00	9.21
	56.70	g	98	10.9	0.9	627.67	122.47	150.82	5.22
	2.00	slices							
bacon, turkey, cooked	100.00	g	382	29.6	3.1	2,285	395.00	460.00	27.90
	28.35	g	108	8.4	0.9	647.80	111.98	130.41	7.91
	1.00	oz							
bacon, turkey, low sodium	100.00	g	253	13.3	4.8	900.00	156.00	145.00	20.00
	15.00	g	38	2.0	0.7	135.00	23.40	21.75	3.00
	1.00	svg							
sausage, turkey, cooked	100.00	g	196	23.9	0.0	665.00	298.00	202.00	10.44
	56.70	g	111	13.6	0.0	377.06	168.97	114.53	5.92
	2.00	oz							

EGG

	SERVING QUANTITY	UNIT	CALORIES (kcal)	PROTEIN (g)	CARBOHYDRATES (g)	SODIUM (mg)	POTASSIUM (mg)	PHOSPHORUS (mg)	TOTAL FAT (g)
chicken, raw, large	100.00 50.00 1.00	g g pc	143 72	12.6 6.3	0.7 0.4	142.00 71.00	138.00 69.00	198.00 99.00	9.51 4.76
chicken, fried, large	100.00 46.00 1.00	g g pc	196 90	13.6 6.3	0.8 0.4	207.00 95.22	152.00 69.92	215.00 98.90	14.84 6.83
chicken, poached, large	100.00 50.00 1.00	g g pc	143 72	12.5 6.3	0.7 0.4	297.00 148.50	138.00 69.00	197.00 98.50	9.47 4.74
chicken, hard boiled, large	100.00 50.00 1.00	g g pc	155 78	12.6 6.3	1.1 0.6	124.00 62.00	126.00 63.00	172.00 86.00	10.61 5.31
scrambled, fast food	100.00 94.00 2.00	g g pc	212 199	13.8 13.0	2.1 2.0	187.00 175.78	147.00 138.18	242.00 227.48	16.18 15.21
substitute, liquid	100.00 251.00 1.00	g g c	84 211	12.0 30.1	0.6 1.6	177.00 444.27	330.00 828.30	121.00 303.71	3.31 8.31
substitute, powder	100.00 9.92 0.35	g g oz	443 44	55.8 5.5	22 2.2	798.19 79.20	742.31 73.66	476.92 47.32	12.97 1.29
substitute, frozen	100.00 60.00 0.25	g g c	160 96	11.3 6.8	3.2 1.9	199.00 119.40	213.00 127.80	72.00 43.20	11.11 6.67
chicken, egg whites only, raw large egg	100.00 33.00 1.00	g g pc	52 17	10.9 3.6	0.7 0.2	166.00 54.78	163.00 53.79	15.00 4.95	0.17 0.06
chicken, yolk only, raw large egg	100.00 17.00 1.00	g g pc	322 55	15.9 2.7	3.6 0.6	48.00 8.16	109.00 18.53	390.00 66.30	26.54 4.51
chicken, whole, raw, frozen	100.00 56.70 2.00	g g oz	147 83	12.3 7.0	1.0 0.6	128.00 72.57	135.00 76.54	193.00 109.43	9.95 5.64
yolk only, frozen, raw	100.00 56.70 2.00	g g oz	296 168	15.5 8.8	0.8 0.5	67.00 37.99	121.00 68.61	419.99 238.14	25.60 14.51
whites, frozen, raw	100.00 56.70 2.00	g g oz	48 27	10.2 5.8	1.0 0.6	169.00 95.82	169.00 95.82	13.00 7.37	0.00 0.00
duck, raw	100.00 70.00 1.00	g g pc	185 130	12.8 9.0	1.5 1.0	146.00 102.20	222.00 155.40	220.00 154.00	13.77 9.64
quail, raw	100.00 9.00 1.00	g g pc	158 14	13.1 1.2	0.4 0.0	141.00 12.69	132.00 11.88	226.00 20.34	11.09 1.00

PORK

	SERVING QUANTITY	UNIT	CALORIES (kcal)	PROTEIN (g)	TOTAL CARBOHYDRATE (g)	SODIUM (mg)	POTASSIUM (mg)	PHOSPHORUS (mg)	TOTAL FAT (g)
ground, cooked	100.00	g	297	25.7	0.0	73.00	362.00	226.00	20.77
	85.05	g	253	21.9	0.0	62.09	307.88	192.21	17.66
	3.00	oz							
ground, raw	100.00	g	263	16.9	0.0	56.00	287.00	175.00	21.19
	113.40	g	298	19.1	0.0	63.50	325.46	198.45	24.03
	4.00	oz							
loin, sirloin, roasts, separable lean roasted	100.00	g	204	27.8	0.0	59.00	352.00	235.00	9.44
	85.05	g	174	23.6	0.0	50.18	299.37	199.87	8.03
	3.00	oz							
loin, center rib, separable lean, roasted	100.00	g	206	28.8	0.0	95.00	287.00	244.00	9.21
	85.05	g	175	24.5	0.0	80.80	244.09	207.52	7.83
	3.00	oz							
loin, sirloin, boneless, separable lean roasted	100.00	g	178	30.4	0.0	66.00	408.00	311.00	5.31
	85.05	g	151	25.9	0.0	56.13	347.00	264.50	4.52
	3.00	oz							
loin, center rib, boneless roasted	100.00	g	214	28.8	0.0	50.00	363.00	222.00	10.13
	85.05	g	182	24.5	0.0	42.52	308.73	188.81	8.62
	3.00	oz							
shoulder blade, boston roasts roasted turkey, salt.	100.00	g	232	24.2	0.0	88.00	427.00	235.00	14.30
	85.05	g	197	20.6	0.0	74.84	363.16	199.87	12.16
	3.00	oz							
shoulder, whole, roasted	100.00	g	230	25.3	0.0	74.96	345.80	220.87	13.53
	85.05	g	196	21.5	0.0	63.75	294.10	187.85	11.51
	3.00	oz							
loin, whole, roasted	100.00	g	209	28.6	0.0	58.00	425.00	249.00	9.63
	85.05	g	178	24.3	0.0	49.33	361.46	211.77	8.19
	3.00	oz							
leg or ham, whole, roasted	100.00	g	211	29.4	0.0	64.00	373.00	281.00	9.44
	85.05	g	179	25.0	0.0	54.43	317.23	238.99	8.03
	3.00	oz							
loin, tenderloin, separable lean & fat roasted	100.00	g	147	26.0	0.0	57.00	419.00	265.00	3.96
	85.05	g	125	22.2	0.0	48.48	356.36	225.38	3.37
	3.00	oz							
ground, cooked	100.00	g	297	25.7	0.0	73.00	362.00	226.00	20.77
	85.05	g	253	21.9	0.0	62.09	307.88	192.21	17.66
	3.00	oz							

PORK	SERVING QUANTITY	UNIT	CALORIES (kcal)	PROTEIN (g)	TOTAL CARBOHYDRATES (g)	SODIUM (mg)	POTASSIUM (mg)	PHOSPHORUS (mg)	TOTAL FAT (g)
bacon, cured, broiled, panfried or roasted	100.00	g	541	37.0	1.4	1,717.0	565.0	533.0	41.78
	8.00	g	43	3.0	0.1	137.36	45.20	42.64	3.34
	1.00	slice							
bacon, reduced sodium, cured broiled, panfried or roasted	100.00	g	541	37.0	1.4	1,030.0	565.0	533.0	41.78
	56.70	g	307	21.0	0.8	584.01	320.4	302.2	23.69
	2.00	oz							
country style ribs, separable lean & fat roasted	100.00	g	359	21.8	0.0	52.00	322.0	214.0	29.46
	85.05	g	305	18.5	0.0	44.23	273.9	182.0	25.06
	3.00	oz							
sirloin, chops or roasts, boneless, raw	100.00	g	121	22.8	0.0	63.00	354.0	251.0	2.59
	113.40	g	137	25.9	0.0	71.44	401.4	284.6	2.94
	4.00	oz							
kidney, braised	100.00	g	151	25.4	0.0	80.00	143.0	240.0	4.70
	85.05	g	128	21.6	0.0	68.04	121.6	204.1	4.00
	3.00	oz							
liver, braised	100.00	g	165	26.0	3.8	49.00	150.0	241.0	4.40
	85.05	g	140	22.1	3.2	41.67	127.6	205.0	3.74
	3.00	oz							
ham, minced, sliced	100.00	g	263	16.3	1.8	1,245.0	311.0	157.0	20.68
	21.00	g	55	3.4	0.4	261.45	65.31	32.97	4.34
	1.00	slice							
ham, extra lean, 5% fat	100.00	g	107	16.9	0.7	944.99	463.0	252.0	4.04
	85.05	g	91	14.3	0.6	803.71	393.8	214.3	3.44
	3.00	oz							
ham, low sodium, cured, cooked	100.00	g	165	22.0	0.5	969.00	362.0	248.0	7.70
	85.05	g	140	18.7	0.4	824.13	307.9	210.9	6.55
	3.00	oz							
sausages, Kielbasa, grilled	100.00	g	337	12.5	5.0	1,062	306.0	204.0	29.68
	85.05	g	287	10.6	4.3	903.22	260.3	173.5	25.24
	3.00	oz							
Kielbasa, panfried	100.00	g	333	12.4	4.8	1,046	304.0	199.0	29.43
	85.05	g	283	10.5	4.1	889.61	258.6	169.3	25.03
	3.00	oz							
Beerwurst, pork/beef	100.00	g	276	14.0	4.3	732.00	244.0	135.0	22.53
	56.70	g	156	7.9	2.4	415.04	138.4	76.6	12.77
	2.00	oz							

PORK	SERVING QUANTITY	UNIT	CALORIES (kcal)	PROTEIN (g)	TOTAL CARBOHYDRATE (g)	SODIUM (mg)	POTASSIUM (mg)	PHOSPHORUS (mg)	TOTAL FAT (g)
Italian Sweet, links	100	g	149	16.1	2.1	570.00	194.00	103.00	8.42
	85.053	oz	127	13.7	1.8	484.79	165.00	87.60	7.16
Polish, pork, cooked	100	g	326	14.1	1.6	875.99	237.00	136.00	28.72
	56.702	oz	185	8.0	0.9	496.68	134.38	77.11	16.28
Bratwurst, pork, cooked	100	g	333	13.7	2.9	845.99	347.99	208.00	29.18
	56.702	oz	189	7.8	1.6	479.67	197.31	117.93	16.54
meatloaf/ luncheon meat pork/beef	100	g	260	15.4	1.6	1,182	245.00	122.00	20.90
	21	g slice	60	3.5	0.4	271.86	56.35	28.06	4.81
peperoni, beef/pork	100	g	504	19.3	1.2	1,582	274.00	158.00	46.28
	56.702	oz	286	11.0	0.7	896.98	155.36	89.58	26.24
salami, italian, pork	100	g	425	21.7	1.2	1,890	340.00	229.00	37.00
	28.351	g oz	120	6.2	0.3	535.82	96.39	64.92	10.49

BEEF	SERVING QUANTITY	UNIT	CALORIES (kcal)	PROTEIN (g)	TOTAL CARBOHYDRATES (g)	SODIUM (mg)	POTASSIUM (mg)	PHOSPHORUS (mg)	TOTAL FAT (g)
chuck eyeroast, boneless, all grades 0" fat, separable lean only, roasted	3 85.05 3.00	g g oz	183 156	26.7 22.7	0.0 0.0	68.04 80.00	344.00 292.57	210.00 178.61	8.46 7.20
chuck eyeroast, boneless, all grades separable lean only, 0", raw	100.00 85.05 3.00	g g oz	137 117	20.6 17.5	0.0 0.0	85.00 72.29	357.00 303.63	204.00 173.50	6.01 5.11
chuck eyeroast, boneless, all grades sep lean & fat, 0" fat, roasted	100.00 85.05 3.00	g g oz	236 201	24.6 21.0	0.0 0.0	76.00 64.64	308.00 261.95	187.00 159.04	15.29 13.00
chuck eyeroast, boneless, all grades sep lean & fat, 0" fat, raw	100.00 85.05 3.00	g g oz	173 147	19.3 16.4	0.0 0.0	82.00 69.74	367.00 312.13	187.00 159.04	10.67 9.07
jerky	100.00 28.35 1.00	g g oz	410 116	33.2 9.4	11 3.1	1,785 506.05	597.00 169.25	407.00 115.38	25.60 7.26
corned beef, brisket, raw	100.00 113.40 4.00	g g oz	198 225	14.7 16.7	0.1 0.2	1,217 1,380	297.00 336.80	117.00 132.68	14.90 16.90
corned beef, brisket, cooked	100.00 85.05 3.00	g g oz	251 213	18.2 15.5	0.5 0.4	927.99 827.53	145.00 123.32	125.00 106.31	18.98 16.14
broth cube 1 cube, 6 fl. oz prepared	100.00 3.60 1.00	g g cube	170 6	17.3 0.6	16 0.6	24,000 864.00	403.00 14.51	225.00 8.10	4.00 0.14
liver, pan fried	100.00 81.00 1.00	g g slice	175 142	26.5 21.5	5.2 4.2	77.00 62.37	351.00 284.31	485.00 392.85	4.68 3.79
liver, braised	100.00 85.05 3.00	g g oz	191 162	29.1 24.7	5.1 4.4	79.00 67.19	352.00 299.37	496.99 422.69	5.26 4.47
tongue, simmered	100.00 85.05 3.00	g g oz	284 242	19.3 16.4	0.0 0.0	65.00 55.28	184.00 156.49	145.00 123.32	22.30 18.97
kidney simmered	100.00 85.05 3.00	g g oz	158 134	27.3 23.2	0.0 0.0	94.00 79.95	135.00 114.82	304.00 258.55	4.65 3.95
tripe, simmered	100.00 85.05 3.00	g g oz	94 80	11.7 10.0	2.0 1.7	68.00 57.83	42.00 35.72	66.00 56.13	4.05 3.44

LAMB	SERVING QUANTITY	UNIT	CALORIES (kcal)	PROTEIN (g)	TOTAL CARBOHYDRATES (g)	SODIUM (mg)	POTASSIUM (mg)	PHOSPHORUS (mg)	TOTAL FAT (g)
tenderloin, New Zealand, separable lean only, raw	100.00	g	116	20.5	0.0	49.00	381.00	222.00	3.81
	85.05	g	99	17.5	0.0	41.67	324.04	188.81	3.24
	3.00	oz							
loin, NZ, separable lean, frozen, broiled	100.00	g	199	29.3	0.0	55.00	189.00	240.00	8.24
	85.05	g	169	24.9	0.0	46.78	160.74	204.12	7.01
	3.00	oz							
australian, separable lean, 1/8" fat, cooked	100.00	g	201	26.7	0.0	80.00	318.00	207.00	9.63
	85.05	g	171	22.7	0.0	68.04	270.46	176.05	8.19
	3.00	oz							
Australian, separable lean, 1/8" fat, raw	100.00	g	142	20.3	0.0	83.00	320.00	188.00	6.18
	113.40	g	161	23.0	0.0	94.12	362.88	213.19	7.01
	4.00	oz							
Australian, ground, 85%Lean/15%fat, raw	100.00	g	255	17.1	0.0	65.49	na	na	20.17
	85.05	g	217	14.6	0.0	77.00	na	na	17.61
	3.00	oz							
NZ, rib, separable lean, frozen, raw	100.00	g	160	20.7	0.0	67.00	309.00	185.00	8.61
	113.40	g	181	23.4	0.0	75.98	350.41	209.79	9.76
	4.00	oz							
NZ, rib, separable lean, frozen, roasted	100.00	g	193	24.4	0.0	72.00	323.00	209.00	10.63
	85.05	g	164	20.8	0.0	61.24	274.71	177.75	9.04
	3.00	oz							
VEAL									
separable lean, cooked	100.00	g	196	32.0	0.0	89.00	338.00	250.00	6.58
	85.05	g	167	27.1	0.0	75.69	287.47	212.62	5.60
	3.00	oz							
liver, pan fried	100.00	g	193	27.4	4.5	85.00	353.00	482.99	6.51
	85.05	g	164	23.3	3.8	72.29	300.22	410.79	5.54
	3.00	oz							
sausage, bratwurst, veal, cooked	100.00	g	341	14.0	0.0	60.00	231.00	150.00	31.70
	83.92	g	286	11.7	0.0	50.35	193.85	125.87	26.60
	2.96	oz							
ground, pan fried	100.00	g	503	8.9	0.9	89.00	107.00	133.00	51.60
	85.05	g	428	7.5	0.8	75.69	91.00	113.12	43.89
	3.00	oz							

VEAL	SERVING QUANTITY	UNIT	CALORIES (kcal)	PROTEIN (g)	TOTAL CARBOHYDRATE (g)	SODIUM (mg)	POTASSIUM (mg)	PHOSPHORUS (mg)	TOTAL FAT (g)
sirloin, separable, lean, braised	100.00	g	204	34.0	0.0	81.00	339.00	259.00	6.51
	85.05	g	174	28.9	0.0	68.89	288.32	220.28	5.54
	3.00	oz							
sirloin separable lean, roasted	100.00	g	168	26.3	0.0	85.00	365.00	231.00	6.22
	85.05	g	143	22.4	0.0	72.29	310.43	196.46	5.29
	3.00	oz							
sirloin, lean, raw	100.00	g	110	20.2	0.0	80.00	348.00	220.00	2.59
	113.40	g	125	22.9	0.0	90.72	394.63	249.48	2.94
	4.00	oz							
loin, lean and fat, braised	100.00	g	284	30.2	0.0	80.00	280.00	220.00	17.21
	85.05	g	242	25.7	0.0	68.04	238.14	187.11	14.64
	3.00	oz							
loin, lean and fat, roasted	100.00	g	217	25.0	0.0	93.00	325.00	212.00	12.32
	85.05	g	185	21.1	0.0	79.10	276.41	180.30	10.48
	3.00	oz							
loin, lean, braised	100.00	g	226	33.6	0.0	84.00	297.00	237.00	9.15
	85.05	g	192	28.6	0.0	71.44	252.60	201.57	7.78
	3.00	oz							
loin, lean, roasted	100.00	g	175	26.3	0.0	96.00	340.00	222.00	6.94
	85.05	g	149	22.4	0.0	81.65	289.17	188.81	5.90
	3.00	oz							
loin, lean, raw	100.00	g	114	21.9	0.0	99.00	260.00	237.00	2.90
	113.40	g	129	24.8	0.0	112.27	294.84	268.76	3.29
	4.00	oz							
loin, chop, lean and fat, grilled	100.00	g	198	28.0	0.2	86.00	229.00	208.00	9.48
	85.05	g	168	23.9	0.1	73.14	194.76	176.90	8.06
	3.00	oz							
bratwwurst, veal, cooked	100.00	g	341	14.0	0.0	60.00	231.00	150.00	31.70
	83.92	g	286	11.7	0.0	50.35	193.85	125.87	26.60
	2.96	oz							

SALMON

	SERVING QUANTITY	UNIT	CALORIES (kcal)	PROTEIN (g)	TOTAL CARBOHYDRATES (g)	SODIUM (mg)	POTASSIUM (mg)	PHOSPHORUS (mg)	TOTAL FAT (g)
pink, raw	100.00	g	127	20.5	0.0	74.99	365.96	260.98	4.40
	113.40	g	144	23.2	0.0	85.04	415.00	295.95	4.99
	4.00	oz							
atlantic, wild, raw	100.00	g	142	19.8	0.0	44.00	489.95	199.98	0.98
	113.40	g	161	22.5	0.0	49.89	555.61	226.78	1.11
	4.00	oz							
atlantic, farmed, raw	100.00	g	208	20.4	0.0	58.99	362.97	239.98	13.42
	113.39	g	236	23.2	0.0	66.90	411.60	272.13	15.22
	4.00	oz							
pink, canned, drained solids, w/ bone	100.00	g	138	23.1	0.0	380.78	332.80	378.78	5.02
	85.05	g	117	19.6	0.0	323.85	283.05	322.15	4.27
	3.00	oz							
pink, canned, with bone and liquid no salt	100.00	g	139	19.8	0.0	75.00	325.99	328.99	6.05
	56.70	g	79	11.2	0.0	42.52	184.84	186.54	3.43
	2.00	oz							
pink, canned, drained solids without skin and bones	100.00	g	136	24.6	0.0	378.00	326.00	253.00	4.21
	85.05	g	116	20.9	0.0	321.49	277.26	215.18	3.58
	3.00	oz							
chum, canned, drained, with bone no salt	100.00	g	141	21.4	0.0	75.00	300.00	353.99	5.50
	56.70	g	80	12.2	0.0	42.52	170.10	200.71	3.12
	2.00	oz							
nuggets, breaded, frozen, heated	100.00	g	212	12.7	14	173.00	165.00	176.00	11.72

TUNA

	SERVING QUANTITY	UNIT	CALORIES	PROTEIN	TOTAL CARBS	SODIUM	POTASSIUM	PHOSPHORUS	TOTAL FAT
bluefin, raw	100.00	g	144	23.3	0.0	39.00	251.98	253.98	4.90
	113.40	g	163	26.5	0.0	44.22	285.74	288.01	5.56
	4.00	oz							
yellowfin or Ahi, raw	100.00	g	109	24.4	0.0	45.00	440.96	277.97	0.49
	113.40	g	124	27.7	0.0	51.03	500.05	315.22	0.56
	4.00	oz							
canned in oil, drained, light no salt	100.00	g	198	29.1	0.0	50.00	207.00	311.00	8.21
	56.70	g	112	16.5	0.0	28.35	117.37	176.33	4.65
	2.00	oz							
white, canned in water, drained no salt	100.00	g	128	23.6	0.0	50.00	237.00	217.00	2.97
	56.70	g	73	13.4	0.0	28.35	134.38	123.04	1.68
	2.00	oz							
canned in water, drained, light no salt	100.00	g	116	25.5	0.0	50.00	237.00	163.00	0.82
	56.70	g	66	14.5	0.0	28.35	134.38	92.42	0.46
	2.00	oz							
white, canned in oil, drained, no salt	100.00	g	186	26.5	0.0	50.00	332.99	267.00	8.08
	56.70	g	105	15.0	0.0	28.35	188.81	151.39	4.58
	2.00	oz							

	SERVING QUANTITY	UNIT	CALORIES (kcal)	PROTEIN (g)	TOTAL CARBOHYDRATES (g)	SODIUM (mg)	POTASSIUM (mg)	PHOSPHORUS (mg)	TOTAL FAT (g)
SARDINES									
spanish	100.00	g	212	6.2	14.2	310.00	0.00	na	14.16
	113.00	g	240	7.0	16.0	350.00	0.00	na	16.00
	4.00	oz							
atlantic, canned in oil, with bones	100.00	g	208	24.6	0.0	307.00	397.0	490.0	11.45
	24.00	g	50	5.9	0.0	73.68	95.28	117.6	2.75
	2.00	oz							
portuguese	100.00	g	236	25.5	0.0	500.00	na	na	12.73
	55.00	g	130	14.0	0.0	275.00	na	na	7.00
	0.50	c							
fillets, canned	100.00	g	338	18.2	7.3	364.00	na	na	28.36
	55.00	g	186	10.0	4.0	200.00	na	na	14.50
	0.25	c							
TILAPIA									
raw	100.00	g	96	20.1	0.0	52.00	302.0	170.0	1.70
	113.40	g	107	22.8	0.0	58.97	342.5	192.8	1.93
	4.00	oz							
cooked, dry heat	100.00	g	128	26.2	0.0	55.97	379.8	203.9	2.65
	85.05	g	109	22.2	0.0	47.60	323.0	173.4	2.25
	3.00	oz							
POLLOCK									
atlantic, raw	100.00	g	92	19.4	0.0	85.99	355.9	220.9	0.98
	113.40	g	104	22.0	0.0	97.51	403.7	250.6	1.11
	4.00	oz							
atlantic, cooked, dry heat	100.00	g	118	24.9	0.0	110.00	456.0	283.0	1.26
	85.05	g	100	21.2	0.0	93.55	387.8	240.7	1.07
	3.00	oz							
alaska, untreated, cooked	100.00	g	87	19.4	0.0	166.00	364.0	206.0	1.00
	85.05	g	74	16.5	0.0	141.18	309.6	175.2	0.85
	3.00	oz							
PANGASIUS (CREAM DORY/SWAI)									
fillets, boneless	100.00	g	71	14.2	0.0	186.00	na	na	1.77
	113.00	g	80	16.0	0.0	210.00	na	na	2.00
	4.00	oz							
fillets, skinless, boneless	100.00	g	177	20.4	0.0	52.00	na	na	1.77
	113.00	g	200	23.0	0.0	58.80	na	na	2.00
	4.00	oz							

	SERVING QUANTITY	UNIT	CALORIES (kcal)	PROTEIN (g)	TOTAL CARBOHYDRATES (g)	SODIUM (mg)	POTASSIUM (mg)	PHOSPHORUS (mg)	TOTAL FAT (g)
MUSSELS									
blue, raw	100.00	g	86	11.9	3.7	286.00	320.00	197.00	2.24
	113.40	g	98	13.5	4.2	324.32	362.88	223.40	2.54
	4.00	oz							
blue, cooked, moist heat	100.00	g	172	23.8	7.4	369.00	268.00	285.00	4.48
	85.05	g	146	20.2	6.3	313.83	227.93	242.39	3.81
	3.00	oz							
atlantic or pacific, meat only	100.00	g	197	8.8	11.6	415.25	243.87	159.06	12.56
	85.05	g	167	7.5	9.9	353.17	207.41	1,315	10.69
	3.00	oz							
MACKEREL									
Atlantic or Boston, raw fillet	100.00	g	205	18.6	0.0	89.99	313.97	216.98	13.89
	113.40	g	232	21.1	0.0	102.05	356.04	246.05	15.75
	4.00	oz							
pacific and Jack, raw fillet	100.00	g	158	20.1	0.0	85.99	405.96	124.99	7.89
	113.40	g	179	22.8	0.0	97.51	460.36	141.71	8.95
	4.00	oz							
Atlantic Spanish, raw fillet	100.00	g	139	19.3	0.0	58.99	445.96	204.98	6.30
	113.40	g	158	21.9	0.0	66.90	505.71	232.45	7.14
	4.00	oz							
Jack, canned, solids, drained	100.00	g	156	23.2	0.0	378.99	194.00	301.00	6.30
	56.70	g	88	13.2	0.0	214.89	110.00	170.66	3.57
	2.00	oz							
Atlantic or Boston, cooked, dry heat	100.00	g	262	23.9	0.0	83.00	401.00	278.00	17.81
	85.05	g	223	20.3	0.0	70.59	341.05	236.44	15.15
	3.00	oz							
Atlantic, Spanish, cooked, dry heat	100.00	g	158	23.6	0.0	66.00	553.99	271.00	6.32
	85.05	g	134	20.1	0.0	56.13	471.17	230.48	5.38
	3.00	oz							
Pacific and Jack, mixed species, cooked	100.00	g	201	25.7	0.0	110.00	520.99	160.00	10.12
	85.05	g	171	21.9	0.0	93.55	443.11	136.08	8.61
	3.00	oz							

	SERVING QUANTITY	UNIT	CALORIES (kcal)	PROTEIN (g)	TOTAL CARBOHYDRATES (g)	SODIUM (mg)	POTASSIUM (mg)	PHOSPHORUS (mg)	TOTAL
TROUT									
rainbow, wild, raw, fillet	100.00	g	119	20.5	0.0	31.00	481.00	271.00	3.
	113.40	g	135	23.2	0.0	35.15	545.45	307.31	3.
	4.00	oz							
rainbow, farmed, raw, fillet	100.00	g	141	19.9	0.0	51.00	376.96	225.98	6.
	113.40	g	160	22.6	0.0	57.83	427.48	256.26	7.
	4.00	oz							
mixed species, raw fillet	100.00	g	148	20.8	0.0	52.00	360.97	244.98	6.
	113.40	g	168	23.6	0.0	58.96	409.33	277.80	7.
	4.00	oz							
sea trout, mixed species, raw	100.00	g	104	16.7	0.0	57.99	340.97	249.98	3.
	113.40	g	118	19.0	0.0	65.77	386.66	283.47	4.
	4.00	oz							
rainbow, wild, cooked, dry heat	100.00	g	150	22.9	0.0	56.00	448.00	269.00	5.
	85.05	g	128	19.5	0.0	47.63	381.02	228.78	4.
	3.00	oz							
rainbow, farmed, cooked, dry heat	100.00	g	168	23.8	0.0	61.00	450.00	270.00	7.
	85.05	g	143	20.2	0.0	51.88	382.72	229.63	6.
	3.00	oz							
mixed species, cooked, dry heat	100.00	g	190	26.6	0.0	67.00	463.00	314.00	8.
	85.05	g	162	22.7	0.0	56.98	393.78	267.05	7.
	3.00	oz							
sea trout, mixed species, cooked, dry heat	100.00	g	133	21.5	0.0	74.00	437.00	321.00	4.
	85.05	g	113	18.3	0.0	62.94	371.66	273.01	3.
	3.00	oz							
CARP									
raw	100.00	g	127	17.8	0.0	49.00	332.97	414.96	5.
	113.40	g	144	20.2	0.0	55.56	377.59	470.56	6.
	4.00	oz							
cooked, dry heat	100.00	g	162	22.9	0.0	63.00	427.00	530.99	7.
	85.05	g	138	19.4	0.0	53.58	363.16	451.61	6.
	3.00	oz							
MAHI-MAHI									
Dorado or Dolphinfish, raw	100.00	g	85	18.5	0.0	87.99	415.96	142.99	0.
	113.40	g	96	21.0	0.0	99.78	471.70	162.15	0.
	4.00	oz							
Doradao or Dolphinfish, cooked, dry heat	100.00	g	109	23.7	0.0	113.00	532.99	183.00	0.
	85.05	g	93	20.2	0.0	96.11	452.31	155.64	0.
	3.00	oz							

	SERVING QUANTITY	UNIT	CALORIES kcal	PROTEIN (g)	TOTAL CARBOHYDRATES (g)	SODIUM (mg)	POTASSIUM (mg)	PHOSPHORUS (mg)	TOTAL FAT (g)
FLATFISH									
raw	100.00	g	70	12.4	0.0	295.97	159.98	251.98	1.93
	113.40	g	79	14.1	0.0	335.63	181.42	285.74	2.19
	4.00	oz							
cooked, dry	100.00	g	86	15.2	0.0	363.00	197.00	309.00	2.37
heat	85.05	g	73	13.0	0.0	308.73	167.55	262.80	2.02
	3.00	oz							
HALIBUT									
greenland, raw	100.00	g	186	14.4	0.0	79.99	267.97	163.98	13.84
	113.40	g	211	16.3	0.0	90.71	303.88	185.96	15.69
	4.00	oz							
atlantic and	100.00	g	91	18.6	0.0	67.99	434.96	235.98	1.33
pacific, raw	113.40	g	103	21.0	0.0	77.10	493.24	267.60	1.51
	4.00	oz							
greenland, cooked, dry heat	100.00	g	239	18.4	0.0	103.00	344.00	210.00	17.71
	85.05	g	203	15.7	0.0	87.60	292.57	178.60	15.09
	3.00	oz							
atlantic and pacific, cooked, dry heat	100.00	g	111	22.5	0.0	82.00	527.99	287.00	1.61
	85.05	g	94	19.2	0.0	69.74	449.06	244.09	1.37
	3.00	oz							
LOBSTER									
Northern, raw (Langoustine)	100.00	g	77	16.5	0.0	423.00	200.00	161.00	0.75
	113.40	g	87	18.7	0.0	479.68	226.80	182.57	0.85
	4.00	Oz							
Spiny, mixed species, raw	100.00	g	112	20.6	2.4	177.00	180.00	238.00	1.51
	113.40	g	127	23.4	2.8	200.72	104.12	269.89	1.71
	4.00	oz							
Northern, cooked, moist heat (Langoustine)	100.00	g	89	19.0	0.0	485.99	230.00	185.00	0.86
	85.05	g	76	16.2	0.0	413.34	195.61	157.34	0.73
	3.00	oz							
Spiny, mixed species, cooked, moist heat	100.00	g	143	26.4	3.1	227.00	208.00	229.00	1.94
	85.05	g	122	22.5	2.7	193.08	176.90	194.76	1.65
	3.00	oz							

	SERVING QUANTITY	UNIT	CALORIES (kcal)	PROTEIN (g)	TOTAL CARBOHYDRATES (g)	SODIUM (mg)	POTASSIUM (mg)	PHOSPHORUS (mg)	TOTAL FAT (g)
COD									
atlantic, raw	100.00	g	82	17.8	0.0	54.00	412.96	202.98	0.67
	113.40	g	93	20.2	0.0	61.23	468.30	230.18	0.76
	4.00	oz							
atlantic, canned	100.00	g	105	22.8	0.0	218.00	527.99	260.00	0.86
	56.70	g	60	12.9	0.0	123.60	299.37	147.42	0.49
	2.00	oz							
atlantic, cooked, dry heat	100.00	g	105	22.8	0.0	78.00	244.00	138.00	0.86
	85.05	g	89	19.4	0.0	66.34	207.52	117.37	0.73
	3.00	oz							
pacific, raw	100.00	g	69	15.3	0.0	302.97	234.98	280.97	0.41
	113.40	g	78	17.3	0.0	343.57	266.46	318.62	0.46
	4.00	oz							
pacific, cooked, dry heat	100.00	g	85	18.7	0.0	372.00	289.00	345.00	0.50
	85.05	g	72	15.9	0.0	316.38	245.79	293.42	0.43
	3.00	oz							
ANCHOVIES									
Raw	100.00	g	131	20.4	0.0	103.99	382.96	173.98	4.84
	113.40	g	149	23.1	0.0	117.92	434.28	197.30	5.49
	4.00	oz							
canned, in oil, drained	100.00	g	210	28.9	0.0	3,668	544.00	252.00	9.71
	16.00	g	34	4.6	0.0	586.88	87.04	40.32	1.55
	4.00	pcs							
SHRIMP									
mixed species, raw	100.00	g	71	13.6	0.9	566.00	113.00	244.00	1.01
	113.40	g	81	15.4	1.0	641.84	128.14	276.40	1.15
	4.00	oz							
mixed species, breaded, fried	100.00	g	242	21.4	12	343.80	224.87	217.87	12.27
	85.05	g	206	18.2	9.8	292.40	191.25	185.30	10.44
	3.00	oz							
mixed species, cooked, moist heat	100.00	g	119	22.8	1.5	946.99	170.00	306.00	1.70
	85.05	g	101	19.4	1.3	805.41	144.58	260.25	1.45
	3.00	oz							
cracker	100.00	g	426	7.1	59	571.00	193.00	191.00	17.86

CRAB	SERVING QUANTITY	UNIT	CALORIES (kcal)	PROTEIN (g)	TOTAL CARBOHYDRATE (g)	SODIUM (mg)	POTASSIUM (mg)	PHOSPHORUS (mg)	TOTAL FAT (g)
blue, raw	100.0	g	87	18.1	0.0	293.00	329.00	229.00	1.08
	113.4	g	99	20.5	0.5	332.26	373.09	259.69	1.22
	4.00	oz							
blue, canned	100.0	g	83	17.9	0.0	562.99	259.00	234.00	0.74
	56.70	g	47	10.1	0.0	319.22	146.85	132.68	0.42
	2.00	oz							
dungeness, raw	100.0	g	86	17.4	0.7	295.00	354.00	182.00	0.97
	113.4	g	98	19.7	0.8	334.53	401.44	206.39	1.10
	4.00	oz							
dungeness, cooked, moist heat	100.0	g	110	22.3	1.0	378.00	408.00	175.00	1.24
	85.05	g	94	19.0	0.8	321.49	347.00	148.84	1.05
	3.00	oz							
alaska king, raw	100.0	g	84	18.3	0.0	836.00	204.00	219.00	0.60
	113.4	g	95	20.7	0.0	948.02	231.34	248.35	0.68
	4.00	oz							
alaska king, cooked, moist heat	100.0	g	97	19.4	0.0	1,072	262.00	280.00	1.54
	85.05	g	83	16.5	0.0	911.73	222.83	238.14	1.31
	3.00	oz							
imitation, crabmeat (Kani)	100.0	g	95	7.6	15.0	528.99	90.00	282.00	0.46
	85.05	g	81	6.5	12.8	449.91	76.54	239.84	0.39
	3.00	oz							
cakes	100.0	g	266	18.8	8.5	819.00	270.00	378.00	17.25
	60.00	g	160	11.3	5.1	491.00	162.00	226.80	10.35
	1.00	pc							

CATFISH

	SERVING QUANTITY	UNIT	CALORIES	PROTEIN (g)	TOTAL CARBOHYDRATE (g)	SODIUM (mg)	POTASSIUM (mg)	PHOSPHORUS (mg)	TOTAL FAT (g)
channel, wild, raw	100.0	g	95	16.4	0.0	43.00	405.93	208.98	2.82
	113.4	g	108	18.6	0.0	48.76	357.97	236.98	3.20
	4.00	oz							
channel, farmed, raw	100.0	g	119	15.2	0.0	97.94	301.82	203.88	5.94
	85.05	g	101	13.0	0.0	83.30	256.70	173.40	5.05
	3.00	oz							
breaded, fried	100.0	g	229	18.1	8.0	280.00	340.00	216.00	13.33
	85.05	g	195	15.4	6.8	238.14	289.17	183.71	11.34
	3.00	oz							
wild, cooked, dry heat	100.0	g	105	18.5	0.0	50.00	419.00	304.00	2.85
	85.05	g	89	15.7	0.0	42.52	356.36	258.55	2.42
	3.00	oz							
farmed, cooked, dry heat	100.0	g	144	18.4	0.0	119.00	366.00	247.00	7.19
	85.05	g	122	15.7	0.0	101.21	311.28	210.07	6.12
	3.00	oz							

CRAYFISH/ CRAWFISH	SERVING QUANTITY	UNIT	CALORIES (kcal)	PROTEIN (g)	TOTAL CARBOHYDRATES (g)	SODIUM (mg)	POTASSIUM (mg)	PHOSPHORUS (mg)	TOTAL FAT (g)
Mixed species, farmed, raw	100.00	g	72	14.9	0.0	62.00	261.00	218.00	0.97
	113.40 4.00	g oz	82	16.8	0.0	70.31	295.97	247.21	1.10
Mixed species, wild, raw	100.00	g	77	16.0	0.0	58.00	302.00	256.00	0.95
	113.40 4.00	g oz	87	18.1	0.0	65.77	342.47	290.30	1.08
Mixed species, farmed, cooked, moist heat	100.00	g	87	17.5	0.0	97.00	238.00	241.00	0.22
	85.05 3.00	g oz	74	14.9	0.0	82.50	202.42	204.97	0.18
mixed species, wild, cooked, moist heat	100.00	g	82	16.8	0.0	94.00	296.00	270.00	1.20
	85.05 3.00	g oz	70	14.3	0.0	79.95	251.75	229.63	1.02
SQUID (CALAMARI)									
mixed species, fried	100.00	g	175	17.9	7.8	306.0	279.00	251.00	7.48
	85.05 3.00	g oz	149	15.3	6.6	260.3	237.29	213.47	6.36
mixed species, raw boneless	100.00	g	92	15.6	3.1	44.00	246.00	221.00	1.38
	113.40 4.00	g oz	104	17.7	3.5	49.90	278.96	250.61	1.56

	SERVING QUANTITY	UNIT	CALORIES (kcal)	PROTEIN (g)	TOTAL CARBOHYDRATE (g)	SODIUM (mg)	POTASSIUM (mg)	PHOSPHORUS (mg)	TOTAL FAT (g)
CLAMS									
mixed species, raw	100	g	86	14.7	3.6	601.00	46.00	198.00	0.96
	85.05	g	73	12.5	3.0	511.15	39.12	168.40	0.82
	3.00	oz							
mixed species, breaded, fried	100.00	g	202	14.2	10.3	364.00	326.00	188.00	11.15
	85.05	g	172	12.1	8.8	309.58	277.26	159.89	9.48
	3.00	oz							
mixed species, canned, with liquid	100.00	g	2	0.4	0.1	215.00	149.00	114.00	0.02
	28.35	g	1	0.1	0.0	60.95	42.24	32.32	0.01
	1.00	oz							
mixed species, canned, drained	100.00	g	142	24.3	5.9	112.00	627.99	326.99	1.59
	56.70	g	81	13.8	3.4	63.50	356.07	185.41	0.90
	2.00	oz							
OYSTERS									
ostrich, raw	100.00	g	125	21.6	0.0	83.00	297.00	204.00	3.67
	85.05	g	106	18.3	0.0	70.59	252.60	173.50	3.12
	3.00	oz							
ostrich, cooked	100.00	g	159	28.8	0.0	81.00	409.00	281.00	3.97
	85.05	g	135	24.5	0.0	68.89	347.85	238.99	3.38
	3.00	oz							
pacific, raw	100.00	g	81	9.5	5.0	106.00	168.00	162.00	2.30
	113.40	g	92	10.7	5.6	120.20	190.51	183.71	2.61
	4.00	oz							
pacific, cooked, moist heat	100.00	g	163	18.9	9.9	212.00	302.00	243.00	4.60
	85.05	g	139	16.1	8.4	180.30	256.85	206.67	3.91
	3.00	oz							
eastern, canned	100.00	g	68	7.1	3.9	112.00	229.00	139.00	2.47
	56.70	g	39	4.0	2.2	63.50	129.84	78.81	1.40
	2.00	oz							
eastern, farmed, raw	100.00	g	59	5.2	5.5	178.00	124.00	93.00	1.55
	85.05	g	50	4.4	4.7	151.39	105.46	79.10	1.32
	3.00	oz							
eastern, wild, raw	100.00	g	51	5.7	2.7	85.00	156.00	97.00	1.71
	113.40	g	58	6.5	3.1	96.39	176.90	110.00	1.94
	4.00	oz							
eastern, wild, breaded, fried	100.00	g	199	8.8	11.6	417.00	244.00	159.00	12.58
	85.05	g	169	7.5	9.9	354.65	207.52	135.23	10.70
	3.00	oz							
battered, breaded, fried, fast food	100.00	g	265	9.0	28.7	486.99	131.00	141.00	12.90
	85.05	g	225	7.7	24.4	414.19	111.41	119.92	10.97
	3.00	oz							

	SERVING QUANTITY	UNIT	CALORIES (kcal)	PROTEIN (g)	TOTAL CARBOHYDRATE (g)	SODIUM (mg)	POTASSIUM (mg)	PHOSPHORUS (mg)
SCALLOPS								
Mixed species, raw	100.00	g	69	12.1	3.2	392.00	205.00	12.80
	113.40 4.00	g oz	78	13.7	3.6	444.53	232.47	14.52
Bay and Sea, steamed	100.00	g	111	20.5	5.4	667.00	314.00	426.00
	85.05 3.00	g oz	94	17.5	4.6	567.28	267.06	362.31
mixed species, breaded and fried	100.00	g	216	18.1	10.1	464.00	333.00	236.00
	46.50 3.00	g pcs	100	8.4	4.7	215.76	15.85	109.74
breaded, fried, fast food	100.00	g	268	10.9	26.7	637.99	204.00	203.00
	85.05 3.00	g oz	228	9.3	22.7	542.61	173.50	172.65
HERRING								
Pacific, raw	100.00	g	195	16.4	0.0	73.99	422.96	227.98
	113.40 4.00	g oz	221	18.6	0.0	83.91	479.64	258.53
Atlantic, raw	100.00	g	158	18.0	0.0	89.99	326.97	235.98
	113.40 4.00	g oz	179	20.4	0.0	102.05	370.78	267.60
Pacific, cooked, dry heat	100.00	g	250	21.0	0.0	95.00	541.99	292.00
	85.05 3.00	g oz	213	17.9	0.0	80.80	460.97	248.34
Atlantic, cooked, dry heat	100.00	g	203	23.0	0.0	115.00	419.00	303.00
	85.05 3.00	g oz	173	19.6	0.0	97.81	356.36	257.70
Roe or eggs, Pacific (Alaska Native)	100.00	g	74	9.6	4.5	61.00	na	na
	85.05 3.00	g oz	63	8.2	3.8	51.88	na	na

C. Milk and Cheeses

(Dairy and Non-Dairy)

Hey there!

Do you need to print out this Food List?

You can download a printable version of this chart by scanning the QR code below or copying the link on your computer browser.

https://go.renaltracker.com/printfoodlist

MILK	SERVING QUANTITY	SERVING UNIT	CALORIES (kcal)	PROTEIN (g)	TOTAL CARBOHYDRATES (g)	SODIUM (mg)	POTASSIUM (mg)	PHOSPHORUS (mg)	TOTAL FAT (g)
(cow) whole	100	g	60	3.3	4.7	38.0	150.0	101.0	3.20
	244	g	146	8.0	11.4	92.7	366.0	246.0	7.81
	1	c							
2% reduced fat	100	g	50	3.4	4.9	39.0	159.0	103.0	1.90
	244	g	122	8.2	12.0	95.2	388.0	251.0	4.64
	1	c							
low fat (1%)	100	g	43	3.4	5.2	39.0	159.0	103.0	0.95
	244	g	105	8.3	12.7	95.2	388.0	251.0	2.32
	1	c							
skim, fat free	100	g	34	3.4	4.9	41.0	167.0	107.0	0.08
	244	g	83	8.4	11.9	100.0	407.0	261.0	0.20
	1	c							
lactose free, from whole milk	100	g	60	3.3	4.7	38.0	150.0	101.0	3.20
	244	g	146	8.0	11.4	92.7	366.0	246.0	7.81
	1	c							
Buttermilk, dried	100	g	387	34.3	49.0	517.0	1592	933	5.78
	6.5	g	25	2.2	3.2	33.6	103.0	60.60	0.38
	1	tbsp							
buttermilk, fluid, whole	100	g	62	3.2	4.9	105.0	135.0	85.00	3.31
	245	g	152	7.9	12.0	257.0	331.0	208.0	8.11
	1	c							
condensed, sweetened	100	g	321	7.9	54.4	127.0	371.0	253.0	8.70
	38	g	122	3.0	20.7	48.3	141.0	96.10	3.31
	1	fl oz							
evaporated, whole	100	g	134	6.8	10.0	106.0	303.0	203.0	7.56
	31.5	g	42	2.1	3.2	33.4	95.40	63.90	2.38
	1	fl oz							
malted	100	g	64	3.2	8.7	60.0	150.0	98.00	1.91
	256	g	164	8.2	22.2	154.0	384.0	251.0	4.89
	1	c							
chocolate	100	g	67	3.4	13.5	79.0	182.0	101.0	0.00
	248	g	166	8.4	33.4	196.0	451.0	250.0	0.00
	1	c							
strawberry (whole milk)	100	g	85	3.0	11.8	38.0	139.0	94.00	2.97
	248	g	211	7.5	29.3	94.2	345.0	233.0	7.37
	1	c							

MILK

	SERVING QUANTITY	SERVING UNIT	CALORIES (kcal)	PROTEIN (g)	TOTAL CARBOHYDRATE (g)	SODIUM (mg)	POTASSIUM (mg)	PHOSPHORUS (mg)	TOTAL FAT
SOY	100	g	43	2.6	4.9	47.0	122.0	43.00	1.4
	244	g	105	6.3	12.0	115.0	298.0	105.0	3.5
	1	c							
soy, light	100	g	30	2.4	3.5	48.0	117.0	87.00	0.7
	244	g	73	5.8	8.6	117.0	285.0	212.0	1.8
	1	c							
soy, chocolate	100	g	63	2.3	10.0	53.0	143.0	51.00	1.5
	244	g	154	5.5	24.3	129.0	349.0	124.0	3.7
	1	c							
soy, non-fat	100	g	28	2.5	4.1	57.0	105.0	87.00	0.0
	244	g	68	6.0	10.1	139.0	256.0	212.0	0.1
	1	c							
RICE	100	g	47	0.3	9.2	39.0	27.00	56.00	0.9
	244	g	115	0.7	22.4	95.2	65.90	137.0	2.3
	1	c							
rice milk, unsweetened	100	g	47	0.3	9.2	39.0	27.00	56.00	0.9
	240	g	113	0.7	22.0	93.6	64.80	134.0	2.3
	8	fl oz							
ALMOND, unsweetened	100	g	15	0.4	1.3	72.0	67.00	9.00	0.9
	244	g	37	1.0	3.2	176.0	163.0	22.00	2.3
	1	c							
almond, unsweetened, chocolate	100	g	16	0.5	1.5	72.0	71.00	11.00	1.0
	244	g	39	1.1	3.6	176.0	173.0	26.80	2.4
	1	c							
almond milk, sweetened	100	g	30	0.4	5.2	69.0	64.00	9.00	0.9
	244	g	73	0.9	12.8	168.0	156.0	22.00	2.2
	1	c							
almond, sweetened, chocolate	100	g	41	0.4	8.3	67.0	67.00	11.00	0.9
	244	g	100	1.1	20.4	163.0	163.0	26.80	2.3
	1	c							
COCONUT	100	g	31	0.2	2.9	19.0	19.00	0.00	2.0
	244	g	76	0.5	7.1	46.4	46.40	0.00	5.0
	1	c							
GOAT, whole	100	g	69	3.6	4.5	50.0	204.0	111.0	4.1
	244	g	168	8.7	10.9	122.0	498.0	271.0	10.
	1	c							

MILK SUBSTITUTE

	SERVING QUANTITY	SERVING UNIT	CALORIES (kcal)	PROTEIN (g)	TOTAL CARBOHYDRATES (g)	SODIUM (mg)	POTASSIUM (mg)	PHOSPHORUS (mg)	TOTAL FAT (g)
Non-dairy milk/creamer	100	g	29	1.0	3.8	60.0	80.00	19.00	1.17
	30.5	g	9	0.3	1.1	18.3	24.40	5.80	0.36
	1	fl oz							
imitation, non-soy	100	g	46	1.6	5.3	55.0	150.0	100.0	2.00
	244	g	112	3.9	12.9	134.0	366.0	244.0	4.88
	1	cup							
Kefir	100	g	52	3.6	7.5	38.0	159.0	100.0	0.96
	244	g	127	8.8	18.3	92.7	388.0	244	2.34
	1	c							
Sorbet	100	g	110	0.8	27.1	13.0	28.00	3.00	0.05
	80	g	88	0.6	21.7	10.4	22.40	2.40	0.04
	1	bar							

YOGURT

	SERVING QUANTITY	SERVING UNIT	CALORIES (kcal)	PROTEIN (g)	TOTAL CARBOHYDRATES (g)	SODIUM (mg)	POTASSIUM (mg)	PHOSPHORUS (mg)	TOTAL FAT (g)
coconut milk, yogurt	100	g	64	0.3	8.0	21.0	27.00	2.00	3.50
	170	g	109	0.5	13.5	35.7	45.90	3.40	5.95
	6	oz							
dressing	100	g	220	3.5	11.8	43.0	146.0	85.00	18.27
	15.4	g	34	0.5	1.8	6.6	22.50	13.10	2.81
	1	tbsp							
liquid	100	g	72	3.7	11.8	53.0	171.0	103.0	1.09
	245	g	176	9.1	28.9	130.0	419.0	252.0	2.67
	1	c							
plain, whole milk	100	g	61	3.5	4.7	46.0	155.0	95.00	3.25
	227	g	138	7.9	10.6	104.0	352.0	216.0	7.38
	8	oz							
Whole milk with fruit	100	g	87	3.1	12.4	44.0	146.0	86.00	2.87
	170	g	14 8	5.3	21.0	74.8	248.0	146.0	4.88
	6	oz							

YOGURT	SERVING QUANTITY	SERVING UNIT	CALORIES (kcal)	PROTEIN (g)	TOTAL CARBOHYDRATES (g)	SODIUM (mg)	POTASSIUM (mg)	PHOSPHORUS (mg)	TOTAL FAT (g)
whole milk, flavored (non-fruit)	100	g	77	3.3	9.4	44.0	147.0	90.00	3.10
	170	g	131	5.6	16.0	74.8	250.0	153.0	5.27
	6	oz							
non-fat milk, plain, vanilla	100	g	78	2.9	17.0	47.0	141.0	88.00	0.00
	227	g	177	6.7	38.7	107.0	320.0	200.0	0.00
	8	oz							
non-fat milk, fruit	100	g	83	5.1	15.0	72.0	234.0	140.0	0.17
	170	g	141	8.7	25.5	122.0	398.0	238.0	0.29
	6	oz							
Soy, yogurt, plain	100	g	94	3.5	16.0	35.0	47.00	38.00	1.80
	170	g	160	6.0	27.1	59.5	79.90	64.60	3.06
	6	oz							
Greek, plain, whole milk	100	g	97	9.0	4.0	35.0	141.0	135.0	5.00
	170	g	165	15.3	6.8	59.5	240.0	230.0	8.50
	6	oz							
Greek, fruit, whole milk	100	g	106	7.3	12.3	37.0	113.0	109.0	3.00
	170	g	180	12.5	20.9	62.9	192.0	185.0	5.10
	6	oz							
Greek, flavored, other than fruit	100	g	111	8.5	9.4	39.0	121.0	117.0	4.44
	170	g	189	14.4	15.9	66.3	206.0	199.0	7.55
	6	oz							
Greek, plain, low fat	100	g	73	10.0	3.9	34.0	141.0	137.0	1.92
	170	g	124	16.9	6.7	57.8	240.0	233.0	3.26
	6	oz							
Greek, LF, flavors other than fruit	100	g	95	8.6	9.5	40.0	123.0	119.0	2.50
	170	g	162	14.7	16.2	68.0	209.0	202.0	4.25
	6	oz							
Greek, non-fat (NF), plain	100	g	59	10.2	3.6	36.0	141.0	135.0	0.39
	170	g	100	17.3	6.1	61.2	240.0	230.0	0.66
	6	oz							
Greek, NF, flavors other than fruit	100	g	78	8.6	10.4	34.0	123.0	119.0	0.18
	170	g	133	14.7	17.6	57.8	209.0	202.0	0.31
	6	oz							
Frozen yogurt, chocolate 1 scoop small cup	100	g	131	3.0	21.6	63.0	234.0	89.00	3.60
	160	g	210	4.8	34.6	101.0	374.0	142.0	5.76
	1	scoop							

YOGURT	SERVING QUANTITY	SERVING UNIT	CALORIES (kcal)	PROTEIN (g)	TOTAL CARBOHYDRATES (g)	SODIUM (mg)	POTASSIUM (mg)	PHOSPHORUS (mg)	TOTAL FAT (g)
Frozen yogurt, vanilla	100	g	127	3.0	21.6	63.0	156.0	89.00	3.60
	160	g	203	4.8	34.6	101.0	250.0	142.0	5.76
1 scoop= small cup	1	scoop							
Frozen yogurt, soft serve, chocolate	100	g	160	4.3	24.9	86.0	237.0	141.0	5.76
	175	g	280	7.5	43.5	150.0	415.0	247.0	10.10
	1	c							
Frozn yogurt, soft serve, vanilla	100	g	159	4.0	24.2	87.0	211.0	129.0	5.60
	175	g	278	7.0	42.4	152.0	369.0	226.0	9.80
	1	c							
Frozn yogurt bar, vanilla	100	g	127	3.0	21.6	63.0	156.0	89.00	3.60
	65	g	83	2.0	14.0	41.0	101.0	57.80	2.34
	1	bar							
Frozn yogurt bar, chocolate	100	g	131	3.0	21.6	63.0	234.0	89.00	3.60
	65	g	85	2.0	14.0	41.0	152.0	57.80	2.34
	1	bar							
Frozn yogurt cone, vanilla	100	g	139	3.2	23.9	71.0	154.0	89.00	3.73
	125	g	174	4.0	29.9	88.8	192.0	111.0	4.66
	1	cone							
Frozn yogurt cone, chocolate	100	g	142	3.2	23.9	71.0	229.0	89.00	3.73
	125	g	178	4.0	29.9	88.8	286.0	111.0	4.66
	1	cone							
Frozn yogurt, waffle cone, vanilla	100	g	143	3.3	25.3	77.0	155.0	90.00	3.61
	255	g	365	8.4	64.5	196.0	395.0	230.0	9.20
	1	cone							
Frozn yogurt, waffle cone, choco	100	g	147	3.3	25.3	77.0	229.0	90.00	3.61
	255	g	375	8.4	64.5	196.0	584.0	230.0	9.20
	1	cone							

CHEESE

	SERVING QUANTITY	SERVING UNIT	CALORIES (kcal)	PROTEIN (g)	TOTAL CARBOHYDRATES (g)	SODIUM (mg)	POTASSIUM (mg)	PHOSPHORUS (mg)	TOTAL FAT (g)
mozzarella, from whole milk shredded	100	g	299	22.2	2.4	486.0	76.00	354.0	22.14
	112	g	335	24.8	2.7	544.0	85.10	396.0	24.80
	1	c							
mozzarella, part skim milk	100	g	254	24.3	2.8	619.0	84.00	463.0	15.92
	28.35	g	72	6.9	0.8	175.0	23.80	131.0	4.51
	1	oz							
Mozzarella, reduced sodium (shredded)	100	g	280	27.5	3.1	16.0	95.00	524.0	17.10
	113	g	316	31.1	3.5	18.1	107.0	592.0	19.30
	1	cup							
ricotta, from whole milk	100	g	158	7.8	6.9	105.0	230.0	162.0	11.00
	129	g	204	10.1	8.9	135.0	297.0	209.0	14.20
	0.5	c							
riccota, part skim milk	100	g	138	11.4	5.1	99.0	125.0	183.0	7.91
	124	g	171	14.1	6.4	123.0	155.0	227.0	9.81
	0.5	c							
cream cheese, regular	100	g	295	7.1	3.5	436.0	112.0	91.00	28.60
	28.35	g	84	2.0	1.0	124.0	31.80	25.80	8.11
	1	oz							
cream cheese, light	100	g	201	7.9	8.1	359.0	247.0	152.0	15.28
	28.35	g	57	2.2	2.3	102.0	70.00	43.10	4.33
	1	oz							
processed cheese food	100	g	307	16.1	8.9	1279.0	295.0	768.0	23.06
	21	g	65	3.4	1.9	269.0	62.00	161.0	4.84
	1	slice							
Cottage cheese	100	g	84	11.0	4.3	321.0	120.0	148.0	2.30
	210	g	176	23.1	9.1	674.0	252.0	311.0	4.83
	1	cup							
cottage cheese, low fat	100	g	84	11.0	4.3	321.0	120.0	148.0	2.30
	226	g	190	24.9	9.7	725.0	271.0	334.0	5.20
	1	cup							
Monterey shredded	100	g	373	24.5	0.7	600.0	81.00	444.0	30.28
	113	g	421	27.7	0.8	678.0	91.50	502.0	34.20
	1	cup							
Cheddar	100	g	408	23.3	2.4	654.0	77.00	458.0	34.00
	21	g	86	4.9	0.5	137.0	16.20	96.20	7.14
	1	slice							

CHEESE	SERVING QUANTITY	SERVING UNIT	CALORIES (kcal)	PROTEIN (g)	TOTAL CARBOHYDRATES (g)	SODIUM (mg)	POTASSIUM (mg)	PHOSPHORUS (mg)	TOTAL FAT (g)
Cheddar, reduced sodium	100	g	398	24.4	1.9	21.0	112.00	484.0	32.62
	21	g	84	5.1	0.4	4.4	23.50	102.0	6.85
	1	slice							
Cheddar, sharp sliced	100	g	410	24.3	2.1	644.0	76.00	460.0	33.82
	28	g	115	6.8	0.6	180.0	21.30	129.0	9.47
	1	oz							
Cheddar/ American cheese spread	100	g	290	16.4	8.7	1625	242.00	875.0	21.23
	21	g	61	3.5	1.8	341.0	50.80	184.0	4.46
	1	wedge							
American	100	g	307	16.1	8.9	1279.	295.00	768.0	23.06
	21	g	65	3.4	1.9	269.0	62.00	161.0	4.84
	1	slice							
Brick	100	g	371	23.2	2.8	560.0	136.00	451.0	29.68
	17.2	g	64	4.0	0.5	96.3	23.40	77.60	5.10
	1	cubic inch							
Brie	100	g	334	20.8	0.5	629.0	152.00	188.0	27.68
	17	g	57	3.5	0.1	107.0	25.80	32.00	4.71
	1	cubic inch							
blue	100	g	353	21.4	2.3	1146	256.00	387.0	28.74
	28.35	g	100	6.1	0.7	325.0	72.60	110.0	8.15
	1	oz							
Camembert	100	g	300	19.8	0.5	842.0	187.00	347.0	24.26
	38	g	114	7.5	0.2	320.0	71.10	132.0	9.22
1 wedge = 1.33 oz	1	wedge							
Colby	100	g	394	23.8	2.6	604.0	127.00	457.0	32.11
	21	g	83	5.0	0.5	127.0	26.70	96.00	6.74
	1	slice							
Caraway	100	g	376	25.2	1.1	690.0	93.00	490.0	29.20
	28.35	g	107	7.1	0.9	196.0	26.40	139.0	8.28
	1	oz							
Edam	100	g	356	24.9	2.2	819.0	121.00	546.0	27.44
	21	g	75	5.2	0.5	172.0	25.40	115.0	5.76
	1	slice							
Feta	100	g	265	14.2	3.9	1139.	62.00	337.0	21.49
	17	g	45	2.4	0.7	194.0	10.50	57.30	3.62
	1	cubic inch							
Fontina	100	g	389	25.6	1.6	800.0	64.00	346.0	31.14
	21	g	82	5.4	0.3	168.0	13.40	72.70	6.54
	1	slice							
goat	100	g	364	21.6	0.1	415.0	158.00	375.0	29.84
	25	g	91	5.4	0.0	104.0	39.50	93.80	7.46
	1	cubic inch							

CHEESE

	SERVING QUANTITY	SERVING UNIT	CALORIES (kcal)	PROTEIN (g)	TOTAL CARBOHYDRATES (g)	SODIUM (mg)	POTASSIUM (mg)	PHOSPHORUS (mg)	TOTAL FAT (g)
Gouda	100	g	356	24.9	2.2	819.0	121.0	546.0	27.44
	28.35	g	101	7.0	0.6	232.0	34.30	155.0	7.78
	1	oz							
Gruyere	100	g	413	29.8	0.4	714.0	81.00	605.0	32.34
	21	g	87	6.3	0.1	150.0	17.00	127.0	6.70
	1	slice							
Blue or Roquefort	100	g	353	21.4	2.3	1146.0	256.0	387.0	28.74
	17.3	g	61	3.7	0.4	198.0	44.30	67.00	4.97
	1	cubic inch							
Colby Jack	100	g	384	24.1	1.6	602.0	104.0	450.0	31.20
	21	g	81	5.1	0.3	126.0	21.80	94.50	6.55
	1	slice							
Parmesan, grated	100	g	420	29.6	12.4	1750.0	184.0	634.0	28.00
	7.6	g	32	2.3	0.9	133.0	14.00	48.20	1.82
	1	tbsp							
Parmesan, hard	100	g	421	29.6	12.4	1750.0	184.0	634.0	28.00
	10.3	g	43	3.1	1.3	180.0	19.00	65.30	2.88
	1	cubic inch							
Mexican blend shredded	100	g	358	23.5	1.8	607.0	85.00	438.0	28.51
	113	g	405	26.6	2.0	686.0	96.00	495.0	32.20
	1	cup							
Mexican blend, reduced fat shredded	100	g	282	24.7	3.4	776.0	93.00	583.0	19.40
	113	g	319	27.9	3.9	877.0	105.0	659.0	21.90
	1	cup							
Muenster	100	g	368	23.4	1.1	628.0	134.0	468.0	30.04
	21	g	77	5.0	0.2	132.0	28.10	98.30	6.31
	1	slice							
Neufchatel	100	g	253	9.2	3.6	334.0	152.0	138.0	22.78
	28.35	g	72	2.6	1.0	94.7	43.10	39.10	6.46
	1	oz							
Provolone	100	g	351	25.6	2.1	727.0	138.0	496.0	26.62
	21	g	74	5.4	0.4	153.0	29.00	104.0	5.59
	1	slice							
Romano	100	g	387	31.8	3.6	1433.0	86.00	760.0	26.94
	28.35	g	110	9.0	1.0	406.0	24.40	215.0	7.64
	1	oz							
Swiss	100	g	393	27.0	1.4	185.0	71.00	574.0	31.00
	21	g	83	5.7	0.3	38.8	14.90	121.0	6.51
	1	slice							
Tilsiter/Tilsit	100	g	340	24.4	1.9	753.0	65.00	500.0	25.98
	28.35	g	96	6.9	0.5	213.0	18.40	142.0	7.36
	1	oz							

CREAM

	SERVING QUANTITY	SERVING UNIT	CALORIES (kcal)	PROTEIN (g)	TOTAL CARBOHYDRATES (g)	SODIUM (mg)	POTASSIUM (mg)	PHOSPHORUS (mg)	TOTAL FAT (g)
sour cream, regular	100	g	198	2.4	4.6	31.0	125.00	76.00	19.35
	30	g	59	0.7	1.4	9.3	37.50	22.80	5.80
	1	container							
sour cream, light	100	g	136	3.5	7.1	83.0	212.00	71.00	10.60
	240	g	326	8.4	17.0	199.0	509.00	170.0	25.40
	1	cup							
sour cream, imitation	100	g	208	2.4	6.6	102.0	161.00	45.00	19.52
	240	g	499	5.8	15.9	245.0	386.00	108.0	46.80
	1	cup							
sour cream, fat free	100	g	74	3.1	15.6	141.0	129.00	95.00	0.00
	240	g	178	7.4	37.4	338.0	310.00	228.0	0.00
	1	cup							
heavy full cream	100	g	340	2.8	2.8	27.0	95.00	58.00	36.08
	30	g	102	0.9	1.0	8.1	28.50	17.40	10.80
	1	fl oz							
whipped	100	g	343	2.7	8.6	26.0	89.00	55.00	33.94
	40	g	137	1.1	3.4	10.4	35.60	22.00	13.60
	1	cup							
half and half	100	g	131	3.1	4.3	61.0	132.00	95.00	11.50
	30	g	39	0.9	1.3	18.3	39.60	28.50	3.45
	1	fl oz							
coffee, light cream	100	g	195	3.0	3.7	72.0	136.00	92.00	19.10
	11	g	21	0.3	0.4	7.9	15.00	10.10	2.10
	1	ind. container							

D. Fats

(Oils, Nuts, & Seeds)

Hey there!

Do you need to print out this Food List?

You can download a printable version of this chart by scanning the QR code below or copying the link on your computer browser.

https://go.renaltracker.com/printfoodlist

ALMOND	SERVING QUANTITY	UNIT	CALORIES (kcal)	PROTEIN (g)	TOTAL CARBOHYDRATE (g)	SODIUM (mg)	POTASSIUM (mg)	PHOSPHORUS (mg)	TOTAL FAT (g)
whole	100	g	579	21.2	21.6	1.00	733.00	481.00	49.9
	35.75	g	207	7.6	7.7	0.36	262.05	171.96	17.9
	0.25	c							
slivered	100	g	579	21.2	21.6	1.00	733.00	481.00	49.9
	27	g	156	5.7	5.8	0.27	197.91	129.87	13.5
	0.25	c							
ground	100	g	579	21.2	21.6	1.00	733.00	481.00	49.9
	23.75	g	138	5.0	5.1	0.24	174.09	114.42	11.9
	0.25	c							
paste (marzipan)	100	g	458	9.0	47.8	9.00	314.00	258.00	27.7
	28.38	g	130	2.6	13.6	2.55	89.10	73.21	7.9
	2	tbsp							
oil	100	g	884	0.0	0.0	0.00	0.00	0.00	100
	13.6	g	120	0.0	0.0	0.00	0.00	0.00	13.6
	1	tbsp							
butter, without salt added	100	g	614	21.0	18.8	227.0	748.00	508.00	55.5
	16	g	98	3.4	3.0	1.12	119.68	81.28	8.9
	1	tbsp							
dry roasted, without salt added	100	g	598	3.0	21.0	3.00	713.00	471.00	52.5
	34.5	g	206	7.2	7.3	1.04	245.99	162.50	18.1
	0.25	c							
oil roasted, without salt	100	g	607	21.2	17.7	1.00	699.00	466.00	55.2
	39.25	g	238	8.3	6.9	0.39	274.36	182.91	21.7
	0.25	c							
milk, unsweetened, shelf stable	100	g	15	0.4	1.3	72.00	67.00	9.00	1.0
	262	g	39	1.1	3.4	188.6	175.54	23.58	2.5
	1	c							
milk, sweetened, vanilla flavor ready-to-drink	100	g	38	0.4	6.6	63.00	50.00	8.00	1.0
	240	g	91	1.0	15.8	151.2	120.00	19.20	2.5
	1	c							
milk, chocolate flavor, unsweetened fortified Vit. D2 and E	100	g	21	0.8	1.3	75.00	96.00	17.00	1.5
	240	g	50	2.0	3.0	180.0	130.40	40.80	3.5
	1	c							

WALNUT	SERVING QUANTITY	SERVING UNIT	CALORIES (kcal)	PROTEIN (g)	TOTAL CARBOHYDRATES (g)	SODIUM (mg)	POTASSIUM (mg)	PHOSPHORUS (mg)	TOT...
english, halves	100	g	654	15.2	13.7	2.00	441.00	346.0	6...
	25	g	164	3.8	3.4	0.50	110.25	86.50	1...
	0.25	c							
english, ground	100	g	654	15.2	13.7	2.00	441.00	346.0	6...
	20	g	131	3.1	2.7	0.40	88.20	69.20	1...
	0.25	c							
english, chopped	100	g	654	15.2	13.7	2.00	441.00	346.0	6...
	29.25	g	191	4.5	4.0	0.59	128.99	101.2	1...
	0.25	c							
butternut or white walnut, dried	100	g	612	24.9	12.1	1.00	421.00	446.0	5...
	120	g	734	29.9	14.5	1.20	505.20	535.2	6...
	1	c							
black or american, dried, chopped	100	g	619	24.1	9.6	2.00	523.00	513.0	5...
	31.25	g	193	7.5	3.0	0.63	163.44	160.3	1...
	0.25	c							
black or american, dried, ground	100	g	604	23.5	9.3	1.95	509.92	500.2	5...
	26.67	g	161	6.3	2.5	0.52	135.98	133.4	1...
	0.33	c							
glazed	100	g	500	8.3	47.6	446.0	232.00	na	3...
	28.35	g	142	2.4	13.5	126.5	65.77	na	1...
	1	oz							
oil	100	g	884	0.0	0.0	0.0	0.00	0.00	1...
	13.6	g	120	0.0	0.0	0.0	0.00	0.00	1...
	1	tbsp							

	SERVING QUANTITY	SERVING UNIT	CALORIES	PROTEIN (g)	TOTAL CARBOHYDRATES (g)	SODIUM (mg)	POTASSIUM (mg)	PHOSPHORUS (mg)	TOTAL FAT (g)
PINE									
(Pinyon), dried	100	g	629	11.6	19.3	72.00	628.00	35.00	61.0
	28.35	g	178	3.3	5.5	20.41	178.04	9.92	17.3
	1	oz							
(Pignolia), dried	100	g	673	13.7	13.1	2.00	597.00	575.0	68.4
	8.6	g	58	1.2	1.1	0.17	51.34	49.45	5.9
	1	tbsp							
CHESTNUT									
Japanese	100	g	154	2.3	34.9	14.00	329.00	72.00	0.5
	28.35	g	44	0.6	9.9	3.97	93.27	20.41	0.2
	1	oz							
Chinese	100	g	224	4.2	49.1	3.00	447.00	96.00	1.1
	28.35	g	64	1.2	13.9	0.85	126.72	27.22	0.3
	1	oz							
European, unpeeled	100	g	213	2.4	45.5	3.00	518.00	93.00	2.3
	36.25	g	77	0.9	16.5	1.09	187.78	33.71	0.8
	0.25	c							
European, peeled	100	g	196	1.6	44.2	2.00	484.00	38.00	1.3
	28.35	g	56	0.5	12.5	0.57	137.21	10.77	0.4
	1	oz							
European, roasted	100	g	245	3.2	53.0	2.00	592.00	107.0	2.2
	28.35	g	69	0.9	15.0	0.57	167.83	30.33	0.6
	1	oz							
Japanese, roasted	100	g	201	3.0	45.1	19.00	427.00	93.00	0.8
	28.35	g	57	0.8	12.8	5.39	121.05	26.37	0.2
	1	oz							
Chinese, roasted	100	g	239	4.5	52.4	4.00	477.00	102.0	1.2
	28.35	g	68	1.3	14.8	1.13	135.23	28.92	0.3
	1	oz							
Chinese, boiled and steamed	100	g	153	2.9	33.6	2.00	306.00	66.00	0.8
	28.35	g	43	0.8	9.5	0.57	86.75	18.71	0.2
	1	oz							
European, boiled and steamed	100	g	131	2.0	27.8	27.00	715.00	99.00	1.4
	28.35	g	37	0.6	7.9	7.65	202.70	15.31	0.4
	1	oz							
Japanese, boiled and steamed	100	g	56	0.8	12.6	5.00	119.00	26.00	0.2
	28.35	g	16	0.2	3.6	1.42	33.74	7.37	0.1
	1	oz							

PEANUT	SERVING QUANTITY	SERVING UNIT	CALORIES (kcal)	PROTEIN (g)	TOTAL CARBOHYDRATES (g)	SODIUM (mg)	POTASSIUM (mg)	PHOSPHORUS (mg)	TOTAL FAT
oil	100	g	884	0.0	0.0	0.00	0.00	0.00	1
	13.5	g	119	0.0	0.0	0.00	0.00	0.00	1
	1	tbsp							
all types	100	g	567	25.8	16.1	18.00	705.00	376.00	4
	36.5	g	207	9.4	5.9	6.57	257.33	137.24	1
	0.25	c							
all types, dry roasted, no salt added (1 oz = 28.35g)	100	g	587	24.4	21.4	6.00	634.00	363.00	4
	36.5	g	214	8.9	7.8	2.19	231.41	132.50	1
	0.25	c							
all types, oil roasted, no salt	100	g	599	28.0	15.3	6.00	726.00	397.00	5
	133	g	797	37.3	20.3	7.98	965.58	528.01	6
	1	c							
butter, smooth, reduced fat	100	g	520	25.9	36.7	540.0	669.00	369.00	3
	36	g	187	9.3	12.8	194.4	240.84	132.84	1
	2	tbsp							
butter, smooth, no salt added	100	g	598	22.2	22.3	17.00	558.00	335.00	5
	32	g	191	7.1	7.1	5.44	178.56	107.20	1
	2	tbsp							
butter, chunky, no salt added	100	g	589	24.1	21.6	17.00	745.00	319.00	4
	32	g	188	7.7	6.9	5.44	238.40	102.08	1
	2	tbsp							
butter, reduced sodium	100	g	590	24.0	21.8	203.0	747.00	317.00	4
	16	g	94	3.8	3.5	32.48	119.52	50.72	8
	1	tbsp							
sauce, made with PB, water & soy sauce	100	g	257	6.3	22.0	1338	235.00	107.00	1
	18	g	46	1.1	4.0	240.8	42.30	19.26	2
	1	tbsp							
brittle	100	g	486	7.6	71.2	445.0	168.00	106.00	1
	42.5	g	207	3.2	30.3	189.2	71.44	45.08	8
	1.5	oz							
flour, defatted	100	g	327	52.2	34.7	180.0	1,290	760.00	0
	30	g	98	15.7	10.4	54.00	387.00	228.00	0
	0.5	c							

	SERVING QUANTITY	SERVING UNIT	CALORIES (kcal)	PROTEIN (g)	TOTAL CARBOHYDRATES (g)	SODIUM (mg)	POTASSIUM (mg)	PHOSPHORUS (mg)	TOTAL FAT (g)
CASHEW									
raw	100	g	553	18.2	30.2	12.00	660.00	593.0	43.9
	28.35	g	157	5.2	8.6	3.40	187.11	168.1	12.4
	1	oz							
oil roasted, no salt added	100	g	580	16.8	29.9	13.00	632.00	531.0	47.8
	129	g	748	21.7	38.5	16.77	815.28	685	61.6
	1	c							
dry roasted, no salt added (halves and whole)	100	g	574	15.3	32.7	16.00	565.00	490.0	46.4
	137	g	786	21.0	44.8	21.92	774.05	671.3	63.5
	1	c							
butter, without salt added	100	g	587	17.6	27.6	15.00	546.00	457.0	49.4
	32	g	188	5.6	8.8	4.80	174.72	146.3	15.8
	2	tbsp							
HAZELNUT									
oil	100	g	884	0.0	0.0	0.00	0.00	0.00	100.0
	13.6	g	120	0.0	0.0	0.00	0.00	0.00	13.6
	1	tbsp							
whole (1 oz= 21 kernels)	100	g	628	15.0	16.7	0.00	680.00	290.0	60.8
	33.75	g	212	5.1	5.6	0.00	229.50	97.88	20.5
	0.25	c							
blanched	100	g	629	13.7	17.0	0.00	658.00	310.0	61.2
	28.35	g	178	3.9	4.8	0.00	186.54	87.89	17.3
	1	oz							
chopped	100	g	628	15.0	16.7	0.00	680.00	290.0	60.8
	28.75	g	181	4.3	4.8	0.00	195.50	83.38	17.5
	0.25	c							
ground	100	g	628	15.0	16.7	0.00	680.00	290.0	60.8
	18.75	g	118	2.8	3.1	0.00	127.50	54.38	11.4
	0.25	c							
dry roasted, without salt added	100	g	646	15.0	17.6	0.00	755.00	310.0	62.4
	28.35	g	183	4.3	5.0	0.00	214.04	87.89	17.7
	1	oz							
spread, chocolate flavored	100	g	539	5.4	62.4	41.00	407.00	152.0	29.7

	SERVING QUANTITY	SERVING UNIT	CALORIES (kcal)	PROTEIN (g)	TOTAL CARBOHYDRATES (g)	SODIUM (mg)	POTASSIUM (mg)	PHOSPHORUS (mg)	TOTAL FAT (g)
PECANS									
chopped	100	g	691	9.2	13.9	0.00	410.00	277.00	72.0
	109	g	753	10.0	15.1	0.00	446.90	410.00	78.5
	1	c							
halves	100	g	691	9.2	13.9	0.00	410.00	277.00	72.0
	24.75	g	171	2.3	3.4	0.00	101.48	68.56	17.8
	0.25	c							
halves, oil roasted	100	g	715	9.2	13.0	1.00	392.00	263.00	75.2
	110	g	787	10.1	14.3	1.10	431.20	289.30	82.8
	1	c							
dry roasted, without salt added	100	g	710	9.5	13.6	1.00	424.00	293.00	74.3
	28.35	g	201	2.7	3.8	0.28	120.20	83.07	21.1
	1	oz							
PISTACHIO									
raw	100	g	560	20.2	27.2	1.00	1,025	490.00	45.3
(1 oz = 49 kernels)	123	g	689	24.8	33.4	1.23	1,261	602.70	55.7
	1	c							
dry roasted, no salt added	100	g	572	21.1	28.3	6.00	1,007	469.00	45.8
	123	g	704	25.9	34.8	7.38	1,239	576.87	56.4
	1	c							
MACADAMIA									
whole or halves	100	g	718	7.9	13.8	5.00	368.00	188.00	75.8
(1 oz = 10-12 kernels)	134	g	962	10.6	18.5	6.70	493.12	251.92	101.5
	1	c							
dry roasted, without salt added	100	g	718	7.8	13.4	4.00	363.00	198.00	76.1
	33.5	g	241	2.6	4.5	1.34	121.61	66.33	25.5
	0.25	c							

SESAME	SERVING QUANTITY	SERVING UNIT	CALORIES (kcal)	PROTEIN (g)	TOTAL CARBOHYDRATES (g)	SODIUM (mg)	POTASSIUM (mg)	PHOSPHORUS (mg)	TOTAL FAT (g)
seeds, kernels, toasted	100	g	567	17.0	26.0	39.00	406.00	774.00	48.0
	128	g	726	21.7	33.3	49.92	519.68	990.72	61.4
	1	c							
butter or Tahini	100	g	592	17.4	21.5	35.00	459.00	790.00	53.0
	30	g	178	5.2	6.5	10.50	137.70	237.00	15.9
	2	tbsp							
seeds, whole, dried	100	g	573	17.7	23.5	11.00	468.00	629.00	49.7
	9	g	52	1.6	2.1	0.99	42.12	56.61	4.5
	1	tbsp							
butter or Tahini, from roasted/toasted kernels	100	g	595	17.0	21.2	115.00	414.00	732.00	53.8
	30	g	179	5.1	6.4	34.50	124.20	219.60	16.1
	2	tbsp							
SUNFLOWER									
seeds, kernels, toasted	100	g	619	17.2	20.6	3.00	491.00	1,158	56.8
	33.5	g	207	5.8	6.9	1.01	164.49	387.93	19.0
	0.25	c							
seeds, kernels, dried	100	g	584	20.8	20.0	9.00	645.00	660.00	51.5
	36	g	210	7.5	7.2	3.24	232.20	237.60	18.5
	0.25	c							
seeds, kernels, oil roasted	100	g	592	20.1	22.9	3.00	483.00	1,139	51.3
	135	g	799	27.1	31.0	4.05	652.05	1,538	69.3
	1	c							
seeds, kernel, dry roasted	100	g	582	19.3	24.1	3.00	850.00	1,155	49.8
	32	g	186	6.2	7.7	0.96	272.00	369.60	15.9
	0.25	c							
butter, without salt added	100	g	617	17.3	23.3	3.00	576.00	666.00	55.2
	16	g	99	2.8	3.7	0.48	92.16	106.56	8.8
	1	tbsp							
oil, <60% / >60%/ >70% Linoleic	100	g	884	0.0	0.0	0.00	0.00	0.00	100
	13.6	g	120	0.0	0.0	0.00	0.00	0.00	13.6
	1	tbsp							
oil, industrial, mid-oleic for frying and salad dressings	100	g	884	0.0	0.0	0.00	0.00	0.00	100
	13.6	g	120	0.0	0.0	0.00	0.00	0.00	13.6
	1	tbsp							

ACORN	SERVING QUANTITY	SERVING UNIT	CALORIES (kcal)	PROTEIN (g)	TOTAL CARBOHYDRATES (g)	SODIUM (mg)	POTASSIUM (mg)	PHOSPHORUS (mg)	TOTAL FAT
Nuts	100	g	387	6.2	40.8	0.00	539.00	79.00	23
	28.35	g	110	1.7	11.6	0.00	152.81	22.40	6.
	1	oz							
flour	100	g	501	7.5	54.7	0.00	712.00	103.0	30
	28.35	g	142	2.1	15.5	0.00	201.85	29.20	8.
	1	oz							
nuts, dried	100	g	509	8.1	53.7	0.00	709.00	103.0	31
	28.35	g	144	2.3	15.2	0.00	201.00	29.20	8.
	1	oz							
CHIA									
seeds, dried	100	g	486	16.5	42.1	16.00	407.00	860.0	30
	28.35	g	138	4.7	11.9	4.54	115.38	243.8	8.
	1	oz							
HEMP									
seeds, hulled	100	g	553	31.6	8.7	5.00	1,200	1,650	48
	30	g	166	9.5	2.6	1.50	360.00	495.0	14
	3	tbsp							
FLAXSEED									
seeds, whole	100	g	534	18.3	28.9	30.00	813.00	642.0	42
	10.3	g	55	1.9	3.0	3.09	83.70	66.10	4.
	1	tbsp							
seeds, ground	7	g	37	1.3	2.0	2.10	56.90	44.90	3.
	1	tbsp							
oil	100	g	884	0.1	0.0	0.00	0.00	1.00	10
	14	g	124	0.0	0.0	0.00	0.00	0.14	14
	1	tbsp							
oil with added sliced flaxseed	100	g	878	0.4	0.4	6.00	31.00	27.00	99
	13.7	g	120	0.1	0.1	0.82	4.25	3.70	13
	1	tbsp							
oil, cold pressed	100	g	884	0.1	0.0	0.00	0.00	1.00	10
	13.6	g	120	0.0	0.0	0.00	0.00	0.14	13
	1	tbsp							

PUMPKIN	SERVING QUANTITY	UNIT	CALORIES (kcal)	PROTEIN (g)	TOTAL CARBOHYDRATES (g)	SODIUM (mg)	POTASSIUM (mg)	PHOSPHORUS (mg)	TOTAL FAT (g)
meat, 1" cubes	100	g	26	1.0	6.5	1.00	340.00	44.00	0.1
	116	g	30	1.2	7.5	1.16	394.40	51.04	0.1
	1	c							
flowers	100	g	15	1.0	3.3	5.00	173.00	49.00	0.1
	33	g	1	0.0	0.1	0.20	6.92	1.96	0.0
	1	c							
meat, boiled, drained, no salt added	100	g	20	0.7	4.9	1.00	230.00	30.00	0.1
	122.5	g	25	0.9	6.0	1.23	281.75	36.75	0.1
	0.5	c							
pumpkin pie spice powder	100	g	342	5.8	69.3	52.00	663.00	118.0	12.6
	1.7	g	6	0.1	1.2	0.88	11.27	2.01	0.2
	1	tsp							
seed sunfish, cooked dry heat	100	g	114	24.9	0.0	103.0	449.00	231.00	0.9
	85.05	g	97	21.2	0.0	87.60	381.87	196.46	0.8
	3	oz							
seeds, kernels, whole, roasted without salt added	100	g	446	18.6	53.8	18.00	919.00	92.00	19.4
	32	g	143	5.9	17.2	5.76	294.08	29.44	6.2
	0.5	c							
POPPYSEED									
oil	100	g	884	0.0	0.0	0.00	0.00	0.00	100
	13.6	g	120	0.0	0.0	0.00	0.00	0.00	13.6
	1	tbsp							
salad dressing, creamy	100	g	399	0.9	23.7	933.0	61.00	49.00	33.3
	33	g	132	0.3	7.8	307.9	20.13	16.17	11.0
	2	tbsp							

OLIVE

	SERVING QUANTITY	UNIT	CALORIES (kcal)	PROTEIN (g)	TOTAL CARBOHYDRATES (g)	SODIUM (mg)	POTASSIUM (mg)	PHOSPHORUS (mg)	TOTAL FAT
oil, extra virgin, virgin	100	g	884	0.0	0.0	2.00	1.00	0.00	
	14	g	124	0.0	0.0	0.28	0.14	0.00	
	1	tbsp							
black, kalamata	100	g	116	0.8	6.0	735.0	8.00	3.00	
	15	g	17	0.1	0.9	110.0	1.20	0.45	
	3	pcs							
green	100	g	145	1.0	3.8	1556	42.00	4.00	
	15	g	22	0.2	0.6	233	6.30	0.60	
	3	pcs							
spread (tapenade)	100	g	278	0.7	4.2	835	17.00	3.00	
	16	g	45	0.1	0.7	134	2.72	0.48	
	1	tbsp							
stuffed	100	g	128	1.0	4.0	1340	58.00	6.00	
	15	g	19	0.2	0.6	201	8.70	0.90	
	3	pcs							

COCONUT

	SERVING QUANTITY	UNIT	CALORIES	PROTEIN (g)	TOTAL CARBOHYDRATES (g)	SODIUM (mg)	POTASSIUM (mg)	PHOSPHORUS (mg)	TOTAL FAT
fresh	100	g	354	3.3	15.2	20.00	356.00	113.00	
	85	g	301	2.8	12.9	17.00	303.00	96.00	
	1	c							
water, unsweetened	100	g	18	0.2	4.2	26.00	165.00	5.00	
	240	g	43	0.5	10.2	62.40	396.00	12.00	
	1	c							
milk	100	g	31	0.2	2.9	19.00	19.00	0.00	
	244	g	76	0.5	7.1	46.40	46.40	0.00	
	1	c							
milk/cream for cooking	100	g	230	2.3	5.5	15.00	263.00	100.00	
	240	g	552	5.5	13.3	36.00	631.00	240.00	
	1	c							
yogurt	100	g	64	0.3	8.0	21.00	27.00	2.00	
	170	g	109	0.5	13.5	35.70	45.90	3.40	
	6	oz							
cream, canned, sweetened	100	g	357	1.2	53.2	36.00	101.00	22.00	
	37	g	132	0.4	19.7	13.30	37.40	8.14	
	1/4	c							
oil	100	g	833	0.0	0.0	0.00	0.00	0.00	
	14	g	117	0.0	0.0	0.00	0.00	0.00	
	1	tbsp							
flaked, shredded, packed	100	g	456	3.1	51.9	285.00	361.00	100.00	
	28	g	128	1.0	14.5	79.80	101.00	28.00	
	2	tbsp							

	SERVING QUANTITY	UNIT	CALORIES (kcal)	PROTEIN (g)	TOTAL CARBOHYDRATES (g)	SODIUM (mg)	POTASSIUM (mg)	PHOSPHORUS (mg)	TOTAL FAT (g)
SAFFLOWER									
oil	100	g	884	0.0	0.0	0.00	0.00	0.00	100.0
	14	g	124	0.0	0.0	0.00	0.00	0.00	14.0
	1	tbsp							
CANOLA									
oil	100	g	884	0.0	0.0	0.00	0.00	0.00	100.0
	14	g	124	0.0	0.0	0.00	0.00	0.00	14.0
	1	tbsp							
SOYBEAN									
oil	100	g	884	0.0	0.0	0.00	0.00	0.00	100.0
	14	g	124	0.0	0.0	0.00	0.00	0.00	14.0
	1	tbsp							
BUTTER									
stick	100	g	717	0.9	0.1	643.00	24.00	24.00	81.1
	14	g	100	0.1	0.0	90.00	3.36	3.36	11.4
	1	tbsp							
light, stick or tub	100	g	499	3.3	0.0	450.00	71.00	34.00	55.1
	14	g	70	0.5	0.0	63.00	9.94	4.76	7.7
	1	tbsp							
unsalted	100	g	717	0.9	0.1	11.00	24.00	24.00	81.1
	14	g	102	0.1	0.0	1.56	3.41	3.41	11.5
	1	tbsp							
GHEE									
clarified butter	100	g	876	0.3	0.0	2.00	5.00	3.00	99.5
	14	g	123	0.0	0.0	0.28	0.70	0.42	13.9
	1	tbsp							
MARGARINE									
stick	100	g	717	0.2	0.7	751.00	18.00	5.00	80.7
	14	g	100	0.0	0.1	105.00	2.52	0.70	11.3
	1	tbsp							

E. Vegetables

Hey there!

Do you need to print out this Food List?

You can download a printable version of this chart by scanning the QR code below or copying the link on your computer browser.

https://go.renaltracker.com/printfoodlist

TOMATO

	SERVING QUANTITY	SERVING UNIT	CALORIES (kcal)	PROTEIN (g)	TOTAL CARBOHYDRATES (g)	SODIUM (mg)	POTASSIUM (mg)	PHOSPHORUS (mg)	TOTAL FAT (g)
red, whole medium 2.6 in diameter	100.00	g	18	0.9	3.9	5.00	237	24.00	
	123.00	g	22	1.1	4.8	6.15	292	29.52	
	1.00	pc							
diced or chopped	100.00	g	18	0.9	3.9	5.00	237	24.00	
	90.00	g	16	0.8	3.5	4.50	213	21.60	
	0.50	c							
yellow, chopped	100.00	g	15	1.0	3.0	23.00	258	36.00	
	92.67	g	14	0.9	2.8	21.31	239	33.36	
	0.67	c							
orange, chopped	100.00	g	16	1.2	3.2	42.00	212	29.00	
	79.00	g	13	0.9	2.5	33.18	167	22.91	
	0.50	c							
green	100.00	g	23	1.2	5.1	13.00	204	28.00	
	90.00	g	21	1.1	4.6	11.70	183	25.20	
	0.50	c							
whole, canned	100.00	g	16	0.8	3.5	115	191	17.00	
	240.00	g	38	1.9	8.3	276	458	40.80	
	1.00	c							
sauce, canned, no salt	100.00	g	24	1.2	5.3	11.00	297	27.00	
	244.00	g	59	2.9	13.0	26.84	725	65.88	
	1.00	c							
crushed, canned	100.00	g	32	1.6	7.3	186	293	32.00	
	56.70	g	18	0.9	4.1	106	166	18.14	
	2.00	oz							
paste, canned	100.00	g	82	4.3	18.9	790	1,014	83.00	
	32.80	g	27	1.4	6.2	259	333	27.22	
	2.00	tbsp							
puree, canned, no salt	100.00	g	38	1.7	9.0	28.00	439	40.00	
	250.00	g	95	4.1	22.5	70.00	1,098	100.00	
	1.00	c							
sun dried, in oil, drained	100.00	g	213	5.1	23.3	266	1,565	139.00	
	27.50	g	59	1.4	6.4	73.15	430	38.23	
	0.25	c							
Ketchup, low sodium	100.00	g	101	1.0	27.4	20.00	281	26.00	
	15.00	g	15	0.2	4.1	3.00	42.15	3.90	
	1.00	tbsp							
juice, canned	100.00	g	17	0.9	3.5	253	217	19.00	
	243.00	g	41	2.1	8.6	614	527	46.17	
	8.00	fl oz							
cherry, sweet, raw	100.00	g	63	1.1	16.0	0.00	222	21.00	
	138.00	g	87	1.5	22.1	0.00	306	29.00	
	1.00	c							

ASPARAGUS	SERVING QUANTITY	SERVING UNIT	CALORIES (kcal)	PROTEIN (g)	TOTAL CARBOHYDRATE (g)	SODIUM (mg)	POTASSIUM (mg)	PHOSPHORUS (mg)	TOTAL FAT
boiled,	100.00	g	22	2.4	4.1	14.00	224.00	54.00	
drained	90.00	g	20	2.2	3.7	12.60	201.60	48.60	
	0.50	c							
frozen	100.00	g	24	3.2	4.1	8.00	253.00	64.00	
	87.00	g	21	2.8	3.6	6.96	220.11	55.68	
	6.00	pcs							
frozen,	100.00	g	18	3.0	1.9	3.00	172.00	49.00	
boiled,	90.00	g	16	2.7	1.7	2.70	154.80	44.10	
drained	0.50	c							
canned,	100.00	g	19	2.1	2.5	287.00	172.00	43.00	
drained	121.00	g	23	2.6	3.0	347.27	208.12	52.03	
	0.50	c							
BEANS									
green wax,	100.00	g	31	1.8	7.0	6.00	211.00	38.00	
raw	82.50	g	26	1.5	5.8	4.95	174.08	31.35	
	0.75	c							
green wax,	100.00	g	33	1.8	7.5	3.00	186.00	32.00	
frozen	82.67	g	27	1.5	6.2	2.48	153.76	26.45	
	0.67	c							
green wax,	100.00	g	35	1.9	7.9	1.00	146.00	29.00	
boiled, drained	125.00	g	44	2.4	9.9	1.25	182.50	36.25	
	1.00	c							
green wax,	100.00	g	21	1.1	4.2	268.00	96.00	22.00	
canned,	135.00	g	28	1.4	5.7	361.80	129.60	29.70	
drained	1.00	c							
CARROTS									
strips, slices	100.00	g	41	0.9	9.6	69.00	320.00	35.00	
	122.00	g	50	1.1	11.7	84.18	390.40	42.70	
	1.00	c							
grated	100.00	g	41	0.9	9.6	69.00	320.00	35.00	
	82.50	g	34	0.8	7.9	56.93	264.00	28.88	
	0.75	c							
sliced, boiledd	100.00	g	35	0.8	8.2	58.00	235.00	30.00	
rained, no salt	78.00	g	27	0.6	6.4	45.24	183.30	23.40	
	0.50	c							
frozen	100.00	g	36	0.8	7.9	68.00	235.00	33.00	
	85.33	g	31	0.7	6.7	58.03	200.53	28.16	
	0.67	c							
baby	100.00	g	35	0.6	8.2	78.00	237.00	28.00	
	80.00	g	28	0.5	6.6	62.40	189.60	22.40	
	8.00	pcs							
juice, canned	100.00	g	40	1.0	9.3	66.00	292.00	42.00	
	236.00	g	94	2.2	21.9	155.76	689.12	99.12	
	8.00	fl oz							

CORN	SERVING QUANTITY	SERVING UNIT	CALORIES (kcal)	PROTEIN (g)	TOTAL CARBOHYDRATES (g)	SODIUM (mg)	POTASSIUM (mg)	PHOSPHORUS (mg)	TOTAL FAT (g)
white, sweet	100.00	g	390	7.8	86.6	956.00	88.00	39.00	
	25.00	g	98	2.0	21.7	239.00	22.00	9.75	
	1.00	c							
white, steamed (Navajo)	100.00	g	386	9.7	75.2	4.00	532.00	312.00	
	85.05	g	328	8.3	64.0	3.40	452.47	265.36	
	3.00	oz							
white, stew, steamed (Navajo)	100.00	g	112	8.8	10.8	104.00	177.00	107.00	
	85.05	g	95	7.5	9.2	88.45	150.54	91.00	
	3.00	oz							
sweet, boiled, drained	100.00	g	94	3.1	22.3	4.00	251.00	75.00	0.74
	82.00	g	77	2.6	18.3	3.28	205.82	61.50	0.61
	0.50	c							
flour, white, whole grain	100.00	g	361	6.9	76.9	5.00	315.00	272.00	3.86
	29.25	g	106	2.0	22.5	1.46	92.14	79.56	1.13
	0.25	c							
yellow, sweet, boiled, drained	100.00	g	96	3.4	21.0	1.00	218.00	77.00	1.50
	82.00	g	79	2.8	17.2	0.82	178.76	63.14	1.23
	0.50	c							
yellow, sweet, on the cob	100.00	g	86	3.3	18.7	15.00	270.00	89.00	1.35
	154.00	g	77	2.9	16.8	13.50	243.00	80.10	1.22
	1.00	c							
yello, sweet, creamed, canned	100.00	g	72	1.7	18.1	261.00	134.00	51.00	0.42
	128.00	g	92	2.2	23.2	334.08	171.52	65.28	0.54
	0.50	c							
yellow, sweet, kernels, frozen	100.00	g	88	3.0	20.7	3.00	213.00	70.00	0.78
	82.00	g	72	2.5	17.0	2.46	174.66	57.40	0.64
	0.50	c							
yellow, sweet, canned with liquid	100.00	g	61	2.0	13.9	195.00	136.00	46.00	0.77
	128.00	g	78	2.5	17.7	249.60	174.08	58.88	0.99
	0.50	c							
tortilla, no salt added	100.00	g	222	5.7	46.6	11.00	154.00	314.00	2.50
	26.00	g	58	1.5	12.1	2.86	40.04	81.64	0.65
	1.00	pc							

MUSHROOM	SERVING QUANTITY	SERVING UNIT	CALORIES (kcal)	PROTEIN (g)	TOTAL CARBOHYDRATES (g)	SODIUM (mg)	POTASSIUM (mg)	PHOSPHORUS (mg)	TOTAL FAT (g)
Shitake, raw	100.00	g	34	2.2	6.8	9.00	304	112.00	
	19.00	g	6	0.4	1.3	1.71	57.76	21.28	
	1.00	pc							
Shitake, dried	100.00	g	296	9.6	75.4	13.00	1,534	294.00	
	32.40	g	96	3.1	24.4	4.21	497	95.26	
	9.00	pcs							
Shitake, cooked	100.00	g	56	1.6	14.4	4.00	117	29.00	
	72.50	g	41	1.1	10.4	2.90	84.83	21.03	
	0.50	c							
Shitake, stir fried	100.00	g	39	3.5	7.7	5.00	326	111.00	
	108.00	g	42	3.7	8.3	5.40	352	119.88	
	1.00	c							
Portabella/Portabello	100.00	g	22	2.1	3.9	9.00	364	108.00	
Portabello, grilled	100.00	g	29	3.3	4.4	11.00	437	135.00	
White, raw	100.00	g	22	3.0	3.3	5.00	318	86.00	
	96.00	g	21	3.0	3.1	4.80	305	82.56	
	1.00	c							
white, sliced, stir-fried	100.00	g	26	3.6	4.0	12.00	396	105.00	
	108.00	g	28	3.9	4.4	12.96	428	113.40	
	1.00	c							

LETTUCE

	SERVING QUANTITY	SERVING UNIT	CALORIES (kcal)	PROTEIN (g)	TOTAL CARBOHYDRATES (g)	SODIUM (mg)	POTASSIUM (mg)	PHOSPHORUS (mg)	TOTAL FAT (g)
romaine, shredded	100.00	g	17	1.2	3.3		8.00	247.00	30.0
	70.50	g	12	0.9	2.3		5.64	174.14	21.1
	1.50	c							
butterhead, medium leaves	100.00	g	13	1.4	2.2		5.00	238.00	33.0
	82.50	g	11	1.1	1.8		4.13	196.35	27.2
	11.00	pcs							
Red Leaf, shredded	100.00	g	13	1.3	2.3		25	187	28.00
	28.00	g	4	0.4	0.6		7	52.36	7.84
	1.00	c							
Iceberg, shredded or chopped	100.00	g	14	0.9	3.0		10	141	20.00
	108.00	g	15	1.0	3.2		11	152.28	21.60
	1.50	c							
Iceberg, loose leaves, medium	100.00	g	14	0.9	3.0		10	141.00	20.00
	80.00	g	11	0.7	2.4		8	112.80	16.00
	10.00	pcs							

CABBAGE	SERVING QUANTITY	SERVING UNIT	CALORIES (kcal)	PROTEIN (g)	TOTAL CARBOHYDRATES (g)	SODIUM (mg)	POTASSIUM (mg)	PHOSPHORUS (mg)	TOTAL FAT (g)
green, chopped	100.00	g	25	1.3	5.8	18.00	170.00	26.00	
	89.00	g	22	1.1	5.2	16.02	151.30	23.14	
	1.00	c							
green shredded, sliced	100.00	g	25	1.3	5.8	18.00	170.00	26.00	
	87.50	g	22	1.1	5.1	15.75	148.75	22.75	
	1.25	c							
green, shredded, boiled, drained, no salt added	100.00	g	23	1.3	5.5	8.00	196.00	33.00	
	75.00	g	17	1.0	4.1	6.00	147.00	24.75	
	0.50	c							
chinese, shredded, raw	100.00	g							
	76.00	g	12	0.9		6.84	181.00	22.04	
	1.00	c							
chinese, cooked, no salt	100.00	g							
	75.00	g	17	1.0		6.00	147.00	24.75	
	0.50	c							
red, shredded	100.00	g	31	1.4	7.4	27.00	243.00	30.00	
	87.50	g	27	1.3	6.5	23.63	212.63	26.25	
	1.25	c							
red, shredded, boiled, drained, no salt added	100.00	g	29	1.5	6.9	28.00	262.00	33.00	
	75.00	g	27	1.1	5.2	21.00	196.50	24.75	
	0.50	c							
Bok Choy or White Mustard, shredded	100.00	g	13	1.5	2.2	65.00	252.00	37.00	
	87.50	g	11	1.3	1.9	56.88	220.50	32.38	
	1.25	c							
Bok Choy/ Pak Choi, shredded, boiled, drained	100.00	g	12	1.6	1.8	34.00	371.00	29.00	
	85.00	g	10	1.3	1.5	28.90	315.35	24.65	
	0.50	c							
Kimchi	100.00	g	15	1.1	2.4	498.00	151.00	24.00	
	150.00	g	23	1.7	3.6	747.00	226.50	36.00	
	1.00	c							

PEPPER

	SERVING QUANTITY	SERVING UNIT	CALORIES (kcal)	PROTEIN (g)	TOTAL CARBOHYDRATES (g)	SODIUM (mg)	POTASSIUM (mg)	PHOSPHORUS (mg)	TOTAL FAT (g)
bell, sweet yellow, 3 in diameter	100.00 186.00 1.00	g g pc	27 50	1.0 1.9	6.3 11.8	2.00 3.72	212.00 394.32	24.00 44.64	
bell, sweet green, chopped	100.00 74.50 0.50	g g c	20 15	0.9 0.6	4.6 3.5	3.00 2.24	175.00 130.38	20.00 14.90	
bell, sweet green, sauteed	100.00	g	116	0.8	4.2	17.00	134.00	15.00	
bell, sweet red, chopped	100.00 74.50 0.50	g g c	26 19	1.0 0.7	6.0 4.5	4.00 2.98	211.00 157.20	26.00 19.37	
bell, sweet red, sauteed	100.00	g	133	1.0	6.8	21.00	193.00	23.00	
bell, sweet red, chopped, frozen, drained, boiled, no salt added	100.00 85.05 3.00	g g oz	16 14	1.0 0.8	3.3 2.8	4.00 3.40	72.00 61.24	13.00 11.06	
jalapeno, sliced	100.00 22.50 0.13	g g c	29 7	0.9 0.2	6.5 1.5	3.00 0.68	248.00 55.80	26.00 5.85	
serrano, chopped	100.00 26.25 0.25	g g c	32 8	1.7 0.5	6.7 1.8	10.00 2.63	305.00 80.06	40.00 10.50	
black, ground	100.00 2.10 1.00	g g tsp	251 5	10.4 0.2	64.0 1.3	20.00 0.42	1,329.00 27.91	158.00 3.32	
white, ground	100.00 2.40 1.00	g g tsp	296 7	10.4 0.3	68.6 1.7	5.00 0.12	73.00 1.75	176.00 4.22	
hot chilli, red	100.00 45.00 1.00	g g pc	40 18	1.9 0.8	8.8 4.0	9.00 4.05	322.00 144.90	43.00 19.35	

	SERVING QUANTITY	SERVING UNIT	CALORIES (kcal)	PROTEIN (g)	TOTAL CARBOHYDRATES (g)	SODIUM (mg)	POTASSIUM (mg)	PHOSPHORUS (mg)	TOTAL FAT (g)
BROCCOLI									
florets, raw	100.00	g	28	3.0	5.1	27.00	325.00	66.00	0.35
	71.00	g	20	2.1	3.6	19.17	230.75	46.86	0.25
	1.00	c							
Cooked, no salt	100.00	g	35	2.4	7.2	41.00	293.00	67.00	0.41
	78.00	g	27	1.9	5.6	31.98	228.54	52.26	0.32
	0.50	c							
frozen, spears	100.00	g	29	3.1	5.4	17.00	250.00	59.00	0.34
	85.05	g	25	2.6	4.6	14.46	212.62	50.18	0.29
	3.00	oz							
CAULIFLOWER									
green, raw	100.00	g	31	3.0	6.1	23.00	300.00	62.00	0.30
	64.00	g	20	1.9	3.9	14.72	192.00	39.68	0.19
	1.00	c							
cooked, no salt	100.00	g	32	3.0	6.3	23.00	278.00	57.00	0.31
	62.00	g	20	1.9	3.9	14.26	172.36	35.34	0.19
	0.50	c							
CUCUMBER									
sliced, raw	100.00	g	15	0.7	3.6	2.00	147.00	24.00	0.11
	52.00	g	8	0.3	1.9	1.04	76.44	12.48	0.06
	0.50	c							
sliced	100.00	g	15	0.7	3.6	2.00	147.00	24.00	0.11
	78.00	g	12	0.5	2.8	1.56	114.66	18.72	0.09
	0.75	c							
BEETS									
raw	100.00	g	43	1.6	9.6	78.00	325.00	40.00	0.17
	90.67	g	39	1.5	8.7	70.72	294.67	36.27	0.15
	0.67	c							
whole or sliced, boiled, drained, no salt	100.00	g	44	1.7	10.0	77.00	305.00	38.00	0.18
whole, canned	100.00	g	30	0.7	7.1	143.00	159.00	15.00	0.09
	246.00	g	74	1.8	17.6	351.78	391.14	36.90	0.22
	1.00	c							
sliced, canned, drained	100.00	g	31	0.9	7.2	194.00	148.00	17.00	0.14
	85.00	g	26	0.8	6.1	164.90	125.80	14.45	0.12
	0.50	c							

POTATOES	SERVING QUANTITY	SERVING UNIT	CALORIES (kcal)	PROTEIN (g)	TOTAL CARBOHYDRATES (g)	SODIUM (mg)	POTASSIUM (mg)	PHOSPHORUS (mg)	TOTAL FAT (g)
russet, flesh and skin	100.00	g	79	2.1	18.1	5.00	417.00	55.00	0.0
russet, flesh and skin, baked	100.00	g	95	2.6	21.4	14.00	550.00	71.00	0.1
	173.00	g	164	4.6	37.1	24.22	951.50	122.83	0.2
	1.00	pc							
white, flesh and skin	100.00	g	69	1.7	15.7	16.00	407.00	62.00	0.1
white, flesh and skin, baked	100.00	g	92	2.1	21.1	7.00	544.00	75.00	0.1
	173.00	g	159	3.6	36.5	12.11	941.12	129.75	0.2
	1.00	pcs							
french fries, frozen	100.00	g	147	2.2	24.8	332.00	408.00	83.00	4.6
	71.50	g	105	1.6	17.7	237.38	291.72	59.35	3.3
	11.00	pcs							
sweet, cubed	100.00	g	86	1.6	20.1	55.00	337.00	47.00	0.0
	99.75	g	86	1.6	20.1	54.86	336.16	46.88	0.0
	0.75	c							
sweet, boiled, mashed	100.00	g	76	1.4	17.7	27.00	230.00	32.00	0.1
	328.00	g	249	4.5	58.1	88.56	754.40	104.96	0.4
	1.00	c							
sweet, frozen, baked	100.00	g	100	1.7	23.4	8.00	377.00	44.00	0.1
	117.33	g	117	2.0	27.5	9.39	442.35	51.63	0.1
	0.67	c							
sweet, baked, peeled	100.00	g	90	2.0	20.7	36.00	475.00	54.00	0.1
	0.50	c							
chips, unsalted	100.00	g	536	7.0	52.9	8.00	1,275	165.00	34.
	28.35	g	152	2.0	15.0	2.27	361.46	46.78	9.8
	1.00	oz							
hash browns, frozen	100.00	g	82	2.1	17.7	22.00	285.00	47.00	0.6
	70.00	g	57	1.4	12.4	15.40	199.50	32.90	0.4
	0.33	c							
wedges, frozen	100.00	g	129	2.7	25.5	49.00	394.00	87.00	2.2

PEAS

	SERVING QUANTITY	SERVING UNIT	CALORIES (kcal)	PROTEIN (g)	TOTAL CARBOHYDRATES (g)	SODIUM (mg)	POTASSIUM (mg)	PHOSPHORUS (mg)	TOTAL FAT (g)
green	100.00	g	81	5.4	14.5	5.00	244.00	108.00	0.40
	72.50	g	59	3.9	10.5	3.63	176.90	78.30	0.29
	0.50	c							
green, frozen	100.00	g	77	5.2	13.6	108.00	153.00	82.00	0.40
	72.00	g	55	3.8	9.8	77.76	110.16	59.04	0.29
	0.50	c							
green, boiled, drained	100.00	g	84	5.4	15.6	3.00	271.00	117.00	0.22
	80.00	g	67	4.3	12.5	2.40	216.80	93.60	0.18
	0.50	c							
green, canned, drained	100.00	g	68	4.5	11.4	273.00	106.00	67.00	0.80
	87.50	g	60	3.9	9.9	238.88	92.75	58.63	0.70
	0.50	c							
green, frozen, boiled, drained	100.00	g	78	5.2	14.3	72.00	110.00	77.00	0.27
	80.00	g	62	4.1	11.4	57.60	88.00	61.60	0.22
	0.50	c							
split, boiled, no salt added	100.00	g	118	8.3	21.1	2.00	362.00	99.00	0.39
	98.00	g	116	8.2	21.0	1.96	354.76	97.02	0.38
	0.50	c							
sugar or snow peas, whole fresh	100.00	g	42	2.8	7.6	4.00	200.00	53.00	0.20
	78.75	g	33	2.2	6.0	3.15	157.50	41.74	0.16
	1.25	c							
snow/sugar, frozen	100.00	g	42	2.8	7.6	4.00	200.00	53.00	0.20
	78.75	g	33	2.2	6.0	3.15	157.50	41.74	0.16
	1.25	c							
snow/sugar, boiled, drained	100.00	g	42	3.3	7.1	4.00	240.00	55.00	0.23
	80.00	g	34	2.6	5.6	3.20	192.00	44.00	0.18
	0.50	c							
snow/sugar, frozen, boiled, drained	100.00	g	52	3.5	9.0	5.00	217.00	58.00	0.38
	80.00	g	42	2.8	7.2	4.00	173.60	46.40	0.30
	0.50	c							

	SERVING QUANTITY	SERVING UNIT	CALORIES	PROTEIN (g)	TOTAL CARBOHYDRATES (g)	SODIUM (mg)	POTASSIUM (mg)	PHOSPHORUS (mg)	TOTAL FAT
ARTICHOKES									
whole, boiled, drained	100.00	g	53	2.9	12.0	60.00	286	73.00	0
med size	120.00	g	64	3.5	14.3	72.00	343	87.60	0
	1.00	pc							
hearts, boiled, drained	100.00	g	53	2.9	11.9	60.00	286	73.00	0
	84.00	g	45	2.4	10.0	50.40	240	61.32	0
	0.50	c							
Globe or French, frozen	100.00	g	45	3.1	9.2	53.00	264	61.00	0
boiled, drained	80.00	g	36	2.5	7.3	42.40	211	48.80	0
1 svg = 1/3 of 9oz package	1.00	svg							
ALFALFA									
sprouts	100.00	g	23	4.0	2.1	6.00	79.00	70.00	0
	33.00	g	8	1.3	0.7	1.98	26.07	23.10	0
	1.00	c							
CELERY									
stalk	100.00	g	14	0.7	3.0	80.00	260	24.00	0
medium 7.5 - 8 in long	80.00	g	11	0.6	2.4	64.00	208	19.20	0
	2.00	stalks							
diced, chopped	100.00	g	14	0.7	3.0	80.00	260	24.00	0
	101.00	g	14	0.7	3.0	80.80	263	24.24	0
	1.00	c							
celeriac or celery root	100.00	g	42	1.5	9.2	100.00	300	115	0
	78.00	g	33	1.2	7.2	78.00	234	90	0
	0.50	c							
seeds	100.00	g	392	18.1	41.4	160.00	1,400	547	2
	2.00	g	8	0.4	0.8	3.20	28.00	10.94	0
	1.00	tsp							
flakes, dried	100.00	g	319	11.3	68.7	1,435.00	4,388	402	2
	28.35	g	90	3.2	18.1	406.82	1,244	114	0
	1.00	oz							

	SERVING QUANTITY	SERVING UNIT	CALORIES (kcal)	PROTEIN (g)	TOTAL CARBOHYDRATES (g)	SODIUM (mg)	POTASSIUM (mg)	PHOSPHORUS (mg)	TOTAL FAT (g)
COLLARDS									
chopped, raw	100.00	g	32	3.0	5.4	17.00	213.00	25.00	0.61
	90.00	g	29	2.7	4.9	15.30	191.70	22.50	0.55
	2.50	c							
boiled, drained	100.00	g	33	2.7	5.7	15.00	117.00	32.00	0.72
	95.00	g	31	2.6	5.4	14.25	111.15	30.40	0.68
	0.50	c							
frozen, chopped, raw	100.00	g	33	2.7	6.5	48.00	253.00	27.00	0.37
	85.05	g	28	2.3	5.5	40.82	215.17	22.96	0.31
	3.00	oz							
frozen, chopped, boiled/drained	100.00	g	36	3.0	7.1	50.00	251.00	27.00	0.41
	85.00	g	31	2.5	6.0	42.50	213.35	22.95	0.35
	0.50	c							
EGGPLANT/AUBERGINE									
boiled, drained, no salt cut in 1" cubes	100.00	g	35	0.8	8.7	1.00	123.00	15.00	0.23
	99.00	g	35	0.8	8.6	0.99	121.77	14.85	0.23
	1.00	c							
pickled	100.00	g	49	0.9	9.8	1,674	12.00	9.00	0.70
	136	g	67	1.2	13.3	2,276	16.32	12.24	0.95
	1.00	c							
JICAMA (YAMBEAN)									
raw	100.00	g	38	0.7	8.8	4.00	150.00	18.00	0.09
	86.67	g	33	0.6	7.6	3.47	130.00	15.60	0.08
	0.67	c							
boiled, drained, no salt 1 svg= 3oz	100.00	g	38	0.7	8.8	4.00	135.00	16.00	0.09
	85.05	g	32	0.6	7.5	3.40	114.82	13.61	0.08
	3.00	oz							

	SERVING QUANTITY	SERVING UNIT	CALORIES (kcal)	PROTEIN (g)	TOTAL CARBOHYDRATES (g)	SODIUM (mg)	POTASSIUM (mg)	PHOSPHORUS (mg)	TOTAL FAT
ARUGULA									
raw, leaves	100	g	25	2.6	3.7	27.00	369	52.00	0
	80.00	g	20	2.1	2.9	21.60	295	41.60	0
	4.00	c							
salad mixed	100	g	18	1.5	3.3	16.94	299	32.15	0
baby greens	41.25	g	7	0.6	1.4	6.99	123	13.26	0
Arugula, butterhead, endives, Radicchio	1.00	c							
ENDIVE OR ESCAROLE									
raw, chopped	100	g	17	1.3	3.4	22.00	314.00	28.00	0
	87.50	g	15	1.1	2.9	19.25	274.75	24.50	0
	1.75	c							
Chicory, Witlof	100	g	17	0.9	4.0	2.00	211.00	26.00	0
or Belgium	90.00	g	15	0.8	3.6	1.80	189.90	23.40	0
	1.00	c							
OKRA									
raw	100	g	33	1.9	7.5	7.00	299.00	61.00	0
	75.00	g	25	1.5	5.6	5.25	224.25	45.75	0
	0.75	c							
sliced, boiled,	100	g	22	1.9	4.5	6.00	135.00	32.00	0
drained, n.s.	80.00	g	18	1.5	3.6	4.80	108.00	25.60	0
	0.50	c							
frozen	100	g	30	1.7	6.6	3.00	211.00	42.00	0
	85.05	g	26	1.4	5.6	2.55	179.45	35.72	0
	3.00	oz							
frozen, boiled,	100	g	29	1.6	6.4	3.00	184.00	37.00	0
drained, no salt	92.00	g	27	1.5	5.9	2.76	169.28	34.04	0
sliced	0.50	c							
PUMPKIN									
fruit/meat, raw,	100	g	26	1.0	6.5	1.00	340.00	44.00	0
cut 1" cube	116	g	30	1.2	7.5	1.16	394.40	51.04	0
	1.00	c							
boiled, drained,	100	g	20	0.7	4.9	1.00	230.00	30.00	0
mashed, n.s.	122.5	g	25	0.9	6.0	1.23	281.75	36.75	0
	0.50	c							
flowers	100	g	15	0.0	3.3	5.00	173.00	49.00	0
	33.00	g	1	0.0	0.1	0.20	6.92	1.96	0
	1.00	c							
flowers, boiled,	100	g	15	1.1	3.3	6.00	106.00	34.00	0
drained	89.33	g	13	1.0	3.0	5.36	5.36	30.37	0
	0.67	c							
seeds (squash	100	g	559	30.2	10.7	7.00	809.00	1,233	4
kernels), dried	34.50	g	193	10.4	3.7	2.42	279.11	425.4	1
	0.25	c							
seeds	100	g	446	18.6	53.8	18.00	919.00	92.00	1
(pumkin/squash), whole,	32.00	g	143	5.9	17.2	5.76	294.08	29.44	6
roasted no salt added	0.50	c							

	SERVING QUANTITY	SERVING UNIT	CALORIES (kcal)	PROTEIN (g)	TOTAL CARBOHYDRATES (g)	SODIUM (mg)	POTASSIUM (mg)	PHOSPHORUS (mg)	TOTAL FAT (g)
SQUASH									
winter, all varieties cubes	100.00	g	34	1.0	8.6	4.00	350.00	23.00	0.13
	116.00	g	39	1.1	10.0	4.64	406.00	26.68	0.15
	1.00	c							
butternut cubes	100.00	g	45	1.0	11.7	4.00	352.00	33.00	0.10
	140.00	g	63	1.4	16.4	5.60	492.80	46.20	0.14
	1.00	c							
winter, butternut, frozen	100.00	g	57	1.8	14.4	2.00	212.00	22.00	0.10
	85.05	g	48	1.5	12.3	1.70	180.30	18.71	0.09
	3.00	oz							
summer, all varieties sliced	100.00	g	16	1.2	3.4	2.00	262.00	38.00	0.18
	84.75	g	14	1.0	2.8	1.70	222.05	32.21	0.15
	0.75	c							
KOHLRABI									
raw	100.00	g	27	1.7	6.2	20.00	350.00	46.00	0.10
	135.00	g	36	2.3	8.4	27.00	472.50	62.10	0.14
	1.00	c							
boiled, drained, sliced	100.00	g	29	1.8	6.7	21.00	340.00	45.00	0.11
	165.00	g	48	3.0	11.0	34.65	561.00	74.25	0.18
	1.00	c							
LEEKS									
raw	100.00	g	61	1.5	14.2	20.00	180.00	35.00	0.30
	89.00	g	54	1.3	12.6	17.80	160.20	31.15	0.27
	1.00	c							
boiled, drained, chopped or diced	100.00	g	31	0.8	7.6	10.00	87.00	17.00	0.20
	26.00	g	8	0.2	2.0	2.60	22.62	4.42	0.05
	0.25	c							
CASSAVA/YUCCA/MANIOC									
raw	100.00	g	160	1.4	38.1	14.00	271.00	27.00	0.28
	103.00	g	165	1.4	39.2	14.42	279.13	27.81	0.29
	0.50	c							
RADISH									
oriental (Daikon), 7" long	100.00	g	18	0.6	4.1	21.00	227.00	23.00	0.10
	338.00	g	61	2.0	13.9	70.98	767.26	77.74	0.34
	1.00	pc							
oriental, boiled, drained, no salt sliced	100.00	g	17	0.7	3.4	13.00	285.00	24.00	0.24
	73.50	g	13	0.5	2.5	9.56	209.48	17.64	0.18
	0.50	c							
sprouts	100.00	g	43	3.8	3.6	6.00	86.00	113.0	2.53
	38.00	g	16	1.5	1.4	2.28	32.68	42.94	0.96
	1.00	c							

	SERVING QUANTITY	SERVING UNIT	CALORIES	PROTEIN (g)	TOTAL CARBOHYDRATES (g)	SODIUM (mg)	POTASSIUM (mg)	PHOSPHORUS (mg)	TOTAL FAT
TURNIP GREENS									
raw, turnip greens, chopped	100.00	g	32	1.5	7.1	40.00	296.00	42.00	0
	82.50	g	26	1.2	5.9	33.00	244.20	34.65	0
	1.50	c							
frozen	100.00	g	22	2.5	3.7	12.00	184.00	27.00	0
	82.00	g	18	2.0	3.0	9.84	150.88	22.14	0
	0.50	c							
canned	100.00	g	14	1.4	2.4	277.00	141.00	21.00	0
	78.00	g	11	1.1	1.9	216.06	109.98	16.38	0
	0.33	c							
chopped, boiled, drained, no salt	100.00	g	20	1.1	4.4	29.00	203.00	29.00	0
	144.00	g	29	1.6	6.3	41.76	292.32	41.76	0
	1.00	c							
canned, with no salt	100.00	g	19	1.4	2.8	29.00	141.00	21.00	0
	144.00	g	27	2.0	4.1	41.76	203.04	30.24	0
	1.00	c							
frozen, chopped, boiled, drained, no salt added	100.00	g	29	3.4	5.0	15.00	224.00	34.00	0
	164.00	g	48	5.5	8.2	24.60	367.36	55.76	0
	1.00	c							
RUTABAGA									
raw, cubes	100.00	g	37	1.1	8.6	12.00	305.00	53.00	0
	93.33	g	35	1.0	8.1	11.20	284.67	49.47	0
	0.67	c							
boiled, drained, no salt cubed	100.00	g	30	0.9	6.8	5.00	216.00	41.00	0
	170.00	g	51	1.6	11.6	8.50	367.20	69.70	0
	1.00	c							
boiled, drained, mashed	100.00	g	30	0.9	6.8	5.00	216.00	41.00	0
	160.80	g	48	1.5	11.0	8.04	347.33	65.93	0
	0.67	c							
PARSNIPS									
raw, sliced	100.00	g	75	1.2	18.0	10.00	375.00	71.00	0
	88.67	g	67	1.1	16.0	8.87	332.50	62.95	0
	0.67	c							
boiled, drained, sliced, no salt	100.00	g	71	1.3	17.0	10.00	367.00	69.00	0
	78.00	g	55	1.0	13.3	7.80	286.26	53.82	0
	0.50	c							

	SERVING QUANTITY	SERVING UNIT	CALORIES (kcal)	PROTEIN (g)	TOTAL CARBOHYDRATES (g)	SODIUM (mg)	POTASSIUM (mg)	PHOSPHORUS (mg)	TOTAL FAT (g)
WATER CHESTNUTS									
fresh, raw, Chinese (Matai) slices	100.00	g	97	1.4	23.9	14.00	584.00	63.00	0.10
	62.00	g	60	0.9	14.8	8.68	362.08	39.06	0.06
	0.50	c							
canned with liquid Chinese (Matai)	100.00	g	50	0.9	12.3	8.00	118.00	19.00	0.06
	70.00	g	35	0.6	8.6	5.60	82.60	13.30	0.04
	0.50	c							
WATERCRESS									
raw, chopped	100.00	g	11	2.3	1.3	41.00	330.00	60.00	0.10
	34.00	g	4	0.8	0.4	13.94	112.20	20.40	0.03
	1.00	c							
YAM									
raw, in cubes	100.00	g	118	1.5	28.0	9.00	816.00	55.00	0.17
	112.50	g	133	1.7	31.4	10.13	918.00	61.88	0.19
	0.75	c							
baked or broiled, drained, no salt cubed	100.00	g	116	1.5	27.5	8.00	670.00	49.00	0.14
	68.00	g	79	1.0	18.7	5.44	455.60	33.32	0.10
	0.50	c							
Hawaiin Mountain, raw cubed	100.00	g	67	1.3	16.3	13.00	418.00	34.00	0.10
	68.00	g	46	0.9	11.1	8.84	284.24	23.12	0.07
	0.50	c							
Hawaiian Mountain, steamed cubed	100.00	g	82	1.7	20.0	12.00	495.00	40.00	0.08
	145.00	g	119	2.5	29.0	17.40	717.75	58.00	0.12
	1.00	c							
MIXED VEGETABLES									
frozen	100.00	g	72	3.3	13.5	47.00	212.00	59.00	0.52
	72.00	g	52	2.4	9.7	33.84	152.64	42.48	0.37
	0.50	c							
frozen, boiled, drained, no salt added	100.00	g	65	2.9	13.1	35.00	169.00	51.00	0.15
	91.00	g	59	2.6	11.9	31.85	153.79	46.41	0.14
	0.50	c							
canned, drained	100.00	g	49	2.6	9.3	214.00	291.00	42.00	0.25
	163.00	g	80	4.2	15.1	348.82	474.33	68.46	0.41
	1.00	c							
BRUSSEL SPROUTS									
raw	100.00	g	43	33.4	9.0	25.00	389.00	69.00	0.30
	88.00	g	38	3.0	7.9	22.00	342.00	60.70	0.26
	1.00	c							

	SERVING QUANTITY	SERVING UNIT	CALORIES (kcal)	PROTEIN (g)	TOTAL CARBOHYDRATES (g)	SODIUM (mg)	POTASSIUM (mg)	PHOSPHORUS (mg)	TOTAL FAT (g)
SWISS CHARD									
raw	100.00	g	19	1.8	3.7	213.00	379.00	46.00	0.20
	36.00	g	7	0.7	1.4	76.68	136.44	16.56	0.07
	1.00	c							
boiled, drained, no salt	100.00	g	20	1.9	4.1	179.00	549.00	33.00	0.08
	175.00	g	35	3.3	7.2	313.25	960.75	57.75	0.14
	1.00	c							
SPINACH									
raw, chopped	100.00	g	23	2.9	3.6	79.00	558.00	49.00	0.39
	90.00	g	21	2.6	3.3	71.10	502.20	44.10	0.35
	3.00	c							
frozen	100.00	g	29	3.6	4.2	74.00	346.00	49.00	0.57
	78.00	g	23	2.8	3.3	57.72	269.88	38.22	0.44
	0.50	c							
chopped, boiled, drained, no salt	100.00	g	23	3.0	3.8	70.00	466.00	56.00	0.26
	90.00	g	21	2.7	3.4	63.00	419.40	50.40	0.23
	0.50	c							
mustard (Tendergreens)	100.00	g	22	2.2	3.9	21.00	449.00	28.00	0.30
	150.00	g	33	3.3	5.9	31.50	673.50	42.00	0.45
	1.00	c							
mustard, boiled, drained, no salt	100.00	g	16	1.7	2.8	14.00	285.00	18.00	0.20
	180.00	g	29	3.1	5.0	25.20	513.00	32.40	0.36
	1.00	c							
TOMATILLOS									
chopped	100.00	g	32	1.0	5.8	1.00	268.00	39.00	1.02
	132.00	g	42	1.3	7.7	1.32	353.76	51.48	1.35
	1.00	c							
TURNIPS									
raw	100.00	g	28	0.9	6.4	67.00	191.00	27.00	0.10
	130.00	g	34	1.1	7.8	81.74	233.02	32.94	0.12
	1.00	c							
frozen	100.00	g	16	1.0	2.9	25.00	137.00	20.00	0.16
	85.05	g	14	0.9	2.5	21.26	116.52	17.01	0.14
	3.00	oz							
cubed, boiled, drained, no salt	100.00	g	22	0.7	5.1	16.00	177.00	40.56	0.08
	156.00	g	34	1.1	7.9	24.96	276.12	26.00	0.12
	1.00	c							
frozen, boiled, drained, no salt	100.00	g	23	1.5	4.4	36.00	182.00	26.00	0.24
	78.00	g	18	1.2	3.4	28.08	141.96	20.28	0.19
	0.50	c							

	SERVING QUANTITY	SERVING UNIT	CALORIES (kcal)	PROTEIN (g)	TOTAL CARBOHYDRATES (g)	SODIUM (mg)	POTASSIUM (mg)	PHOSPHORUS (mg)	TOTAL FAT (g)
KALE									
raw, chopped	100.00	g	35	2.9	4.4	53.00	348.00	55.00	1.49
	83.75	g	29	2.5	3.7	44.39	291.45	46.06	1.25
	1.25	c							
chopped, boiled, drained, no salt	100.00	g	36	2.9	5.3	16.00	144.00	42.00	1.21
	65.00	g	23	1.9	3.5	10.40	93.60	27.30	0.79
	0.50	c							
scotch, raw, chopped	100.00	g	42	2.8	8.3	70.00	450.00	62.00	0.60
	83.75	g	35	2.4	7.0	58.63	376.88	51.93	0.50
	1.25	c							
scotch, boiled, drained, chopped no salt	100.00	g	28	1.9	5.6	45.00	274.00	38.00	0.41
	86.67	g	24	1.7	4.9	39.00	237.47	32.93	0.36
	0.67	c							
frozen, raw 1 pack=10 oz/284g	100.00	g	28	2.7	4.9	15.00	333.00	29.00	0.46
	85.05	g	24	2.3	4.2	12.76	283.21	24.66	0.39
	3.00	oz							
frozen, chopped, boiled, drained, no salt	100.00	g	36	2.9	5.3	16.00	144.00	42.00	1.21
	65.00	g	23	1.9	3.5	10.40	93.60	27.30	0.79
	0.50	c							
MUSTARD GREENS									
raw, chopped	100.00	g	27	2.9	4.7	20.00	384.00	58.00	0.42
	84.00	g	23	2.4	3.9	16.80	322.56	48.72	0.35
	1.50	c							
boiled, drained, chopped, no salt	100.00	g	26	2.6	4.5	9.00	162.00	42.00	0.47
	70.00	g	18	1.8	3.2	6.30	113.40	29.40	0.33
	0.50	c							
frozen 1 pack=10oz/284g	100.00	g	20	2.5	3.4	29.00	170.00	30.00	0.27
	73.00	g	15	1.8	2.5	21.17	124.10	21.90	0.20
	0.50	c							
frozen, boiled, drained, no salt 1 pack = 10oz/212g	100.00	g	19	2.3	3.1	25.00	139.00	24.00	0.25
	75.00	g	14	1.7	2.3	18.75	104.25	18.00	0.19
	0.50	c							

F. Fruits

Hey there!

Do you need to print out this Food List?

You can download a printable version of this chart by scanning the QR code below or copying the link on your computer browser.

https://go.renaltracker.com/printfoodlist

APPLE	SERVING QUANTITY	SERVING UNIT	CALORIES (kcal)	PROTEIN (g)	TOTAL CARBOHYDRATES (g)	SODIUM (mg)	POTASSIUM (mg)	PHOSPHORUS (mg)	TOTAL FAT (g)
Gala, raw, with skin	100.00	g	57	0.3	13.7	1.00	108.00	11.00	0.12
	172.00	g	98	0.4	23.5	1.72	185.76	18.92	0.21
	1.00	pc, med							
fuji, raw, with skin	100.00	g	63	0.2	15.2	1.00	109.00	13.00	0.18
	192.00	g	121	0.4	29.2	1.92	209.28	24.96	0.35
	1.00	pc, med							
golden delicious, with skin	100.00	g	57	0.3	13.6	2.00	100.00	10.00	0.15
	169.00	g	96	0.5	23.0	3.38	169.00	16.90	0.25
	1.00	pc, med							
granny smith, w/ skin, raw	100.00	g	58	0.4	13.6	1.00	120.00	12.00	0.19
	167.00	g	97	0.7	22.7	1.67	200.40	20.04	0.32
	1.00	pc, med							
juice, frozen concentrate	100.00	g	47	0.1	11.5	7.00	126.00	7.00	0.10
	239.00	g	112	0.3	27.6	16.73	301.14	16.73	0.24
	8.00	fl oz							
applesauce, sweetened, canned	100.00	g	68	0.2	17.5	2.00	75.00	6.00	0.17
	123.00	g	84	0.2	21.5	2.46	92.25	7.38	0.21
	0.50	c							
applesauce, unsweetened, canned	100.00	g	42	0.2	11.3	2.00	74.00	5.00	0.10
	122.00	g	51	0.2	13.8	2.44	90.28	6.10	0.12
	0.50	c							
BLACK BERRIES									
raw	100.00	g	43	1.4	9.6	1.00	162.00	22.00	0.49
	144.00	g	62	2.0	13.8	1.44	233.28	31.68	0.71
	1.00	c							
frozen, unsweetened	100.00	g	64	1.2	15.7	1.00	140.00	30.00	0.43
	151.00	g	97	1.8	23.7	1.51	211.40	45.30	0.65
	1.00	c							
canned, heavy syrup	100.00	g	92	1.3	23.1	3.00	99.00	14.00	0.14
	256.00	g	236	3.4	59.1	7.68	253.44	35.84	0.36
	1.00	c							

RASPBERRIES	SERVING QUANTITY	SERVING UNIT	CALORIES (kcal)	PROTEIN (g)	TOTAL CARBOHYDRATES (g)	SODIUM (mg)	POTASSIUM (mg)	PHOSPHORUS (mg)	TOTAL FAT
raw	100.00	g	52	1.2	11.9	1.00	151.00	29.00	0.
	123.00	g	64	1.5	14.7	1.23	185.73	35.67	0.
	1.00	c							
frozen, unsweetend	100.00	g	56	1.2	12.6	4.00	184.00	30.00	0.
	140.00	g	78	1.6	17.6	5.60	257.60	42.00	1.
	1.00	c							
red, frozen, sweetened, unthawed	100.00	g	103	0.7	26.2	1.00	114.00	17.00	0.
	125.00	g	129	0.9	32.7	1.25	142.50	21.25	0.
	0.50	c							
puree, with seeds	100.00	g	55	na	11.5	4.00	195.00	30.00	0.
juice concentrate	100.00	g	221	3.0	53.2	10.0	1,178.0	100.0	1.
PEARS									
whole, medium (2.5/lb)	100.00	g	57	0.4	15.2	1.00	116.00	16.00	0.
	166.00	g	95	0.6	25.3	1.66	192.56	19.92	0.
	1.00	pc							
halves, canned in water	100.00	g	29	0.2	7.8	2.00	53.00	7.00	0.
	244.00	g	71	0.5	19.1	4.88	129.32	17.08	0.
	1.00	c							
Asian	100.00	g	42	0.5	10.7	0.00	121.00	11.00	0.
	122.00	g	51	0.6	13.0	0.00	147.62	13.42	0.
	1.00	pc							
CRANBERRY									
fresh, chopped	100.00	g	46	0.5	12.0	2.00	80.00	11.00	0.
	55.00	g	25	0.3	6.6	1.10	44.00	6.05	0.
	0.50	c							
dried, sweetened	100.00	g	308	0.2	82.8	5.00	49.00	8.00	1.
	40.00	g	123	0.1	33.1	2.00	19.60	3.20	0.
	0.33	c							
juice, unsweetened	100.00	g	46	0.4	12.2	2.00	77.00	13.00	0.
	253.00	g	116	1.0	30.9	5.06	194.81	32.89	0.
	1.00	c							
juice, cran cocktail	100.00	g	54	0.0	13.5	2.00	14.00	1.00	0.
	253.00	g	137	0.0	34.2	5.06	35.42	2.53	0.
	8.00	fl oz							
sauce, canned, sweetened	100.00	g	159	0.9	40.4	5.00	28.00	4.00	0.
	69.25	g	110	0.6	28.0	3.46	19.39	2.77	0.
	0.25	c							

BLUE BERRIES	SERVING QUANTITY	SERVING UNIT	CALORIES (kcal)	PROTEIN (g)	TOTAL CARBOHYDRATES (g)	SODIUM (mg)	POTASSIUM (mg)	PHOSPHORUS (mg)	TOTAL FAT (g)
fresh	100.00	g	57	0.7	14.5	1.00	77.00	12.00	0.33
	145.00	g	83	1.1	21.0	1.45	111.6	17.40	0.48
	1.00	c							
sweetened, dried	100.00	g	317	2.5	80.0	3.00	214.0	36.00	2.50
	40.00	g	127	1.0	32.0	1.20	85.60	14.40	1.00
	0.25	c							
wild, frozen	100.00	g	57	0.0	13.9	3.00	68.00	13.00	0.16
	140.00	g	80	0.0	19.4	4.20	95.20	18.20	0.22
	1.00	c							
unsweetened, frozen	100.00	g	51	0.4	12.2	1.00	54.00	11.00	0.64
	155.00	g	79	0.7	18.9	1.55	83.70	17.05	0.99
	1.00	c							
canned, light syrup, drained	100.00	g	88	1.0	22.7	3.00	54.00	12.00	0.40
	244.00	g	215	2.5	55.3	7.32	131.7	29.28	0.98
	1.00	c							

STRAWBERRIES

	SERVING QUANTITY	SERVING UNIT	CALORIES (kcal)	PROTEIN (g)	TOTAL CARBOHYDRATES (g)	SODIUM (mg)	POTASSIUM (mg)	PHOSPHORUS (mg)	TOTAL FAT (g)
fresh, whole	100.00	g	32	0.7	7.7	1.00	153.0	24.00	0.30
	144.00	g	46	1.0	11.1	1.44	220.3	34.56	0.43
	1.00	c							
unsweetened, frozen (unthawed)	100.00	g	35	0.4	9.1	2.00	148.0	13.00	0.11
	149.00	g	52	0.6	13.6	2.98	220.5	19.37	0.16
	1.00	c							
sweetened, frozen, thawed	100.00	g	78	0.5	21.0	1.00	98.00	12.00	0.14
	127.50	g	99	0.7	26.8	1.28	124.9	15.30	0.18
	0.50	c							
fruit topping	100.00	g	254	0.2	66.3	21.00	51.00	5.00	0.10
	42.00	g	107	0.1	27.9	8.82	21.42	2.10	0.04
	2.00	tbsp							
pastry, azpprox, enriched	100.00	g	371	5.4	47.8	445.00	83.00	89.00	18.50
	71.00	g	263	3.8	33.9	315.95	58.93	63.19	13.14
	1.00	pc							
Milkshake (fastfood)	100.00	g	113	3.4	18.9	83.00	182.0	100.0	2.80
	226.40	g	256	7.7	42.8	187.91	412.1	226.4	6.34
	8.00	fl oz							
yogurt azppro, low fat 1 item = 1 container	100.00	g	105	8.2	12.3	33.00	129.0	109.0	2.57
	150.00	g	158	12.3	18.4	49.50	193.5	163.5	3.86
	1.00	item							

PINEAPPLE

	SERVING QUANTITY	SERVING UNIT	CALORIES	PROTEIN (g)	TOTAL CARBOHYDRATES (g)	SODIUM (mg)	POTASSIUM (mg)	PHOSPHORUS (mg)	TOTAL FAT
traditional varieties, diced	100.00	g	45	0.6	18.3	1.00	125.00	9.00	
	155.00	g	70	0.9	11.8	1.55	193.75	13.95	
	1.00	c							
sweetened, frozen, chunks	100.00	g	86	0.4	22.2	2.00	100.00	4.00	
	245.00	g	211	1.0	54.4	4.90	245.00	9.80	
	1.00	c							
canned in water crushed, sliced, or chunks	100.00	g	32	0.4	8.3	1.00	127.00	4.00	
	246.00	g	79	1.1	20.4	2.46	312.42	9.84	
	1.00	c							
canned in juice crushed, sliced, or chunks	100.00	g	60	0.4	15.7	1.00	122.00	6.00	
	249.00	g	149	1.1	39.1	2.49	303.78	14.94	
	1.00	c							
extra sweet variety, diced	100.00	g	51	0.5	13.5	1.00	108.00	8.00	
	155.00	g	79	0.8	20.9	1.55	167.40	12.40	
	1.00	c							
juice, unsweetened, canned	100.00	g	53	0.4	12.9	2.00	130.00	8.00	
	250.00	g	133	0.9	32.2	5.00	325.00	20.00	
	8.00	fl oz							
canned in light syrup crushed, sliced, or chunks	100.00	g	52	0.4	13.5	1.00	105.00	7.00	
	126.00	g	66	0.5	17.0	1.26	132.30	8.82	
	0.50	c							
juice, unsweetened, frozen concentrate	100.00	g	179	1.3	44.3	3.00	472.00	28.00	
	288.00	g	387	2.8	95.7	6.48	1,019.5	60.48	
	1.00	c							
juice, 83pprox.83ned with Vit A, C & E	100.00	g	50	0.4	12.2	3.00	132.00	9.00	
	250.00	g	125	0.9	30.5	7.50	330.00	22.50	
	1.00	c							

GRAPE

	SERVING QUANTITY	SERVING UNIT	CALORIES (kcal)	PROTEIN (g)	TOTAL CARBOHYDRATES (g)	SODIUM (mg)	POTASSIUM (mg)	PHOSPHORUS (mg)	TOTAL FAT (g)
red or green, seedless	100.00	g	69	0.7	18.1	2.00	191.00	20.00	0.16
	151.00	g	104	1.1	27.3	3.02	288.41	30.20	0.24
	1.00	c							
juice, unsweetened, plus Vit.C	100.00	g	60	0.4	14.8	5.00	104.00	14.00	0.13
	252.80	g	152	0.9	37.3	12.64	262.90	35.39	0.33
	8.00	fl oz							
fruit mixed/ fruit cocktail, light, drained	100.00	g	55	0.4	14.3	6.00	85.00	13.00	0.08
juice, sweetened, frozen concentrate 6 fl oz can	100.00	g	179	0.7	44.4	7.00	74.00	15.00	0.31
	216.00	g	387	1.4	95.8	15.12	159.84	32.40	0.67
	1.00	can/ item							
seedless, Thompson, canned in water	100.00	g	40	0.5	10.3	6.00	107.00	18.00	0.11
	245.00	g	98	1.2	25.2	14.70	262.15	44.10	0.27
	1.00	c							
jelly 1 packet= 14g (0.5oz)	100.00	g	266	0.2	70.0	30.00	54.00	6.00	0.02
	21.00	g	56	0.0	14.7	6.30	11.34	1.26	0.00
	1	tbsp							

	SERVING QUANTITY	SERVING UNIT	CALORIES (kcal)	PROTEIN (g)	TOTAL CARBOHYDRATES (g)	SODIUM (mg)	POTASSIUM (mg)	PHOSPHORUS (mg)	TOTAL FAT
GRAPEFRUIT									
fresh	100.00	g	32	0.6	8.1	0.00	139.0	8.00	0.1
	153.33	g	49	1.0	12.4	0.00	213.1	12.27	0.1
	0.67	c							
white, fresh, small (3-5 diameter)	100.00	g	33	0.7	8.4	0.00	148.0	8.00	0.1
	118.00	g	39	0.8	9.9	0.00	174.6	9.44	0.1
	0.50	pc							
pink or red	100.00	g	42	0.8	10.7	0.00	135.0	18.00	0.1
	153.33	g	64	1.2	16.4	0.00	207.0	27.60	0.2
	0.67	c							
juice, white	100.00	g	39	0.5	9.2	1.00	162.0	15.00	0.1
	247.00	g	96	1.2	22.7	2.47	400.2	37.05	0.2
	8.00	fl oz							
juice, pink	100.00	g	39	0.5	9.2	1.00	162.0	15.00	0.1
	247.00	g	96	1.2	22.7	2.47	400.2	37.05	0.2
	1.00	c							
juice, unsweetened, pink, canned	100.00	g	37	0.6	7.5	2.00	141.0	17.00	0.6
	247.20	g	91	1.4	18.6	4.94	348.6	42.02	1.6
	8.00	fl oz							
ELDERBERRIES									
	100.00	g	73	7.0	18.4	6.00	280.0	39.00	0.5
fresh	145.00	g	106	1.0	26.7	8.70	406.0	56.55	0.7
	1.00	c							
GOOSEBERRIES									
	100.00	g	44	0.9	10.2	1.00	198.0	27.00	0.5
fresh	150.00	g	66	1.3	15.3	1.50	297.0	40.50	0.8
	1.00	c							
	100.00	g	73	0.7	18.8	2.00	77.00	7.00	0.2
canned in light syrup	252.00	g	184	1.6	47.3	5.04	194.1	17.64	0.5
	1.00	c							
KIWI (Chinese gooseberries)									
fresh, medium, without skin	100.00	g	61	1.1	14.7	3.00	312.0	34.00	0.5
	76.00	g	46	0.9	11.1	2.28	237.1	25.84	0.4
	1.00	pc							
LOGAN BERRIES									
frozen	100.00	g	55	1.5	13.0	1.00	145.0	26.00	0.3
	147.00	g	81	2.2	19.1	1.47	213.2	38.22	0.4
	1.00	c							

CHERRIES

	SERVING QUANTITY	SERVING UNIT	CALORIES (kcal)	PROTEIN (g)	TOTAL CARBOHYDRATES (g)	SODIUM (mg)	POTASSIUM (mg)	PHOSPHORUS (mg)	TOTAL FAT (g)
sweet, without pits	100.00	g	63	1.1	16.0	0.00	222.0	21.00	0.20
	154.00	g	97	1.6	24.7	0.00	341.9	32.34	0.31
	1.00	c							
sour red, without pits	100.00	g	50	1.0	12.2	3.00	173.0	15.00	0.30
	155.00	g	78	1.6	18.9	4.65	268.2	23.25	0.47
	1.00	c							
juice, tart	100.00	g	59	0.3	13.7	4.00	161.0	17.00	0.54
	269.00	g	159	0.8	36.9	10.76	433.1	45.73	1.45
	1.00	c							
Pitanga or Surinam	100.00	g	33	0.8	7.5	3.00	103.0	11.00	0.40
	173.00	g	57	1.4	13.0	5.19	178.2	19.03	0.69
	1.00	c							
tart, dried, sweetened	100.00	g	333	1.3	80.5	13.00	376.0	36.00	0.73
	40.00	g	133	0.5	32.2	5.20	150.4	14.40	0.29
	0.25	c							
maraschino, canned, drained	100.00	g	165	0.2	42.0	4.00	21.0	3.00	0.21
	5.00	g	8	0.0	2.1	0.20	1.05	0.15	0.01
	1.00	pc/ item							
sweet, canned in juice, pitted	100.00	g	54	0.9	13.8	3.00	131.0	22.00	0.02
	250.00	g	135	2.3	34.5	7.50	327.5	55.00	0.05
	1.00	c							
sweet, canned in water	100.00	g	46	0.8	11.8	1.00	131.0	15.00	0.13
	248.00	g	114	1.9	29.2	2.48	324.9	37.20	0.32
	1.00	c							
sweet, frozen, sweetened thawed	100.00	g	89	1.2	22.4	1.00	199.0	16.00	0.13
	259.00	g	231	3.0	57.9	2.59	515.4	41.44	0.34
	1.00	c							
pie filling, canned 1/8 of 21 oz can	100.00	g	115	0.4	28.0	18.00	105.0	15.00	0.07
	74.00	g	85	0.3	20.7	13.32	77.70	11.10	0.05
	1.00	svg							
pie fillings, low calorie	100.00	g	53	0.8	12.0	12.00	118.0	15.00	0.16
	264.00	g	140	2.2	31.6	31.68	311.5	39.60	0.42
	1.00	c							
sour red, canned in water, drained	100.00	g	42	0.7	10.5	4.00	115.0	16.00	0.21
	168.00	g	71	1.2	17.6	6.72	193.2	26.88	0.35
	1.00	c							
sour red, 86pprox.86ned, frozen unthawed	100.00	g	46	0.9	11.0	1.00	124.0	16.00	0.44
	155.00	g	71	1.4	17.1	1.55	192.2	24.80	0.68
	1.00	c							
sour red, canned in light syrup	100.00	g	75	0.7	19.3	7.00	95.00	10.00	0.10
	126.00	g	95	0.9	24.3	8.82	119.7	12.60	0.13
	0.50	c							

PEACHES	SERVING QUANTITY	SERVING UNIT	CALORIES (kcal)	PROTEIN (g)	TOTAL CARBOHYDRATES (g)	SODIUM (mg)	POTASSIUM (mg)	PHOSPHORUS (mg)	TOTAL FAT (g)
raw, medium (87pprox. 4/lb)	100.00	g	39	0.9	9.5	0.00	190.0	20.00	0.25
	150.00	g	59	1.4	14.3	0.00	285.0	30.00	0.38
	1.00	pc/ item							
dried	100.00	g	325	4.9	83.2	10.00	1,351	162.0	1.03
	38.67	g	126	1.9	32.2	3.87	522.4	62.64	0.40
	0.33	c							
slices	100.00	g	39	0.9	9.5	0.00	190.0	20.00	0.25
	154.00	g	60	1.4	14.7	0.00	292.6	30.80	0.39
	1.00	c							
nectar, canned	100.00	g	49	0.1	11.6	11.00	30.00	3.00	0.57
	249.00	g	122	0.3	28.9	27.39	74.70	7.47	1.42
	8.00	fl oz							
pie, prepared 1/6 of 8-in. pie	100.00	g	224	1.9	33.0	217.00	125.0	22.00	10.00
	117.00	g	262	2.2	38.5	253.89	146.3	25.74	11.70
	1.00	slice							
slices, sweetened, frozen	100.00	g	94	0.6	24.0	6.00	130.0	11.00	0.13
	125.00	g	118	0.8	30.0	7.50	162.5	13.75	0.16
	0.50	c							
halves/ slices, canned in water	100.00	g	24	0.4	6.1	3.00	99.00	10.00	0.06
	122.00	g	29	0.5	7.5	3.66	120.8	12.20	0.07
	0.50	c							
halves/ slices, canned in juice	100.00	g	44	0.6	11.6	4.00	128.0	17.00	0.03
	124.00	g	55	0.8	14.4	4.96	158.7	21.08	0.04
	0.50	c							
canned in extra light syrup	100.00	g	42	0.4	11.1	5.00	74.00	11.00	0.10
	123.50	g	52	0.5	13.7	6.18	91.39	13.59	0.12
	0.50	c							
canned in heavy syrup	100.00	g	75	0.4	20.1	4.00	85.00	9.00	0.10
	242.00	g	182	1.0	48.6	9.68	205.7	21.78	0.24
	1.00	c							
canned in light syrup, drained	100.00	g	61	0.6	15.7	7.00	87.00	10.00	0.15
fruit cocktail, canned light syrup with solids and liquid	100.00	g	55	0.4	14.3	6.00	85.00	13.00	0.08

CANTALOUPE MELON	SERVING QUANTITY	SERVING UNIT	CALORIES (kcal)	PROTEIN (g)	TOTAL CARBOHYDRATES (g)	SODIUM (mg)	POTASSIUM (mg)	PHOSPHORUS (mg)	TOTAL FAT
composite, raw	100.00	g	31	0.7	7.5	8.22	202.4	8.67	0
	165.50	g	51	1.1	12.5	13.60	334.9	14.34	0
	1.00	c							
honeydew, balls	100.00	g	36	0.5	9.1	18.00	228.0	11.00	0
1 slice = 125g	132.75	g	48	0.7	12.1	23.90	302.7	14.60	0
	0.75	c							
Navajo	100.00	g	21	0.8	4.1	11.00	140.0	9.00	0
	85.05	g	18	0.7	3.5	9.36	119.1	7.65	0
	3.00	oz							
melon balls,	100.00	g	33	0.8	7.9	31.00	280.0	12.00	0
frozen, unthawed	173.00	g	57	1.5	13.7	53.63	484.4	20.76	0
	1.00	c							

BANANA									
medium, 7.7.8 in long	100.00	g	89	1.1	22.8	1.00	358.0	22.00	0
	118.00	g	105	1.3	27.0	1.18	422.5	25.96	0
	1.00	pc/item							
dehydrated, powder	100.00	g	346	3.9	88.3	3.00	1,491	74.00	1
	6.20	g	21	0.2	5.5	0.19	92.44	4.59	0
	1.00	tbsp							
chips, dried	100.00	g	519	2.3	58.4	6.00	536.0	56.00	1·
	42.53	g	221	1.0	24.8	2.55	227.9	23.81	3
	1.50	oz							
pudding, mix mix to make ½ c 1 package= 88g = 3 ½ oz	100.00	g	366	0.0	93.0	788.00	17.00	5.00	0
	22.00	g	81	0.0	20.5	172.36	3.74	1.10	0
	1.00	svg							
pudding, ready to eat 1 can = 5 oz	100.00	g	127	2.4	21.2	196.00	110	69.00	3
	142.00	g	180	3.4	30.1	278.32	156.2	97.98	5
	5.00	oz							

ORANGE	SERVING QUANTITY	SERVING UNIT	CALORIES (kcal)	PROTEIN (g)	TOTAL CARBOHYDRATES (g)	SODIUM (mg)	POTASSIUM (mg)	PHOSPHORUS (mg)	TOTAL FAT
whole, 2-5/8" diameter	100.00	g	47	0.9	11.8	0.00	181.0	14.00	0.
	131.00	g	62	1.2	15.4	0.00	237.1	18.34	0.
	1.00	pc/ item							
Valencia (California)	100.00	g	49	1.0	11.9	0.00	179.0	17.00	0.
	135.00	g	66	1.4	16.1	0.00	241.7	22.95	0.
	0.75	c							
Navel (California)	100.00	g	49	0.9	12.5	1.00	166.0	28.46	0.
	123.75	g	61	1.1	15.5	1.24	205.4	23.00	0.
	0.75	c							
Clementines	100.00	g	47	0.9	12.0	1.00	177.0	21.00	0.
	74.00	g	35	0.6	8.9	0.74	130.9	15.54	0.
	1.00	pc/ item							
orange sections	100.00	g	47	0.9	11.8	0.00	181.0	14.00	0.
	135.00	g	63	1.3	15.9	0.00	244.4	18.90	0.
	0.75	c							
juice	100.00	g	45	0.7	10.4	1.00	200.0	17.00	0.
	248.00	g	112	1.7	25.8	2.48	496.0	42.16	0.
	8.00	fl oz							
Florida, sections 1 fruit = 141g	100.00	g	46	0.7	11.5	0.00	169.0	12.00	0.
	138.75	g	64	1.0	16.0	0.00	234.5	16.65	0.
	0.75	c							
soda	100.00	g	48	0.0	12.3	12.00	2.00	1.00	0.
	248.00	g	119	0.0	30.5	29.76	4.96	2.48	0.
	8.00	fl oz							
marmalade	100.00	g	246	0.3	66.3	56.00	37.00	4.00	0.
	20.00	g	49	0.1	13.3	11.20	7.40	0.80	0.
	1.00	tbsp							
juice, frozen	100.00	g	95	0.5	23.2	8.00	100.0	13.00	0.
	238.40	g	70	0.4	17.2	5.92	74.00	9.62	0.
	1.00	c							
orange peel zest	100.00	g	97	1.5	25.0	3.00	212.0	21.00	0.
	2.00	g	2	0.0	0.5	0.06	4.24	0.42	0.
	1.00	tsp							
juice, unsweetened, canned	100.00	g	47	0.7	11.0	4.00	184.0	17.00	0.
	249.00	g	117	1.7	27.4	9.96	458.2	42.33	0.
	8.00	fl oz							
Mandarin, canned in juice	100.00	g	37	0.6	9.6	5.00	133.0	1l	
	249.00	g	92	1.5	23.8	12.45	331.2	2.	
	1.00	c							
juice, light, no pulp	100.00	g	21	0.2	5.4	4.00	188.0	4.	
	240.00	g	50	0.5	13.0	9.60	451.2	9.	
	8.00	fl oz							
Mandarin, canned in light syrup	100.00	g	61	0.5	16.2	6.00	78.00	1l	
	252.00	g	154	1.1	40.8	15.12	196.6	2!	
	1.00	c							

LEMON

	SERVING QUANTITY	SERVING UNIT	CALORIES (kcal)	PROTEIN (g)	TOTAL CARBOHYDRATES (g)	SODIUM (mg)	POTASSIUM (mg)	PHOSPHORUS (mg)	TOTAL FAT (g)
whole, without seeds	100	g	20	1.2	10.7	3.00	145.0	15.00	0.30
	108.00	g	22	1.3	11.6	3.24	156.6	16.20	0.32
	1.00	pc/ item							
peeled, 2-1/8" in diameter)	100.00	g	29	1.1	9.3	2.00	138.0	16.00	0.30
	58.00	g	17	0.6	5.4	1.16	80.04	9.28	0.17
	1.00	pc/ item							
juice, fresh	100.00	g	22	0.4	6.9	1.00	103.0	8.00	0.24
	30.50	g	7	0.1	2.1	0.31	31.42	2.44	0.07
	1.00	fl oz							
peel or zest	100.00	g	47	1.5	16.0	6.00	160.0	12.00	0.30
	2.00	g	1	0.0	0.3	0.12	3.20	0.24	0.01
	1.00	tsp							
pudding mix 1 svg = ½ c 1 package = 85g	100.00	g	363	0.1	91.8	506.00	5.00	3.00	0.50
	21.20	g	77	0.0	19.5	107.27	1.06	0.64	0.11
	1.00	svg							
juice, canned	100.00	g	17	0.5	5.6	24.00	109.0	9.00	0.07
	30.50	g	5	0.1	1.7	7.32	33.25	2.75	0.02
	1.00	fl oz							
soda, lemon lime	100.00	g	40	0.1	24.9	9.00	1.00	0.00	0.02
	245.60	g	98	0.1	10.1	22.10	2.46	0.00	0.05
	8.00	fl oz							
juice, unsweetened, frozen	100.00	g	22	0.5	6.5	1.00	89.00	8.00	0.32
	5.08	g	1	0.0	0.3	0.05	4.52	0.41	0.02
	1.00	tsp							
pudding, ready to eat 1 can= 5 oz	100.00	g	125	0.1	25.0	140.00	1.00	5.00	3.00
	142.00	g	178	0.1	35.5	198.80	1.42	7.10	4.26
	1.00	can/ item							
tea, black, sweetened, ready to drink	100.00	g	45	0.0	10.8	3.00	14.00	1.00	0.22
	271.00	g	122	0.0	29.3	8.13	37.94	2.71	0.60
	1.00	c							

	SERVING QUANTITY	SERVING UNIT	CALORIES (kcal)	PROTEIN (g)	TOTAL CARBOHYDRATES (g)	SODIUM (mg)	POTASSIUM (mg)	PHOSPHORUS (mg)	TOTAL FAT
LIME									
whole, 2" in diameter	100.00	g	30	0.7	10.5	2.00	102.0	18.00	
	67.00	g	20	0.5	7.1	1.34	68.34	12.06	
	1.00	pc/ item							
juice, fresh	100.00	g	25	0.4	8.4	2.00	117.0	14.00	
	5.13	g	1	0.0	0.4	0.10	6.01	0.72	
	1.00	tsp							
juice, unsweetened, canned	100.00	g	21	0.3	6.7	16.00	75.00	10.00	
	246.00	g	52	0.6	16.5	39.36	184.5	24.60	
	1.00	c							
frozen ice dessert	100.00	g	128	0.4	32.6	22.00	3.00	1.00	
	99.00	g	127	0.4	32.3	21.78	2.97	0.99	
	0.50	c							
LYCHEE									
whole, fresh	100.00	g	66	0.8	16.5	1.00	171.0	31.00	
	142.50	g	94	1.2	23.6	1.43	243.7	44.18	
	0.75	c							
dried	100.00	g	277	3.8	70.7	3.00	1,110	181.00	
	40.00	g	111	1.5	28.3	1.20	444.0	72.40	
	16.00	pcs/ items							
MANGO									
whole, fresh	100.00	g	60	0.8	15.0	1.00	168.0	14.00	
	207.00	g	124	1.7	31.0	2.07	347.8	28.98	
	1.00	pc/ item							
dired, sweetened	100.00	g	319	2.5	78.6	162.00	279.0	50.00	
nectar, canned	100.00	g	51	0.1	13.1	5.00	24.00	2.00	
	251.00	g	128	0.3	32.9	12.55	60.24	5.02	
	1.00	c							

APRICOT

	SERVING QUANTITY	SERVING UNIT	CALORIES (kcal)	PROTEIN (g)	TOTAL CARBOHYDRATES (g)	SODIUM (mg)	POTASSIUM (mg)	PHOSPHORUS (mg)	TOTAL FAT (g)
whole, fresh	100.00	g	48	1.4	11.1	1.00	259.0	23.00	0.39
	140.00	g	67	2.0	15.6	1.40	362.6	32.20	0.55
	4.00	pcs/ items							
jam or preserves	100.00	g	242	0.7	64.4	40.00	77.00	3.00	0.20
1 packet = 0.5 oz = 14g	20.00	g	48	0.1	12.9	8.00	15.40	0.60	0.04
	1.00	tbsp							
nectar, canned	100.00	g	56	0.2	13.6	8.00	67.00	5.00	0.45
	251.00	g	141	0.4	34.2	20.08	168.2	12.55	1.13
	8.00	fl oz							
sweetened, frozen	100.00	g	98	0.7	25.1	4.00	229.0	19.00	0.10
	242.00	g	237	1.7	60.7	9.68	554.2	45.98	0.24
	1.00	c							
dehydrated, sulfured	100.00	g	320	4.9	82.9	13.00	1,850	157.00	0.62
	30.00	g	96	1.5	24.9	3.90	555.0	47.10	0.19
	0.25	c							
dried, halves, sulfured	100.00	g	241	3.4	62.6	10.00	1,162	71.00	0.51
	43.33	g	104	1.5	27.1	4.33	503.5	30.77	0.22
	0.33	c							
halves w/ skin, canned in juice	100.00	g	48	0.6	12.3	4.00	165.0	20.00	0.04
	244.00	g	117	1.5	30.1	9.76	402.6	48.80	0.10
	1.00	c							
halves with skin, canned in light syrup	100.00	g	63	0.5	16.5	4.00	139.0	32.89	0.05
	253.00	g	159	1.3	41.7	10.12	349.1	13.00	0.13
	1.00	c							

PLUM

	SERVING QUANTITY	SERVING UNIT	CALORIES (kcal)	PROTEIN (g)	TOTAL CARBOHYDRATES (g)	SODIUM (mg)	POTASSIUM (mg)	PHOSPHORUS (mg)	TOTAL FAT (g)
whole, fresh, sliced	100.00	g	46	0.7	11.4	0.00	157.0	16.00	0.28
	165.00	g	76	1.2	18.8	0.00	259.1	26.40	0.46
	1.00	c							
sauce	100.00	g	184	0.9	42.8	538.00	259.0	22.00	1.04
	19.00	g	35	0.2	8.1	102.22	49.21	4.18	0.20
	1.00	tbsp							
purple, pitted, canned in water	100.00	g	41	0.4	11.0	1.00	126.0	13.00	0.01
	249.00	g	102	1.0	27.5	2.49	313.7	32.37	0.02
	1.00	c							
purple, canned in juice	100.00	g	58	0.5	15.2	1.00	154.0	15.00	0.02
	252.00	g	146	1.3	38.2	2.52	388.1	37.80	0.05
	1.00	c							

	SERVING QUANTITY	SERVING UNIT	CALORIES (kcal)	PROTEIN (g)	TOTAL CARBOHYDRATES (g)	SODIUM (mg)	POTASSIUM (mg)	PHOSPHORUS (mg)	TOTAL FAT (g)
PRUNE									
puree	100.00	g	257	2.1	65.1	23.00	852.00	72.00	0.20
	28.35	g	73	0.6	18.5	6.52	241.54	20.41	0.06
	1.00	oz							
dried	100.00	g	240	2.2	63.9	2.00	732.00	69.00	0.38
	42.50	g	102	0.9	27.2	0.85	311.10	29.33	0.16
	0.25	c							
juice, canned	100.00	g	71	0.6	17.5	4.00	276.00	25.00	0.03
	256.00	g	182	1.6	44.7	10.24	706.56	64.00	0.08
	8.00	fl oz							
dehydrated, stewed	100.00	g	113	1.2	29.7	2.00	353.00	37.00	0.24
	36.40	g	41	0.5	10.8	0.73	128.49	13.47	0.09
	0.13	c							
dehydrated, low moisture	100.00	g	339	3.7	89.1	5.00	1,058	112.00	0.73
	33.00	g	112	1.2	29.4	1.65	349.14	36.96	0.24
	0.25	c							
RHUBARB									
whole, fresh, diced	100.00	g	21	0.9	4.5	4.00	288.00	14.00	0.20
	81.33	g	17	0.7	3.7	3.25	234.24	11.39	0.16
	0.67	c							
diced, frozen	100.00	g	21	0.6	5.1	2.00	108.00	12.00	0.11
	137.00	g	29	0.8	7.0	2.74	147.96	16.44	0.15
	1.00	c							
frozen, cooked with sugar	100.00	g	116	0.4	31.2	1.00	96.00	8.00	0.05
	120.00	g	139	0.5	37.4	1.20	115.20	9.60	0.06
	0.50	c							
POMEGRANATE									
whole, fresh, 4" in diameter	100.00	g	83	1.7	18.7	3.00	236.00	36.00	1.17
	282.00	g	234	4.7	52.7	8.46	665.52	101.52	3.30
	1.00	pc/ item							
juice, bottled	100.00	g	54	0.2	13.1	9.00	214.00	11.00	0.29
	251.20	g	136	0.4	33.0	22.61	537.57	27.63	0.73
	8.00	fl oz							

	SERVING QUANTITY	SERVING UNIT	CALORIES (kcal)	PROTEIN (g)	TOTAL CARBOHYDRATES (g)	SODIUM (mg)	POTASSIUM (mg)	PHOSPHORUS (mg)	TOTAL FAT (g)
PLANTAIN									
ripe, raw, fresh	100.00	g	122	1.3	31.9	4.00	487.00	32.00	0.35
	180.00	g	220	2.3	57.4	7.20	877.00	57.60	0.63
	1.00	pc/item							
green, raw, fresh	100.00	g	152	1.3	36.7	2.00	431.00	31.00	0.07
	267.00	g	406	3.3	97.9	5.34	1,150.0	82.80	0.19
	1.00	pc/item							
green, boiled	100.00	g	121	1.1	29.2	2.00	289.00	24.00	0.08
	137.00	g	166	1.5	39.9	2.74	396.00	32.90	0.11
	1.00	c							
green, fried	100.00	g	309	1.5	49.2	2.00	482.00	44.00	11.81
	118.00	g	365	1.8	58.0	2.36	569.00	51.90	13.90
	1.00	c							
yellow, raw, fresh	100.00	g	122	1.3	31.9	4.00	487.00	32.00	0.35
	270.00	g	329	3.5	86.1	10.8	1,310.0	86.40	0.95
	1.00	pc/item							
yellow, baked	100.00	g	155	1.5	41.4	2.00	477.00	37.00	0.16
	139.00	g	215	2.1	57.5	2.78	663.00	51.40	0.22
	1.00	c							
chips	100.00	g	531	2.3	63.8	202	786.00	78.00	29.59
	28.35	g	151	0.6	18.1	57.3	223.00	22.10	8.39
	1.00	oz							
AVOCADO									
fresh, raw	100.00	g	160	2.0	8.5	7.00	485.00	52.00	14.66
mashed/pureed	230.00	g	368	4.6	19.6	16.1	1,120.0	120.0	33.70
	1.00	c							
oil	100.00	g	884	0.0	0.0	0.00	0.00	0.00	100.0
	14.00	g	124	0.0	0.0	0.00	0.00	0.00	14.00
	1.00	tbsp							
dressing	100.00	g	427	1.9	7.4	867	58.00	31.00	43.33
	15.30	g	65	0.3	1.1	133.	8.87	4.74	6.63
	1.00	tbsp							
California, raw/fresh no seed and skin	100.00	g	167	2.0	8.6	8.00	507.00	54.00	15.41
	136.00	g	227	2.7	11.8	10.9	690.00	73.40	21.00
	1.00	pc/item							
Florida, fresh/raw no seed and skin	100.00	g	120	2.2	7.8	2.00	351.00	40.00	10.06
	304.00	g	365	6.8	23.8	6.08	1,070.0	122.0	30.60
	1.00	pc/item							
Guacamole	100.00	g	155	2.0	8.5	344	472.00	51.00	14.18
	15.00	G	23	0.3	1.3	51.6	70.80	7.65	2.13
	1.00	tbsp							

	SERVING QUANTITY	SERVING UNIT	CALORIES	PROTEIN (g)	TOTAL CARBOHYDRATES (g)	SODIUM (mg)	POTASSIUM (mg)	PHOSPHORUS (mg)	TOTAL FAT (g)
PAPAYA									
whole, fresh, cubes	100.00	g	43	0.5	10.8	8.00	182.00	10.00	C
	140.00	g	60	0.7	15.2	11.20	254.80	14.00	C
	1.00	c							
nectar, canned	100.00	g	57	0.2	14.5	5.00	31.00	0.00	C
	250.00	g	143	0.4	36.3	12.50	77.50	0.00	C
	8.00	fl oz							
canned with heavy syrup, drained	100.00	g	206	0.1	55.8	9.00	67.00	6.00	C
	39.00	g	80	0.1	21.8	3.51	26.13	2.34	C
	1.00	pc/ chunk							
NECTARINE									
whole, fresh, slices	100.00	g	44	1.1	10.6	0.00	201.00	26.00	C
	138.00	g	61	1.5	14.7	0.00	277.38	35.88	C
	1.00	c							
PERSIMMON									
whole, fresh	100.00	g	127	0.8	33.5	1.00	310.00	26.00	C
	25.00	g	32	0.2	8.4	0.25	77.50	6.50	C
	1.00	pc/ item							
Japanese, fresh, 2-1/2" in diameter	100.00	g	70	0.6	18.6	1.00	161.00	17.00	C
	168.00	g	118	1.0	31.2	1.68	270.48	28.56	C
	1.00	pc/item							
Japanese, dried	100.00	g	274	1.4	73.4	2.00	802.00	81.00	C
	34.00	g	93	0.5	25.0	0.68	272.68	27.54	C
	1.00	pc/ item							
PURPLE PASSION FRUIT/ GRANADILLA									
whole, fresh – no refuse	100.00	g	97	2.2	23.4	28.00	348.00	68.00	C
	18.00	g	18	0.4	4.2	5.04	62.60	12.20	C
	1.00	pc/ fruit							
nectar, no ice	100.00	g	67	1.2	17.4	4.00	112.00	5.00	C
	31.00	g	21	0.1	5.4	1.24	34.70	1.55	C
	1.00	fl oz							
juice, purple passion fruit	100.00	g	51	0.4	13.6	6.00	278.00	13.00	C
	30.90	g	16	0.1	4.2	1.85	85.90	4.02	C
	1.00	fl oz							
juice, yellow passion fruit	100.00	g	60	0.7	14.5	6.00	278.00	25.00	C
	30.90	g	19	0.2	4.5	1.85	85.90	7.72	C
	1.00	fl oz							

	SERVING QUANTITY	SERVING UNIT	CALORIES (kcal)	PROTEIN (g)	TOTAL CARBOHYDRATES (g)	SODIUM (mg)	POTASSIUM (mg)	PHOSPHORUS (mg)	TOTAL FAT (g)
WATER MELON									
raw, balls	100.00	g	30	0.6	7.6	1.00	112.00	11.00	0.15
	154.00	g	46	0.9	11.6	1.54	172.00	16.00	0.23
	1.00	c							
juice, 100%, no ice	100.00	g	30	0.6	7.6	1.00	112.00	11.00	0.15
	30.00	g	9	0.2	2.3	0.30	33.60	3.30	0.05
	1.00	fl oz							
seeds, kernels, dried	100.00	g	557	28.3	15.3	99.00	648.00	755.0	47.37
	28.35	g	158	8.0	4.3	28.10	184.00	214.0	13.40
	1.00	oz							
FIG									
raw	100.00	g	74	0.8	19.2	1.00	232.00	14.00	0.30
	50.00	g	37	0.4	9.6	0.50	116.00	7.00	0.15
	1.00	pc/ item							
dried	100.00	g	249	3.3	63.9	10.00	680.00	67.00	0.92
	8.00	g	20	0.3	5.1	0.80	54.40	5.36	0.07
	1.00	pc							
canned	100.00	g	75	0.6	19.4	1.00	157.00	10.00	0.24
	250.00	g	188	1.4	48.4	2.50	392.00	25.00	0.60
	1.00	c							
dried, stewed	100.00	g	107	1.4	27.6	4.00	294.00	29.00	0.40
	259.00	g	277	3.7	71.4	10.40	761.00	75.10	1.04
	1.00	c							
canned, water pack, solids/liquids	100.00	g	53	0.4	14.0	1.00	103.00	10.00	0.10
	248.00	g	131	1.0	34.7	2.48	255.00	24.80	0.25
	1.00	c							
canned, light syrup pack, solids/liquids	100.00	g	69	0.4	18.0	1.00	102.00	10.00	0.10
	252.00	g	174	1.0	45.2	2.52	257.00	25.20	0.25
	1.00	c							
GUAVA									
raw	100.00	g	68	2.6	14.3	2.00	417.00	40.00	0.95
	55.00	g	37	1.4	7.9	1.10	229.00	22.00	0.52
	1.00	pc/ item							
nectar no ice	100.00	g	48	0.3	13.3	6.00	33.00	3.00	0.07
	31.00	g	15	0.1	4.1	1.86	10.20	0.93	0.02
	1.00	fl oz							
paste	100.00	g	280	0.1	77.6	2.00	69.00	3.00	0.27
	20.00	g	56	0.0	14.5	0.40	13.80	0.60	0.05
	1.00	tbsp							

	SERVING QUANTITY	SERVING UNIT	CALORIES (kcal)	PROTEIN (g)	TOTAL CARBOHYDRATES (g)	SODIUM (mg)	POTASSIUM (mg)	PHOSPHORUS (mg)	TOTAL FAT
DATES									
whole, dried	100.00	g	282	2.5	75.0	2.00	656.0	62.00	0
	8.00	g	23	0.2	6.0	0.16	52.50	4.96	0
	1.00	pc/item							
Medjool, pitted	100.00	g	277	1.8	75.0	1.00	696.0	62.00	0
	24.00	g	67	0.4	18.0	0.24	167.0	14.90	0
	1.00	pc/item							
candy	100.00	g	379	4.2	58.1	22.00	540.0	117.0	1
	28.35	g	107	1.2	16.5	6.24	153.0	33.20	5
	1.00	oz							
POMELO									
whole, fresh	100.00	g	38	0.8	9.6	1.00	216.0	17.00	0
section	190.00	g	72	1.4	18.3	1.90	410.0	32.30	0
	1.00	c							
MANGOSTEEN									
canned, syrup pack	100.00	g	73	0.4	17.9	7.00	48.00	8.00	0
drained	196.00	g	143	0.8	35.1	13.70	94.10	15.70	1
	1.00	c							
JACKFRUIT									
raw, fresh	100.00	g	95	1.7	23.3	2.00	448.0	21.00	0
slices	165.00	g	157	2.8	38.4	3.30	739.0	34.60	1
	1.00	c							
canned, syrup pack	100.00	g	92	0.4	23.9	11.00	96.00	6.00	0
drained	178.00	g	164	0.6	42.6	19.60	171.0	10.70	0
	1.00	c							
DURIAN									
raw or frozen chopped or diced	100.00	g	147	1.5	27.1	2.00	436.0	39.00	5
	243.00	g	357	3.6	65.8	4.86	1,060	94.80	1
	1.00	c							
SOURSOP									
raw, pulp	100.00	g	66	1.0	16.8	14.00	278.0	27.00	0
	225.00	g	148	2.3	37.9	31.50	626.0	60.80	0
	1.00	c							
nectar	100.00	g	59	0.1	14.9	8.00	25.00	2.00	0
no ice, pure	31.00	g	18	0.0	4.6	2.48	7.75	0.62	0
	1.00	fl oz							

	SERVING QUANTITY	SERVING UNIT	CALORIES (kcal)	PROTEIN (g)	TOTAL CARBOHYDRATES (g)	SODIUM (mg)	POTASSIUM (mg)	PHOSPHORUS (mg)	TOTAL FAT (g)
TAMARIND									
fresh, raw	100.00	g	239	2.8	62.5	28.00	628	113	
	2.00	g	5	0.1	1.3	0.56	12.60	2.26	
	1.00	pc/item							
candy	100.00	g	331	0.0	92.0	1,643	309.0	56.00	
	22.00	g	73	0.0	20.2	361.00	68.00	12.30	
	1.00	tbsp							
dried	100.00	g	254	2.5	66.2	25.00	565	102	
	160.00	g	406	4.0	106	40.00	904	163	
	1.00	c							
SAPODILLA									
fresh/raw	100.00	g	83	0.4	20.0	12.00	193	12.00	
	170.00	g	141	0.8	33.9	20.40	328	20.40	
	1.00	pc/item							
SUGARAPPLE (sweetsop)									
fresh, raw	100.00	g	94	2.1	23.6	9.00	247	32.00	
(2-7/8" in diameter)	155.00	g	146	3.2	36.6	14.00	383	49.60	
	1.00	pc/item							
STARFRUIT									
fresh/raw	100.00	g	31	1.0	6.7	2.00	133	12.00	
	90.00	g	28	0.9	6.1	1.80	120.0	10.80	
	1.00	pc/item							

G. Herbs and Spices

Hey there!

Do you need to print out this Food List?

You can download a printable version of this chart by scanning the QR code below or copying the link on your computer browser.

https://go.renaltracker.com/printfoodlist

	SERVING QUANTITY	UNIT	CALORIES (kcal)	PROTEIN (g)	TOTAL CARBOHYDRATE (g)	SODIUM (mg)	POTASSIUM (mg)	PHOSPHORUS (mg)	TOTAL FAT (g)
SAGE									
ground	100	g	315	10.6	60.7	11	1070	91	12.8
1 Tbsp	2	g	6.3	0.21	1.21	0.22	21.4	1.82	0.256
CINNAMON									
ground	100	g	247	3.99	80.6	10	431	64	1.24
1 Tbsp	7.8	g	19.3	0.31	6.29	0.78	33.6	4.99	0.097
CUMIN									
seed	100	g	375	17.8	44.2	168	1790	499	22.3
1 Tbsp Whole	6	g	22.5	1.07	2.65	10.1	107	29.9	1.34
NUTMEG									
ground	100	g	525	5.84	49.3	16	350	213	36.3
1 tsp	7	g	36.8	0.41	3.45	1.12	24.5	14.9	2.54
CLOVES									
ground	100	g	274	5.97	65.5	277	1020	104	13
1 tsp	6.5	g	17.8	0.39	4.26	18	66.3	6.76	0.845
PARSLEY									
fresh	100	g	36	2.97	6.33	56	554	58	0.79
dried	100	g	292	26.6	50.6	452	2680	436	5.48
CORIANDER									
seed	100	g	298	12.4	55	35	1270	409	17.8
leaves, raw	100	g	23	2.13	3.67	46	521	48	0.52
THYME									
fresh	100	g	101	5.56	24.4	9	609	106	1.68
dried	100	g	276	9.11	63.9	55	814	201	7.43
LEMON GRASS									
citronella, raw	100	g	99	1.82	25.3	6	723	101	0.49

	SERVING QUANTITY	UNIT	CALORIES (kcal)	PROTEIN (g)	TOTAL CARBOHYDRATES (g)	SODIUM (mg)	POTASSIUM (mg)	PHOSPHORUS (mg)	TOT
ONION									
red, raw	100	g	44	0.94	9.93	1	197	41	0
1 onion	197	g	86.7	1.85	19.6	1.97	388	80.8	0
white, raw	100	g	36	0.89	7.68	2	141	29	0
yellow, raw	100	g	38	0.83	8.61	1	182	34	0
1 onion	143	g	54.3	1.19	12.3	1.43	260	48.6	0
GARLIC									
raw	100	g	149	6.36	33.1	17	401	153	0
3 cloves	9	g	13.4	0.572	2.98	1.53	36.1	13.8	0
GINGER									
raw	100	g	80	1.82	17.8	13	415	34	0
SPRING ONIONS									
raw	100	g	32	1.83	7.34	16	276	37	0
1 large	25	g	8	0.458	1.84	4	69	9.25	0
CHIVES									
raw	100	g	30	3.27	4.35	3	296	58	0
BASIL									
fresh	100	g	23	3.15	2.65	4	295	56	0
dried	100	g	233	23	47.8	76	2630	274	4
OREGANO									
dried	100	g	265	9	68.9	25	1260	148	4
ROSEMARY									
fresh	100	g	131	3.31	20.7	26	668	66	5
dried	100	g	331	4.88	64.1	50	995	70	1
MARJORAM									
dried	100	g	271	12.7	60.6	77	1520	306	7

	SERVING QUANTITY	UNIT	CALORIES (kcal)	PROTEIN (g)	TOTAL CARBOHYDRATES (g)	SODIUM (mg)	POTASSIUM (mg)	PHOSPHORUS (mg)	TOTAL FAT (g)
FENNEL									
Bulb, raw	100	g	31	1.24	7.3	52	414	50	0.2
seed	100	g	345	15.8	52.3	88	1690	487	14.9
1 Tbsp	5.8	g	20	0.92	3.03	5.1	98	28	0.864
DILL									
weed, fresh	100	g	43	3.46	7.02	61	738	66	1.12
weed, dried	100	g	253	20	55.8	208	3310	543	4.36
1 Tbsp	3.1	g	7.8	0.62	1.73	6.45	103	16.8	0.135
ANISE									
seed	100	g	337	17.6	50	16	1440	440	15.9
1 Tbsp	6.7	g	22.6	1.18	3.35	1.07	96.5	29.5	1.06
CARDAMOM									
spices	100	g	311	10.8	68.5	18	1120	229	6.7
1 Tbsp	5.8	g	18	0.63	3.97	1.04	65	10.3	0.389
CAYENNE									
pepper, red or cayenne	100	g	318	12	56.6	30	2010	293	17.3
1 tbsp	5.3	g	16.9	0.64	3	1.59	107	15.5	0.917
CURRY POWDER									
	100	g	325	14.3	55.8	52	1170	367	14
1 tbsp	6.3	g	20.5	0.90	3.52	3.28	73.7	23.1	0.882
PAPRIKA									
ground	100	g	282	14.1	54	68	2280	314	12.9
1 tbsp	6.8	g	19.2	0.96	3.67	4.62	155	21.4	0.877
CELERY									
celery, raw	100	g	14	0.69	2.97	80	260	24	0.17

	SERVING QUANTITY	UNIT	CALORIES (kcal)	PROTEIN (g)	TOTAL CARBOHYDRATES (g)	SODIUM (mg)	POTASSIUM (mg)	PHOSPHORUS (mg)	TOTAL FAT (g)
SAFFRON									
	100	g	310	11.4	65.4	148	1720	252	5
1 tbsp	2.1	g	6.51	0.24	1.37	3.11	36.1	5.29	0
PEPPER, BLACK									
ground	100	g	251	10.4	64	20	1330	158	3
1 tbsp	6.9	g	17.3	0.72	4.42	1.38	91.8	10.9	0
PEPPER, WHITE									
ground	100	g	296	10.4	68.6	5	73	176	2
1 tbsp	7.1	g	21	0.74	4.87	0.355	5.18	12.5	0
TARRAGON									
dried	100	g	295	22.8	50.2	62	3020	313	7
1 Tbsp, leaves	1.8	g	5.31	0.41	0.904	1.12	54.4	5.63	0
1 Tbsp, ground	4.8	g	14.2	1.09	2.41	2.98	145	15	0
HORSERADISH									
	100	g	48	1.18	11.3	420	246	31	0
1 tbsp	15	g	7.2	0.18	1.7	63	36.9	4.65	0

H. Carbohydrates

(Grains, Breads, Pasta/Noodles, Cereals)

Hey there!

Do you need to print out this Food List?

You can download a printable version of this chart by scanning the QR code below or copying the link on your computer browser.

https://go.renaltracker.com/printfoodlist

RICE

	SERVING QUANTITY	SERVING UNIT	CALORIES (kcal)	PROTEIN (g)	TOTAL CARBOHYDRATES (g)	SODIUM (mg)	POTASSIUM (mg)	PHOSPHORUS (mg)	TOTAL FAT (g)
white, unenriched	100.00	g	359	6.9	79.8	5.00	75.00	94.00	1.30
white, cooked, glutinous	100.00	g	96	2.0	21.0	5.00	20.00	33.00	0.27
	174.00	g	167	3.5	36.5	6.60	26.40	43.60	0.36
	1.00	c							
white, long-grain, parboiled enriched, cooked	100.00	g	123	2.9	26.1	0.00	29.00	37.00	0.21
	158.00	g	194	4.6	41.2	0.00	53.90	68.80	0.39
	1.00	c							
flour, white, unenriched	100.00	g	359	6.9	79.8	0.00	26.00	33.00	0.19
						0.00	53.30	67.60	0.39
white, steamed, Chinese restaurant cup, loosely packed	100.00	g	151	3.2	33.9				
	132.00	g	199	4.2	44.7	1.00	265.0	319.0	3.85
	1.00	c							
white, medium-grain, cooked unenriched	100.00	g	130	2.4	28.6	201.00	86.00	102.00	0.96
	186.00	g	242	4.4	53.2	394.00	169.0	200.0	1.88
	1.00	c							
white, short-grain, cooked unenriched	100.00	g	130	2.4	28.7	3.00	101.0	82.00	0.34
	205.00	g	266	4.8	58.8	4.92	166.0	134.0	0.56
	1.00	c							
flour, brown,	100.00	g	365	7.2	75.5	7.00	427.0	433.0	1.08
						11.20	683.0	693.0	1.73
brown, cooked, no salt, no fat	100.00	g	122	2.7	25.5				
	196.00	g	239	5.4	49.9	5.00	75.00	94.00	1.30
	1.00	c							
wild, cooked	100.00	g	101	4.0	21.3	5.00	20.00	33.00	0.27
	164.00	g	166	6.5	35.0	6.60	26.40	43.60	0.36
	1.00	c							
wild, raw	100.00	g	357	14.7	74.9	0.00	29.00	37.00	0.21
	160.00	g	571	23.6	120.0	0.00	53.90	68.80	0.39
	1.00	c							

OATS

	SERVING QUANTITY	SERVING UNIT	CALORIES (kcal)	PROTEIN (g)	TOTAL CARBOHYDRATES (g)	SODIUM (mg)	POTASSIUM (mg)	PHOSPHORUS (mg)	TOTAL FAT
raw	100.00	g	379	12.2	67.7	6.00	362.0	410.0	6
	81.00	g	307	10.7	54.8	4.86	293.0	332.0	5
	1.00	c							
cereal, oat,	100.00	g	372	12.4	73.2	497.00	633.0	357.0	6
	33.00	g	123	4.1	24.2	164.00	209.0	118.0	2
	1.00	c							
steel cut	100.00	g	378	13.3	66.7	0.00	356.0	na	6
Brand: ARROWHEAD MILLS	45.00	g	170	6.0	30.0	0.00	160.0	na	3
	1.00	svg							
rolled	100.00	g	350	12.5	67.5	0.00	350.0	na	6
Brand: MILLVILLE by Aldi	40.00	g	140	5.0	27.0	0.00	140.0	na	2
	1.00	svg							
bran, cooked	100.00	g	40	3.2	11.4	1.00	92.00	119.0	0
	219.00	g	88	7.0	25.1	2.19	201.0	261.0	1
	1.00	c							
bran, uncooked (raw)	100.00	g	246	17.3	66.2	4.00	566.0	734.0	7
	94.00	g	231	16.3	62.2	3.76	532.0	690.0	6
	1.00	c							
flour, partially debranned	100.00	g	404	14.7	65.7	19.00	371.0	452.0	9
	104.00	g	420	15.2	68.3	19.80	386.0	470.0	9
	1.00	c							
regular, rolled, not fortified, dry	100.00	g	379	13.2	67.7	6.00	362.0	410.0	6
	81.00	g	307	10.7	54.8	4.86	293.0	332.0	5
	1.00	c							

WHEAT

	SERVING QUANTITY	SERVING UNIT	CALORIES (kcal)	PROTEIN (g)	TOTAL CARBOHYDRATES (g)	SODIUM (mg)	POTASSIUM (mg)	PHOSPHORUS (mg)	TOTAL FAT (g)
durum	100.00	g	399	13.7	71.1	2.00	431.0	508.0	2.47
	192.00	g	651	26.3	137	3.84	828.0	975.0	4.74
	1.00	c							
sprouted	100.00	g	198	7.5	42.5	16.00	169.0	200.0	1.27
	108.00	g	214	8.1	45.9	17.30	183.0	216.0	1.37
	1.00	c							
germ	100.00	g	360	23.2	51.8	12.00	892.0	842.0	9.72
	115.00	g	414	26.7	59.6	13.80	1,030	968	11.20
	1.00	c							
bran	100.00	g	216	15.6	64.5	2.00	1,180	1,010	4.25
	58.00	g	125	9.1	37.4	1.16	684.0	586.0	2.46
	1.00	c							
cream of wheat, instant, dry	100.00	g	366	10.6	75.5	571.00	115.0	103.0	1.40
	11.50	g	42	1.2	8.7	65.70	13.20	11.80	0.16
	1.00	tbsp							
flour, whole wheat, unenriched	100.00	g	370	15.1	71.2	3.00	376.0	352.0	2.73
whole grain, soft wheat	100.00	g	332	9.6	74.5	3.00	394.0	323.0	1.95
bread flour, unenriched unsifted	100.00	g	361	12.0	72.5	2.00	100.0	97.00	1.66
	137.00	g	495	16.4	99.4	2.74	137.0	133.0	2.27
	1.00	c							
flour, bread, white, enriched	100.00	g	361	12.0	72.5	2.00	100.0	97.00	1.66
	137.00	g	495	16.4	99.4	2.74	137.0	133.0	2.27
	1.00	c							
flour, cake, enriched unsifted	100.00	g	362	8.2	78.0	2.00	105.0	85.00	0.86
	137.00	g	496	11.2	107.0	2.74	144.0	116.0	1.18
	1.00	c							

CUOSCUOS

	SERVING QUANTITY	UNIT	CALORIES (kcal)	PROTEIN (g)	TOTAL CARBOHYDRATES (g)	SODIUM (mg)	POTASSIUM (mg)	PHOSPHORUS (mg)	TOTAL FAT
dry	100.00	g	376	12.8	77.4	10.00	166.0	170.0	
	173.00	g	680	22.1	134	17.30	287.0	294.0	
	1.00	c							
cooked	100.00	g	112	3.8	23.2	5.00	58.00	22.00	
	157.00	g	176	6.0	36.4	7.85	91.10	34.50	
	1.00	c							

BARLEY

	SERVING QUANTITY	UNIT	CALORIES (kcal)	PROTEIN (g)	TOTAL CARBOHYDRATES (g)	SODIUM (mg)	POTASSIUM (mg)	PHOSPHORUS (mg)	TOTAL
pearled, cooked	100.00	g	123	2.3	28.2	3.00	93.00	54.00	
	157.00	g	193	3.6	44.3	4.71	146.0	84.80	
	1.00	c							
flour or meal	100.00	g	345	10.5	74.5	4.00	309.0	296.0	
	148.00	g	511	15.5	110.	5.92	457.0	438.0	
	1.00	c							

QUINOA

	SERVING QUANTITY	UNIT	CALORIES (kcal)	PROTEIN (g)	TOTAL CARBOHYDRATES (g)	SODIUM (mg)	POTASSIUM (mg)	PHOSPHORUS (mg)	TOTAL
cooked	100.00	g	120	4.4	21.3	7.00	172.0	152.0	
	185.00	g	222	8.1	39.4	13.00	318.0	281.0	
	1.00	c							
uncooked	100.00	g	368	14.1	64.2	5.00	563.0	457.0	
	170.00	g	626	24.0	109	8.50	957.0	777.0	1
	1.00	c							
pasta from quinoa flour (gluten-free) not packed	100.00	g	152	3.2	31.1	4.00	63.00	91.00	
	132.00	g	201	4.3	41.1	5.28	83.20	120.0	
	1.00	c							

AMARANTH

Grain	100.00	g	102	3.8	18.7	6.00	135.0	148.0	
cooked	246.00	g	251	9.4	46.0	14.80	332.0	364.0	
	1.00	c							

CEREALS	SERVING QUANTITY	SERVING UNIT	CALORIES (kcal)	PROTEIN (g)	TOTAL CARBOHYDRATES (g)	SODIUM (mg)	POTASSIUM (mg)	PHOSPHORUS (mg)	TOTAL FAT (g)
corn flakes, plain (store brands)	100.00	g	357	7.5	84.1	729.00	168.0	102.0	0.40
	25.00	g	89	1.9	21.0	182.00	42.00	25.50	0.10
	1.00	c							
corn flakes, frosted (store brands)	100.00	g	389	4.3	90.2	451.00	82.00	46.00	0.87
	40.00	g	156	1.7	36.1	180.00	32.80	18.40	0.35
	1.00	c							
crsipy rice	100.00	g	383	6.7	86.2	545.00	106.0	98.00	1.26
	26.00	g	100	1.7	22.4	142.00	27.60	25.50	0.33
	1.00	c							
cocoa puffs (General Mills)	100.00	g	383	5.6	83.7	564.00	272.0	222.0	5.20
	36.00	g	138	2.0	30.1	203.00	97.90	79.90	1.87
	1.00	c							
muesli, with fruits & nuts	100.00	g	335	8.6	74.9	239.00	324.0	225.0	5.40
	85.00	g	302	7.3	63.7	203.00	275.0	191.0	4.59
	1.00	c							
muesli Brand: Safeway	100.00	g	386	8.8	73.7	228.00	474.0	175.0	5.26
	57.00	g	220	5.0	42.0	130.00	270.0	99.80	3.00
	1.00	svg							
granola, homemade, ready-to-eat	100.00	g	489	13.7	53.9	26.00	539.0	431.0	24.30
	122.00	g	597	16.7	65.8	31.70	658.0	526.0	29.60
	1.00	c							
granola bars, plain	100.00	g	471	10.1	64.4	294.00	336.0	277.0	19.80
	28.00	g	132	2.8	18.0	82.30	94.10	77.60	5.54
	1.00	bar/oz							
granola bars, almond	100.00	g	495	7.7	62.0	256.00	273.0	228.0	25.50
	28.35	g	140	2.2	17.6	72.60	77.40	64.60	7.23
	1.00	oz							

PANCAKE	SERVING QUANTITY	SERVING UNIT	CALORIES (kcal)	PROTEIN (g)	TOTAL CARBOHYDRATES (g)	SODIUM (mg)	POTASSIUM (mg)	PHOSPHORUS (mg)	TOTAL FAT
buttermilk (from recipe)	100.00	g	227	6.8	28.7	522.00	145.0	139.0	9
	38.00 1- 4" diameter	g pc	86	2.6	10.9	198.00	55.10	52.80	3
plain, (prepared from recipe)	100.00	g	227	6.4	28.3	439.00	132.0	159.0	9
	38.00 1- 4" diameter	g pc	86	2.4	10.8	167.00	50.20	60.40	3
plain, reduced fat	100.00	g	269	5.7	57.3	429.00	97.00	190.0	1
	105.00 3.00	g pcs	282	6.0	60.2	450.00	102.0	200.0	2
plain, frozen, ready to heat includes buttermilk	100.00	g	233	5.2	37.8	461.00	90.00	215.0	6
	40.00 1 (4")	g pc	93	2.1	15.1	184.00	36.00	86.00	2
gluten-free, frozen, ready to heat	100.00	g	215	3.3	40.3	331.00	127.0	306.0	4
	48.00 1.00	g pc	103	1.6	19.3	159.00	61.00	147.0	2
WAFFLE									
plain, prepared from recipe	100.00	g	291	7.9	32.9	511.00	159.0	190.0	1
	75.00 1 (7")	g pc	218	5.9	24.7	383.00	119.0	142.0	1

BREADS	SERVING QUANTITY	SERVING UNIT	CALORIES (kcal)	PROTEIN (g)	TOTAL CARBOHYDRATES (g)	SODIUM (mg)	POTASSIUM (mg)	PHOSPHORUS (mg)	TOTAL FAT (g)
whole wheat	100.00	g	252	12.5	42.7	455.0	254	212.0	3.50
	50.00	g	126	6.2	21.4	227.5	127.0	106.0	1.75
	2.00	slices							
white	100.00	g	266	8.9	49.4	490.0	126.0	98.00	490
	50.00	g	133	4.4	24.7	245.0	63.00	49.00	245
	2.00	slices							
french, small (2"x2.5"x1.75")	100.00	g	272	10.8	51.9	602.0	117.0	105.0	2.42
	32.00	g	87	3.4	16.6	192.6	37.44	33.60	0.77
	1.00	slice							
pita, 6.5"	100.00	g	275	9.1	55.7	536.0	120.0	97.00	1.20
	60.00	g	165	5.5	33.4	321.6	72.00	58.20	0.72
	1.00	pc							
sourdough	100.00	g	272	10.8	51.9	602.0	117.0	105.0	2.42
	50.00	g	136	5.4	25.9	301.0	58.50	52.50	1.21
	2.00	slices							
rye	100.00	g	259	8.5	48.3	603.0	166.0	125.0	33.00
	32.00	g	83	2.7	15.5	192.9	53.12	40.00	1.06
	1.00	slice							
bagels, wheat	100.00	g	250	10.2	48.9	439.0	165.0	142.0	1.53
	105.00	g	262	10.7	51.3	461.0	173.0	149.0	1.61
	1.00	reg pc							
biscuits	100.00	g	362	7.5	43.9	930.0	184.0	501.0	18.19
	45.00	g	163	3.4	19.8	418.0	82.80	225.0	8.19
	1.00	pc							
sprouted, wheat	100.00	g	188	13.2	33.9	474.0	198.0	176.0	0.00
	26.00	g	49	3.4	8.8	123.0	51.50	45.80	0.00
	1.00	slice							
cracked, wheat	100.00	g	274	10.7	47.5	473.0	141.0	129.0	4.53
	28.00	g	77	3.0	13.3	132.0	39.50	36.10	1.27
	1.00	reg slice							
tortillas, corn ready-to-bake or fry	100.00	g	218	5.7	44.6	45.00	186.0	314.0	2.85
	24.00	g	52	1.4	10.7	10.80	44.60	75.40	0.68
	1.00	Pc							
tortillas, flour approx. 6" diameter ready-to-bake or fry, refrigerated	100.00	g	306	8.2	49.4	736.0	125.0	206.0	7.99
	30.00	g	92	2.5	14.8	221.0	37.50	61.80	2.40
	1.00	pc							

BREADS

	SERVING QUANTITY	SERVING UNIT	CALORIES (kcal)	PROTEIN (g)	TOTAL CARBOHYDRATES (g)	SODIUM (mg)	POTASSIUM (mg)	PHOSPHORUS (mg)	TOTAL FAT (g)
tortilla, whole wheat	100.00	g	310	9.8	45.9	617.00	262.0	346.0	9.76
ready-to-bake or fry	41.00	g	127	4.0	18.8	253.00	107.0	142.0	4.00
	1.00	pc							
ciabatta (yeast bread) Italian, grecian, armenian thick slice	100.00	g	259	9.5	48.1	618.00	124.0	95.00	2.73
	43.00	g	111	4.1	20.7	266.00	53.30	40.80	1.17
	1.00	pc							
focaccia, plain (Italian flatbread)	100.00	g	249	8.8	35.8	561.00	114.0	128.0	7.89
	57.00	g	142	5.0	20.4	320.00	65.00	73.00	4.50
	1.00	pc							
Pita, medium	100.00	g	275	9.1	55.7	536.00	120.0	97.00	1.20
	57.00	g	157	5.2	31.7	306.00	68.40	55.30	0.68
	1.00	pc							
Naan, plain	100.00	g	291	9.6	50.4	465.00	125.0	100.0	5.65
	90.00	g	262	8.7	45.4	418.00	112.0	90.00	5.08
	1.00	pc							
Paratha, whole wheat, frozen	100.00	g	326	6.4	45.4	467.00	185.0	188.0	6.70
	79.00	g	258	5.0	35.9	495.00	196.0	199.0	7.10
	1.00	pc							
brioche	100.00	g	418	8.8	35.8	452.00	139.0	120.0	13.20
	77.00	g	322	6.7	27.6	357.00	110.0	94.80	10.40
	1.00	pc							
croissants, plain medium	100.00	g	406	8.2	45.8	440.00	120.0	125.0	26.80
	57.00	g	231	4.7	26.1	339.00	92.40	96.20	20.60
	1.00	pc							
croissants, chocolate	100.00	g	421	7.4	49.4	384.00	118.0	105.0	21.00
	57.00	g	240	4.2	28.2	219.00	67.30	59.80	12.00
	1.00	pc							
croissants, cheese	100.00	g	414	9.2	47.0	361.00	132.0	130.0	20.90
	57.00	g	236	5.2	26.8	206.00	75.22	74.10	11.90
	1.00	pc							
muffins, english, whole grain white	100.00	g	245	7.0	50.2	386.00	130.0	127.0	1.75
	57.00	g	140	4.0	28.6	220.00	74.10	72.40	1.00
	1.00	pc							
muffins, english, whole wheat	100.00	g	203	8.8	40.4	364.00	210.0	282.0	2.10
	66.00	g	134	5.8	26.7	240.00	139.0	186.0	1.39
	1.00	pc							

BREADS

	SERVING QUANTITY	SERVING UNIT	CALORIES (kcal)	PROTEIN (g)	TOTAL CARBOHYDRATES (g)	SODIUM (mg)	POTASSIUM (mg)	PHOSPHORUS (mg)	TOTAL FAT (g)
muffins, english,	100.00	g	235	9.1	46.3	298.00	156.0	81.00	1.80
mixed grain includes granola	66.00	g	155	6.0	30.6	197.00	103.0	53.40	1.19
	1.00	pc							
pumpernickle,	100.00	g	250	8.7	47.5	596.00	208.0	178.0	3.10
med or regular slice	32.00	g	80	2.8	15.2	191.00	66.60	57.00	0.99
	1.00	pc							
cinammon, medium or regular slice	100.00	g	253	7.1	44.4	388.00	74.00	57.00	5.29
	28.00	g	71	2.0	12.4	109.00	20.70	16.00	1.48
	1.00	pc							
raisin, med or regular slice	100.00	g	273	8.8	52.2	432.00	180.0	112.0	3.26
	28.00	g	76	2.5	14.6	121.00	50.40	31.40	0.91
	1.00	pc							
roll, multigrain med, reg, sandwich size	100.00	g	263	9.6	44.6	458.00	160.0	122.0	6.00
	43.00	g	113	4.1	19.2	197.00	68.80	52.50	2.58
	1.00	pc							
bread stuffing, homemade dry mix, prepared	100.00	g	177	3.1	21.7	471.00	72.00	41.00	8.51
	228.00	g	404	7.2	49.5	1,070	164.0	93.50	19.40
	1.00	pc							

GRITS

	SERVING QUANTITY	SERVING UNIT	CALORIES (kcal)	PROTEIN (g)	TOTAL CARBOHYDRATES (g)	SODIUM (mg)	POTASSIUM (mg)	PHOSPHORUS (mg)	TOTAL FAT (g)
corn, yellow, quick, unenriched cooked with water, no salt	100.00	g	59	1.4	12.9	2.00	21.00	11.00	0.19
	242.00	g	143	3.4	31.2	4.84	50.82	26.62	0.46
	1.00	c							
corn, white, quick, unenriched cooked with water	100.00	g	59	1.4	12.9	2.00	21.00	11.00	0.19
	242.00	g	143	3.4	31.2	4.84	50.82	26.62	0.46
	1.00	c							
POLENTA (cornmeal)	100.00	g							
	240.00	g	139	2.7	30.	170.00	50.40	36.00	0.67
	1	c							

PASTA

	SERVING QUANTITY	SERVING UNIT	CALORIES (kcal)	PROTEIN (g)	TOTAL CARBOHYDRATES (g)	SODIUM (mg)	POTASSIUM (mg)	PHOSPHORUS (mg)	TOTAL FAT (g)
spaghetti, unenriched, cooked	100.00	g	158	5.8	30.9	1.00	44.00	58.00	0.93
	70.00	g	111	4.1	21.6	0.70	30.80	40.60	0.65
	0.50	c							
spaghetti, enriched, cooked	100.00	g	158	5.8	30.9	1.00	44.00	58.00	0.93
	140.00	g	221	8.1	43.2	1.40	61.60	81.20	1.30
	1.00	c							
spaghetti, whole wheat, cooked	100.00	g	149	6.0	30.1	4.00	96.00	127.0	1.71
	140.00	g	209	8.4	42.1	5.60	134.4	177.8	2.39
	1.00	c							
bowtie/farfalle, enriched, cooked	100.00	g	136	4.8	27.4	1.10	24.51	-na-	0.55
	154.79	g	210	7.4	42.3	0.16	37.93	-na-	0.86
	1.00	c							
fusilli, enriched, cooked	100.00	g	161	5.7	32.5	1.30	29.09	-na-	0.66
	130.41	g	210	7.4	42.3	1.70	37.93	-na-	0.86
	1.00	c							
penne, enriched, cooked	100.00	g	169	6.0	34.1	1.37	30.55	-na-	0.69
	124.17	g	210	7.4	42.3	1.70	37.93	-na-	0.86
	1.00	c							
macaroni, enriched, cooked	100.00	g	133	4.7	26.8	1.08	24.04	-na-	0.54
	157.79	g	210	7.4	42.3	1.70	37.93	-na-	0.86
	1.00	c							
lasagna, enriched, boiled/drained	100.00	g	150	5.3	30.1	1.21	26.98	-na-	0.61
	140.62	g	210	7.4	42.3	1.70	37.93	-na-	0.86
	1.00	c							
whole grain, 51% whole wheat rest enriched semolina, cooked spaghetti, unenriched, cooked	100.00	g	156	5.7	30.9	4.00	71.00	97.00	1.48

CRACKERS	SERVING QUANTITY	SERVING UNIT	CALORIES (kcal)	PROTEIN (g)	TOTAL CARBOHYDRATES (g)	SODIUM (mg)	POTASSIUM (mg)	PHOSPHORUS (mg)	TOTAL FAT (g)
melba toast, rye	100.00	g	389	11.6	77.3	899.00	193.0	183.0	3.40
3 3/4" x 1 3/4" x 1/8"	15.00	g	58	1.7	11.6	134.85	28.95	27.45	0.51
	3.00	pcs							
melba toast, wheat	100.00	g	374	12.9	76.4	837.00	148.0	165.0	2.30
	15.00	g	56	1.9	11.5	125.55	22.20	24.75	0.35
	3.00	pcs							
saltine, low salt	100.00	g	421	9.5	74.3	198.00	724.0	111.0	8.85
(square)	15.00	g	63	1.4	11.2	29.70	108.6	16.65	1.33
	5.00	pcs							
saltine, fat-free, low sodium	100.00	g	393	10.5	82.3	849.00	115.0	113.0	1.60
	15.00	g	59	1.6	12.4	127.35	17.25	16.95	0.24
	3.00	pcs							
saltines, whole wheat/multi-grain	100.00	g	398	7.1	68.3	1,214	221.0	196.0	10.71
	14.00	g	56	1.0	9.6	169.96	30.94	27.44	1.50
	1.00	svg							
whole wheat, low salt	100.00	g	443	8.8	68.6	186.00	297.0	295.0	17.20
	28.00	g	124	2.5	19.2	52.08	83.16	82.60	4.82
	7.00	pcs							
whole wheat, reduced fat	100.00	g	416	11.3	75.5	745.00	373.0	364.0	7.59
1 svg = 29g	4.20	g	17	0.5	3.2	31.29	15.67	15.29	0.32
	1.00	pcs							
graham, plain or honey, low fat	100.00	g	386	5.7	78.0	629.00	171.0	163.0	5.71
	35.00	g	135	2.0	27.3	220.15	59.85	57.05	2.00
	1.00	svg							
goldfish (fish-shaped), flavored	100.00	g	463	10.2	65.7	970.00	224.0	167.0	17.71
	5.20	g	24	0.5	3.4	50.44	11.65	8.68	0.92
	10.00	pcs							
toast thins, low sodium	100.00	g	442	6.5	67.7	177.00	306.0	266.0	16.13
	31.00	g	137	2.0	21.0	54.87	94.86	82.46	5.00
	1.00	svg							

Part II: Kidney-Friendly Food Lists

Chapter 4: Foods to Avoid or Limit

Now that you have a comprehensive food list to guide your dietary choices, you may wonder which foods you should actively avoid or limit to align with your kidney health goals. Understanding what to steer clear of is essential for successful CKD management.

High-Potassium Foods

What is Potassium and Why is It Important?

Potassium is a vital mineral found in many foods, playing a crucial role in maintaining a regular heartbeat and ensuring proper muscle function. Healthy kidneys regulate potassium levels in the body, but when kidney function declines, you may need to limit foods that can elevate potassium levels to dangerous heights.

Certain medications, such as ACE inhibitors, ARBs, or diuretics like spironolactone, can also raise potassium levels. If you have high blood pressure and take these medications, keeping your potassium levels in check is critical. Symptoms of elevated potassium may include weakness, numbness, and tingling. In severe cases, dangerously high potassium can lead to irregular heartbeats or even heart attacks.

How Can You Keep Your Potassium Levels in Check?

- Limit High-Potassium Foods: Work with your renal dietitian to develop a meal plan that ensures you're getting the right amount of potassium.

- Moderation is Key: Aim for a variety of foods but in appropriate portions.
- Avoid Canned Liquid: Do not consume the liquid from canned fruits or vegetables, or juices from meats.
- Prepare Potatoes Wisely: If you want to include potatoes (which are high in potassium), peel, cut them into small pieces, soak them in water, boil, and then drain to reduce their potassium content.
- Consider Serving Sizes: Remember that nearly all foods contain some potassium; portion sizes significantly impact your overall intake. Eating a large quantity of low-potassium foods can inadvertently lead to a high-potassium meal.

What is a Safe Level of Potassium in Your Blood?

Consult your doctor or dietitian about your recent blood potassium level and record it here: _____

- SAFE Zone: 3.5 – 5.0 mg/dL
- CAUTION Zone: 5.1 – 6.0 mg/dL
- DANGER Zone: Above 6.0 mg/dL

High and Low Potassium Foods

Very High Potassium (Avoid as Much as Possible)	High Potassium (Consume Occasionally)	Low Potassium (Safe to Eat Daily)
Banana	Avocado	Apple
Orange juice	Cantaloupe, honeydew melon	Berries (strawberry, raspberries)
Prune juice	Dates, dried fruits, prunes, raisins	Cherries
Coconut milk	Kiwi, mango, orange	Grapes
Potato (white and sweet)	Artichoke, broccoli, Brussels sprouts	Peaches

Tomato and products	Dried beans, lima beans	Pear
Vegetable juice	Mushroom (canned)	Pineapple
Raisin bran cereal	Winter squash and pumpkin	Watermelon
Salt substitute (Lite salt)	Spinach and most greens (except kale)	Juices (cranberry, apple, grape)
	Organ meat	Asparagus, cucumber, eggplant
	Chocolate	Bean sprouts, green beans, green peas
		Cabbage, cauliflower, kale, lettuce
		Celery, onions, radish
		Corn, rice, noodles, pasta
		Bread and bread products
		Cereals (except raisin bran)
		Cakes, cookies (without nuts and chocolates)
		Coffee and tea

Note: High potassium foods contain more than 200 mg of potassium per serving. The serving size is typically 1/2 cup unless otherwise noted.

- Avoid very high potassium foods entirely.
- Limit high-potassium foods to two times per week, and do not consume them together on the same day.
- While meats, fish, and poultry are high in potassium, they are essential for maintaining good nutritional status, so include them in your diet as needed.

Low potassium foods contain less than 200 mg of potassium per serving (1/2 cup unless otherwise noted). You can enjoy these foods daily, but always be mindful of portion sizes.

High-Phosphorus Foods

What is Phosphorus?

Phosphorus is a mineral crucial for building strong bones and maintaining overall health, working alongside calcium.

Why is Phosphorus Important?

Healthy kidneys can effectively remove excess phosphorus from your blood. However, when you have chronic kidney disease, your kidneys struggle to eliminate phosphorus, leading to elevated levels that can cause significant health issues. High phosphorus can pull calcium from your bones, weakening them and causing dangerous deposits in your blood vessels, lungs, eyes, and heart. Therefore, managing phosphorus levels is vital for your overall health.

What is a Safe Blood Level of Phosphorus?

A normal phosphorus level ranges from 2.1 to 4.6 mg/dL. Consult your doctor or dietitian regarding your last phosphorus level and record it here: _____.

How Can I Control My Phosphorus Level?

You can maintain normal phosphorus levels through dietary management and medications. Work closely with your dietitian and doctor to create a plan. Below is a list of foods high in phosphorus that you should limit or avoid:

High Phosphorus Foods to Limit or Avoid:

Food Category	Foods to Avoid
Beverages	Ale, beer, chocolate drinks, cocoa, milk-based drinks, canned iced tea, dark colas
Dairy Products	Cheese, custard, milk, cream soups, cottage cheese, ice cream, pudding, yogurt

Protein	Beef liver, fish roe, oysters, crayfish, chicken liver, organ meats, sardines
Vegetables	Dried beans and peas (baked beans, black beans, chickpeas, kidney beans, lima beans, lentils, northern beans, split peas, soybeans)
Others	Bran cereals, brewer's yeast, caramels, nuts, seeds, wheat germ, whole grain products

What Should I Do If My Phosphorus Level is Too High?

If your phosphorus level is elevated, consider selecting foods from the low-phosphorus list. Discuss dietary changes with your dietitian and doctor, and inquire about phosphate binder prescriptions.

High Phosphorus Foods and Alternatives:

Instead of	Phos (mg)	Low Phosphorus Foods	Phos (mg)
8 oz milk	230	8 oz non-dairy creamer or 4 oz milk	110 115
8 oz cream soup (with milk)	275	8 oz cream soup (with water)	90
1 oz hard cheese	145	1 oz cream cheese	30
1/2 cup ice cream	80	1/2 cup sorbet or 1 popsicle	0
1/2 cup lima or pinto beans	100	1/2 cup mixed vegetables (green beans)	35
12 oz can cola	55	12 oz ginger ale or lemon soda	3
1/2 cup custard (with milk)	150	1/2 cup pudding (made with non-dairy creamer)	50
2 oz peanuts	200	1 1/2 cup light or low-fat popcorn	35

1 1/2 oz chocolate bar	125	1 1/2 oz hard candy (fruit flavors or jelly beans)	3
2/3 cup oatmeal	130	2/3 cup cream of wheat or grits	40
1/2 cup bran cereal	140-260	1/2 cup non-bran cereal (shredded wheat, rice cereals, or cornflakes)	50-100

High-Sodium Foods

What is Sodium?

Sodium is a mineral that naturally occurs in foods and is the primary component of table salt.

Why Should I Limit My Sodium Intake?

While some sodium is necessary for maintaining water balance in the body, excessive sodium intake can exacerbate conditions like high blood pressure and congestive heart failure, leading to:

- Increased thirst
- Fluid retention
- Elevated blood pressure

Reducing sodium in your diet can help manage these issues.

Tips to Cut Down Sodium Intake

- Cook with Herbs and Spices: Replace salt with herbs and spices for flavor.
- Read Food Labels: Choose foods low in sodium.
- Avoid Salt Substitutes: Steer clear of low-sodium products made with salt substitutes, as they often contain high potassium levels.

- Dining Out: Request meats or fish without added salt, and ask for sauces or gravies on the side, as they may contain large amounts of salt.

Food	Avoid	Choose
Dairy	Buttermilk, Cottage cheese, regular cheese	2%, 1% or skim milk, low fat yogurt, low sodium cheese
Meats	**Processed and luncheon meats** Ham, bacon, salt pork, sausage Hotdogs, corned beef, Spam, Pastrami **Breaded or fried meats** Chicken, fish pork or beef **Canned meats in oil** Sardines, salmon, tuna	Fresh beef, veal, pork, poultry, fish, eggs Low-salt deli meat
Starches	Salted crackers or bread, Pretzels Potato chips, corn chips, tortilla chips, popcorn Instant mashed potatoes Mixed muffins, pancakes, potatoes, noodles, some dry cereals	Fresh bread, most commercial bread Unsalted chips, crackers, pretzels Read labels for dry cereals Unsalted popcorn
Vegetables	Canned vegetables Pickles, sauerkraut, olives, relish, vegetable juice, vegetable soup tomato products Frozen vegetables with cheese or cream sauces	All plain fresh and frozen vegetables Low-sodium canned vegetables Low-sodium tomato sauces Homemade or low-sodium soups
Fruits	None	All
Condiments	Table salt, garlic salt, celery salt Lite salt, Bouillon cubes, seasoning	Fresh garlic, fresh onion, garlic

	salt, onion salt, lemon pepper, meat tenderizer, flavored enhancers, salt substitutes, catsup/ketchup, mustard, salad dressing, soy sauce, steak sauce, barbecue sauce, teriyaki sauce, oyster sauce, hot sauce, Worcestershire sauce	powder, onion powder, black pepper, lemon juice, low-sodium or salt-free seasoning blends, vinegar, homemade or low sodium sauces and salad dressings, dry mustard
Others	**Convenience foods** TV dinners, Chili, spaghetti, frozen prepared foods, fast foods, canned raviolis, macaroni & cheese **Most Chinese, Mexican, and Pizza restaurants**	Low sodium frozen dinner, home-made casseroles without added salt, soups made with fresh or raw vegetables, fresh meat, rice, pasta or unsalted canned vegetables Request no salt on foods when eating out. Ask for sauces on the side when dinning out.

Understanding Nutrition Labels

To help you keep sodium in check, understanding nutrition labels is essential. This knowledge will also assist you in monitoring potassium and protein content.

1. Portion Check: Look at the serving size and the number of servings per container. For example, if one serving is ⅔ cup, eating the entire package amounts to about 5 cups.

2. Calorie Control: Calories reflect the energy you receive per serving. For instance, if one serving provides 230 calories, consuming the entire package results in 1840 calories.

    • General Guidelines: Low = 50 calories per serving; High = 400 calories per serving.

3. Limit These Nutrients:

    • Saturated fat, trans fat, sodium, and added sugars.

    • Low Fat: 3 g or less of total fat per serving.

    • Low Sodium: 140 mg or less per serving; it's acceptable to choose items with less than 200 mg.

4. Get Enough of These Nutrients:

    - Look for foods rich in fiber, protein, and essential vitamins and minerals.
    - Key nutrients include:
        - Vitamin D, Calcium, and Iron
        - Fiber: 3 g or more per serving is good; 5 g or more is high.
        - Protein: Vital for energy, muscle maintenance, and wound healing. Consult your doctor or dietitian regarding your specific protein needs.

5. Watch for Potassium:

    - Based on your individual requirements, aim for low-potassium choices (less than 200 mg per serving). Discuss your potassium needs with your dietitian.

Part III: Meal Planning and Recipes

Chapter 5: Meal Planning for Kidney Health

Creating a Balanced Meal Plan

Developing a balanced meal plan for individuals with Chronic Kidney Disease (CKD) can be challenging due to the varying dietary requirements at each stage of the disease. However, it's essential to remember that every patient is unique, and these guidelines should be customized to meet individual needs and circumstances. Always consult with a healthcare provider or a renal dietitian before making any changes to your diet. In the following chapters, I will provide carefully selected CKD recipes, but for now, here are general daily meal plan guidelines for each CKD stage:

Stage 1 and 2 Chronic Kidney Disease (CKD) Daily Meal Plan Guidelines

Patients with Stage 1 and 2 CKD typically do not need to follow a strict renal diet. Instead, they should focus on a healthy, balanced diet that promotes overall health and slows disease progression.

The dietary guidelines below are general in nature, as individual needs can vary greatly based on age, sex, weight, physical activity level, and other health conditions. It's crucial to consult with a healthcare provider or a registered dietitian for personalized advice.

Caloric Intake

Maintaining a balanced caloric intake is vital for sustaining a healthy weight. The daily caloric requirement varies based on individual factors, but here is a general guideline:

- For Men: 2000 - 2500 calories per day
- For Women: 1600 - 2000 calories per day

Proteins

Protein is essential for growth, repair, and overall health. However, excessive protein intake can put additional strain on the kidneys. The recommended daily protein intake for CKD Stage 1 and 2 is approximately:

- 0.8 grams of protein per kilogram of body weight.

Carbohydrates

Carbohydrates serve as the body's primary energy source. Choose complex carbohydrates such as whole grains, fruits, and vegetables over simple sugars.

- Aim for about 45-65% of your daily caloric intake from carbohydrates.

Fats

Healthy fats are vital for heart health. Opt for unsaturated fats found in fish, nuts, seeds, avocados, and olives.

- Aim for about 20-35% of your daily caloric intake from fats.

Sample Meal Plan for Stages 1 and 2

Here's a sample meal plan that aligns with these guidelines:

Breakfast:

- 1 cup cooked oatmeal topped with a sprinkle of nuts
- 1 medium-sized banana
- 1 cup of skim milk or a dairy alternative

Lunch:

- 2 oz grilled chicken breast
- 1 cup steamed vegetables (such as broccoli or cauliflower)
- 1/2 cup cooked brown rice

Afternoon Snack:

- 1 small apple
- A handful of unsalted almonds

Dinner:

- 3 oz baked salmon
- 1 cup roasted sweet potato
- Side salad with mixed greens, tomatoes, cucumber, and a drizzle of olive oil dressing

Evening Snack:

- 1 cup low-fat yogurt topped with a sprinkle of berries

Remember to stay hydrated and limit your sodium intake, as excessive sodium can raise blood pressure and cause fluid retention, both of which can exacerbate kidney disease.

As CKD progresses to later stages (3 to 5), dietary needs will change significantly, often requiring decreased intake of protein, potassium, phosphorus, and sodium. Regular monitoring and consultation with healthcare providers are crucial.

Stage 3-5 Chronic Kidney Disease (CKD) Daily Meal Plan Guidelines

As kidney function declines in the later stages of CKD (Stages 3 to 5), the kidneys struggle to remove waste products from protein metabolism, necessitating a reduction in protein intake. Additionally, potassium, phosphorus, and sodium levels must be carefully monitored and limited.

These meal plans are general guidelines. Individual needs can vary greatly, so always consult with a healthcare provider or a registered dietitian for personalized advice.

Stage 3 CKD Daily Nutrient Requirements

- Caloric Intake:
    - For Men: 2000 - 2500 calories per day
    - For Women: 1600 - 2000 calories per day
- Proteins:
    - Approximately 0.8 grams per kilogram of body weight.
- Carbohydrates:
    - Aim for about 45-65% of your daily caloric intake from carbohydrates.
- Fats:
    - Aim for about 20-35% of your daily caloric intake from fats.
- Sodium:
    - Aim for less than 2000 mg per day.
- Potassium and Phosphorus:
    - Your healthcare provider will advise you based on your blood levels.

Stage 3 CKD Sample Meal Plan

Breakfast:

- 1 cup of cream of wheat
- 1 slice of toast with 1 tablespoon of jelly
- 1 small apple
- 1 cup of coffee or tea

Lunch:

- Turkey sandwich: 2 oz turkey on whole grain bread with lettuce and mayonnaise
- 15 grapes
- Water or unsweetened iced tea

Afternoon Snack:

- 1 medium-sized peach
- A handful of rice cakes

Dinner:

- 3 oz grilled chicken breast
- 1 cup of cooked zucchini
- 1/2 cup of white rice
- Water or homemade lemonade (watching for sugar content)

Evening Snack:

- 1 cup of low-fat vanilla yogurt

Stage 4 CKD Daily Nutrient Requirements

- Caloric Intake:
    - For Men: 2000 - 2500 calories per day
    - For Women: 1600 - 2000 calories per day
- Proteins:
    - Approximately 0.6 grams per kilogram of body weight.
- Carbohydrates:
    - Aim for about 45-65% of your daily caloric intake from carbohydrates.
- Fats:
    - Aim for about 20-35% of your daily caloric intake from fats.
- Sodium:
    - Aim for less than 2000 mg per day.
- Potassium and Phosphorus:
    - Your healthcare provider will advise you based on your blood levels, often recommending potassium to be limited to 2000-3000 mg per day and phosphorus to less than 800-1000 mg per day.

Stage 4 CKD Sample Meal Plan

Breakfast:

- 1/2 cup high-protein cereal with almond milk
- 1 slice of toast with margarine
- 1/2 cup fresh blueberries
- Coffee or tea

Lunch:

- Tuna salad (made with low-sodium canned tuna) on a bed of lettuce

- Sliced cucumber and cherry tomatoes
- 1/2 cup applesauce
- Water or unsweetened iced tea

Afternoon Snack:
- Rice cakes with a thin layer of cream cheese
- 1/2 cup fresh pineapple chunks

Dinner:
- 3 oz baked fish (like cod)
- 1 cup steamed green beans
- 1/2 cup mashed cauliflower
- Water or cranberry juice (unsweetened)

Evening Snack:
- 2 cups air-popped popcorn

Stage 5 CKD Daily Nutrient Requirements (Not on Dialysis)

- Caloric Intake:
    - For Men: 2000 - 2500 calories per day
    - For Women: 1600 - 2000 calories per day
- Proteins:
    - Approximately 0.6 grams per kilogram of body weight.
- Carbohydrates:
    - Aim for about 45-65% of your daily caloric intake from carbohydrates.
- Fats:
    - Aim for about 20-35% of your daily caloric intake from fats.
- Sodium:
    - Aim for less than 2000 mg per day.
- Potassium and Phosphorus:
    - Your healthcare provider will advise you based on your blood levels, often recommending potassium to be limited to 2000-3000 mg per day and phosphorus to less than 800-1000 mg per day.

Stage 5 CKD Sample Meal Plan

Breakfast:
- 1/2 cup cream of wheat
- White toast with jelly
- 1/2 cup sliced peaches (canned in juice, not syrup)
- Coffee or tea

Lunch:
- Egg salad sandwich: 1 boiled egg on white bread with lettuce and mayonnaise
- Apple slices
- Water or homemade lemonade (watching for sugar content)

Afternoon Snack:
- Rice cakes
- 15 fresh grapes

Dinner:
- 2 oz roasted chicken
- 1/2 cup cooked carrots
- 1/2 cup white rice
- Water or cranberry juice (unsweetened)

Evening Snack:
- 5 vanilla wafers

These meal plans aim to restrict protein, potassium, phosphorus, and sodium intake while providing adequate calories and other nutrients. However, dietary restrictions may vary based on specific lab results. Remember, these are general guidelines, and individual needs can differ significantly based on factors like age, sex, weight, physical activity level, and overall health. Always consult with a healthcare provider for personalized advice.

Portion Control and Serving Sizes

What Distinguishes a Portion from a Serving?

A portion refers to the quantity of food you choose to consume in one sitting, whether at a restaurant, from a packaged product, or at your own dining table. In contrast, a serving size is the specific amount of food defined on a product's Nutrition Facts label.

Serving sizes can vary across different products and may be measured in various units such as cups, ounces, grams, or countable units (like three crackers). Your chosen portion size may align with or differ from the listed serving size based on your appetite.

To determine how many servings are in a container, check the top of the label where "Servings per container" is stated just above "Serving size." For instance, if a frozen lasagna lists 1 cup as the serving size and contains four servings per container, consuming 2 cups (or half the package) means you're eating two servings, which would double the calories and other nutrients listed on the food label.

- Example Calculation:
    - 1 serving = 280 calories
    - 2 servings = 280 × 2 = 560 calories

It's crucial to consult with your doctor and dietitian to determine your daily requirements for protein, sodium, potassium, and phosphorus. Your needs may vary based on:

- Age
- Current weight and height
- Metabolism
- Gender
- Activity level
- Lab numbers

As a CKD patient, always compare general guidelines with what your healthcare team prescribes. To aid in this process, I've created a "Handy" food portioning guide in collaboration with Covenant Home Care to assist my patients.

Tips For Grocery Shopping

The grocery store is your gateway to a diverse selection of food that can contribute to your well-being, especially when living with chronic kidney disease (CKD). Making informed choices here can significantly influence your health. Here are eight tips to help you navigate your grocery shopping experience:

1. Check the Quality Before Buying: Fresh and nutritious foods tend to last longer than their less healthy counterparts. Examine fruits and vegetables for quality before purchasing. If they appear wilted or unusually discolored, opt for fresher options. Seasonal produce often provides the best flavor and affordability.

2. Avoid Processed Foods: Grocery stores offer a mix of healthful and less healthful options. To avoid processed foods, bypass candy and sugary snacks in favor of fresh fruits and vegetables.

Look for minimally processed alternatives, typically found in the natural food sections.

3. Don't Shop on an Empty Stomach: Hunger can influence your shopping habits, leading you to purchase items you wouldn't normally choose due to diminished willpower. Try to avoid shopping when you're feeling hungry.

4. Write Down a Grocery List and Stick with It: Creating a detailed grocery list before you shop can help ensure that you only buy what you need, preventing impulse purchases of unhealthy items. Use paper or a digital note-taking app for convenience. With a meal plan in place, your shopping list is already prepared!

5. Buy Whole Foods: Whole foods—those in their most natural state without added artificial flavors, sweeteners, or preservatives—are the best choice. Studies indicate that individuals who consume more whole foods have a lower body mass index (BMI) and are less likely to develop heart disease and diabetes. Avoid processed and packaged foods that contain unnecessary additives and fillers, which can add calories without contributing nutritional value.

Chapter 6. Renal Diet Recipes

Breakfast Dishes

Kidney Friendly Smoothies

GREEN DETOX SMOOTHIE

Servings:	2	Preparation Time	10 minutes

INGREDIENTS	DIRECTIONS
1 cup Romaine lettuce 1 cucumber (chopped) 1/2 lemon (juiced) 1 pears (peeled and chopped) 1 tbsp ginger (grated) 1 tbsp ground flax seed 1 1/2 cups water 5 Ice cubes	1. Place all ingredients together in a blender. Blend until smooth. Be patient! No one likes clumps in their smoothies. It may take 1 minute or longer to get a great, smoothie-consistency. 2. Divide between glasses and enjoy!

NUTRIENT FACTS	TOTAL	PER SERVING
Calories (kCal):	164	**82**
Proteins (g):	4	**2**
Carbohydrates (g):	38	**19**
Fats (g):	2	**1**
Potassium (mg):	647	**323.5**
Phosphorus (mg):	100	**50**
Sodium (mg):	11.24	**5.62**

FRESH MANGO SMOOTHIE

Servings:	2	Preparation Time	10 minutes

INGREDIENTS

1/2 cup frozen mango
1/2 cup frozen cauliflower
1 banana (medium)
1 1/2 cup water
1 1/2 tsp apple cider vinegar

DIRECTIONS

1. Place all ingredients in your blender and blend until smooth. Pour into a glass and enjoy!

NUTRIENT FACTS

	TOTAL	PER SERVING
Calories (kCal):	173	**86.5**
Proteins (g):	3	**1.5**
Carbohydrates (g):	43	**21.5**
Fats (g):	1	**0.5**
Potassium (mg):	648	**324**
Phosphorus (mg):	57	**28.5**
Sodium (mg):	17	**8.5**

Low Potassium Breakfast Bowls

BREAKFAST TRAIL MIX

Servings:	3	Preparation Time	5 mins or less

INGREDIENTS	DIRECTIONS
1 cup Corn cereal 1 cup Rice cereal 1/2 cup Cocoa cereal 1/2 cup mini rice cakes (plain or apple cinnamon)	1. Mix all ingredients together in a medium bowl then divide into 1 cup portions. 2. Serve dry or with your preferred milk.

NUTRIENT FACTS	TOTAL	PER SERVING
Calories (kCal):	*145*	**48.33**
Proteins (g):	*2*	**0.67**
Carbohydrates (g):	*32*	**10.67**
Fats (g):	*1*	**0.33**
Potassium (mg):	*210*	**70**
Phosphorus (mg):	*150*	**50**
Sodium (mg):	*600*	**200**

GRANOLA IN YOGURT & APPLESAUCE

| Servings: | 1 | Preparation Time | 5 mins |

INGREDIENTS

1/2 cup plain greek yogurt
1/4 cup unsweetened applesauce
1/4 cup granola
2 tbsps. pumpkin seeds

DIRECTIONS

1. Mix the yogurt and apple sauce together in a bowl.

2. Top with granola and pumpkin seeds. Enjoy!

NUTRIENT FACTS

	TOTAL	PER SERVING
Calories (kCal):	355	**355**
Proteins (g):	20	**20**
Carbohydrates (g):	31	**31**
Fats (g):	18	**18**
Potassium (mg):	336	**336**
Phosphorus (mg):	347	**347**
Sodium (mg):	196	**196**

Healthy Breakfast Sides

GUACAMOLE DIP & PLANTAIN CHIPS

Servings:	4	Preparation Time	10 mins

INGREDIENTS	DIRECTIONS
1 avocado (medium, ripe) 2 tbsps. nutritional yeast 1 tbsp lemon juice 1/4 tsp sea salt 1/2 cup plantain chips (store-bought or homemade)	1. In a bowl, mash together the avocado, nutritional yeast, lemon juice, and sea salt with a fork. 2. Place the guacamole in a bowl and serve with plantain chips. Enjoy!

NUTRIENT FACTS	TOTAL	PER SERVING
Calories (kCal):	247	**61.75**
Proteins (g):	7	**1.75**
Carbohydrates (g):	18	**4.5**
Fats (g):	18	**4.5**
Potassium (mg):	1470	**367.5**
Phosphorus (mg):	98	**24.5**
Sodium (mg):	611	**152.75**

Note:

1/2 cup plantain chips (store-bought or homemade): The content can vary greatly depending on the brand used. On average it might contain approximately 400mg of potassium, negligible amounts of phosphorus, and ~10-20mg of sodium.

Lunch Dishes

Light and Nourishing Salads

FARRO AND CHICKPEA BOWL

Servings:	3	Preparation Time	25 mins

INGREDIENTS	DIRECTIONS
1 1/2 cup chickpeas (cooked) 2 tbsps. balsamic vinegar 1 tbsp maple syrup (to taste) 1/2 cup chives (chopped) pinch of sea salt & black pepper (to taste) 1/2 cup farro (rinsed) 1/4 cup pesto 1 cup cherry tomatoes 1 tbsp avocado oil	1. Combine the chickpeas, balsamic vinegar, maple syrup, chives, salt, and pepper in a bowl. Set aside. 2. Meanwhile, cook the farro according to the package directions. 3. Stir in the pesto. Set aside. 4. Toss the tomatoes in oil, salt, and pepper on a baking sheet. 5. Broil for six to eight minutes on the middle rack. 6. Divide the farro, chickpeas, and tomatoes evenly between bowls. Enjoy!

NUTRIENT FACTS	*TOTAL*	PER SERVING
Calories (kCal):	*415*	**138.33**
Proteins (g):	*15*	**5**
Carbohydrates (g):	*54*	**18**
Fats (g):	*16*	**5.33**
Potassium (mg):	*1090*	**363.33**
Phosphorus (mg):	*382*	**127.33**
Sodium (mg):	*512*	**170.67**

PASTA SALAD NIÇOISE

Servings:	6	Preparation Time	25 mins
		Chill Time	1-2 hrs

INGREDIENTS

4 cups cooked small shell macaroni
1 tablespoon olive oil
2 cups fresh green beans, cut in 1-inch pieces
1/2 cup lemon juice
1/3 cup olive oil
2 teaspoons dry mustard
1 tablespoon chopped fresh parsley
1 teaspoon basil
1 7-3/4-oz can tuna packed in water, drained
5 green onions, chopped, including tops
1/4 teaspoon pepper

DIRECTIONS

1. Combine the chickpeas, balsamic vinegar, maple syrup, chives, salt, and pepper in a bowl. Set aside.

2. Meanwhile, cook the farro according to the package directions.

3. Stir in the pesto. Set aside.

4. Toss the tomatoes in oil, salt, and pepper on a baking sheet.

5. Broil for six to eight minutes on the middle rack.

6. Divide the farro, chickpeas, and tomatoes evenly between bowls. Enjoy!

NUTRIENT FACTS	TOTAL	PER SERVING
Calories (kCal):	304	**50.67**
Proteins (g):	15	**2.50**
Carbohydrates (g):	25	**4.17**
Fats (g):	16	**2.67**
Potassium (mg):	1545	**257.50**
Phosphorus (mg):	519	**86.50**
Sodium (mg):	381	**63.50**

Kidney Friendly Sandwich/Wraps

BLUEBERRY COCONUT CREPES

| Servings: | 3 | Preparation Time | 15 mins |

INGREDIENTS

1/4 cup canned coconut milk
1/4 cup frozen blueberries
4 eggs (large)
3 tbsps. coconut flour
1/8 tsp sea salt
2 tbsps. coconut oil (divided)

DIRECTIONS

1. Add the coconut milk, blueberries, eggs, coconut flour, and salt to a blender. Blend until smooth.

2. Heat a bit of the coconut oil in a skillet over medium heat.

3. Pour 1/4 cup of the batter at a time and gently swirl to spread it into a thin layer. Cook each side for about 30 seconds to one minute.

4. Repeat with the remaining batter and coconut oil.

5. Divide the crepes onto plates and enjoy!

NUTRIENT FACTS	TOTAL	PER SERVING
Calories (kCal):	248.01	**82.67**
Proteins (g):	9.99	**3.33**
Carbohydrates (g):	6.99	**2.33**
Fats (g):	20.01	**6.67**
Potassium (mg):	373.98	**124.66**
Phosphorus (mg):	567.99	**189.33**
Sodium (mg):	604.02	**201.34**

STACKED VEGETABLE SANDWICH

Servings:	1	Preparation Time	5 mins

INGREDIENTS

2 tbsps. hummus
2 slices whole grain bread
1/16 green lettuce (leaves separated)
1/4 tomato (medium, sliced)
1/4 cup radishes (trimmed, sliced)
1 tbsp red onion (sliced)
1/2 carrot (small, shredded)

DIRECTIONS

1. Spread the hummus on the bread.

2. Add the remaining sandwich toppings.

3. Close the sandwich and enjoy!

NUTRIENT FACTS	TOTAL	PER SERVING
Calories (kCal):	317	**317**
Proteins (g):	14	**14**
Carbohydrates (g):	46	**46**
Fats (g):	9	**9**
Potassium (mg):	567	**567**
Phosphorus (mg):	177	**177**
Sodium (mg):	476	**476**

Dinner Dishes

Main Course

LEMON, GARLIC, & HERB PASTA

Servings:	3	Preparation Time	20 mins

INGREDIENTS	DIRECTIONS
2 cups brown rice penne (uncooked) 2 cups chickpeas (cooked, drained) 1 tbsp extra virgin olive oil 1 1/2 tbsp lemon juice 2 garlic cloves (minced) 1/2 tsp oregano pinch of sea salt & black pepper (to taste) 2 tbsps. parsley (chopped) 2 tbsps. basil leaves (chopped) 2 tbsps. fresh dill (chopped) Note: Pinch = 1/16 teaspoon	1. Cook pasta according to the package. 2. While the pasta is cooking, in a bowl, add the chickpeas, olive oil, lemon juice, garlic, oregano, salt and pepper. Mix to combine and set aside to marinate. 3. Add the pasta to a serving bowl followed by the chickpea mix (including the liquid). 4. Toss to combine. Add the parsley, basil, dill and toss again. Divide into bowls and enjoy!

NUTRIENT FACTS	TOTAL	PER SERVING
Calories (kCal):	506	**168.67**
Proteins (g):	15	**5**
Carbohydrates (g):	89	**29.67**
Fats (g):	10	**3.33**
Potassium (mg):	1087	**362.33**
Phosphorus (mg):	622	**207.33**
Sodium (mg):	182	**60.67**

COUSCOUS & MUSHROOM BOWL

Servings: 2 Preparation Time 25 mins

INGREDIENTS

2 eggs
2 tsps. extra virgin olive oil (divided)
1 cup Israeli couscous
2 cups water
2 tbsps. shallots (peeled, chopped)
2 garlic cloves (minced)
6 cremini mushrooms (sliced)
Pinch of sea salt & black pepper (to taste)

Note: Pinch = 1/16 teaspoon

DIRECTIONS

1. Place eggs in a saucepan and cover with water. Bring to a boil over high heat. Once boiling, turn off the heat but keep the saucepan on the hot burner. Cover and let sit for 10 to 12 minutes.
2. Strain the water and fill the saucepan with cold water. Once cooled, peel, halve and set aside.
3. Heat half the oil in a saucepan over medium heat. Add the couscous and toast for one to two minutes, stirring often.
4. Pour in the water and bring to a simmer and cook for 8 to 10 minutes, until cooked through. Drain excess water and set aside.
5. In a skillet over medium-low heat, pour in the remaining oil. Add the shallot and sauté until softened, about three minutes.
6. Then add the garlic and mushrooms and continue cooking until the mushrooms are cooked through and water is released, about five minutes.
7. Divide the couscous into bowls and top with mushrooms and the egg. Season with salt and pepper. Enjoy!

NUTRIENT FACTS

	TOTAL	PER SERVING
Calories (kCal):	*393*	**196.5**
Proteins (g):	*17*	**8.5**
Carbohydrates (g):	*59*	**29.5**
Fats (g):	*9*	**4.5**
Potassium (mg):	*530*	**265**
Phosphorus (mg):	*342*	**171**
Sodium (mg):	*304*	**152**

Side Dish

HALLOUMI MUSHROOM TACOS

Servings:	2	Preparation Time	20 mins

INGREDIENTS	DIRECTIONS
1 tsp extra virgin olive oil 6 cremini mushrooms (sliced) pinch of sea salt & black pepper (to taste) 2.5 ozs halloumi (sliced) 1/2 cup pineapple (chopped) 2 tbsps. cilantro (chopped) 2 tbsps. lime juice 4 corn tortillas Note: Pinch = 1/16 teaspoon	1. Heat the oil in a pan over medium-high heat. Add the mushrooms and cook for three to five minutes or until golden brown. Season with salt and pepper. Remove and set them aside. 2. In a small bowl, mix together the pineapple, cilantro, and lime juice. 3. Divide the mushrooms and halloumi between the tortillas. 4. Top with pineapple salsa, season with additional salt and pepper if needed, and enjoy! 5. In the same pan, cook the halloumi slices until golden brown, about one to two minutes per side.

NUTRIENT FACTS	TOTAL	PER SERVING
Calories (kCal):	475	**237.50**
Proteins (g):	22	**11**
Carbohydrates (g):	36	**18**
Fats (g):	26	**13**
Potassium (mg):	604	**302**
Phosphorus (mg):	809	**404.50**
Sodium (mg):	905	**452.5**

Kidney Friendly Dessert

FRESH FRUIT AND SWEET CRANBERRY DIP

Servings: 24	Preparation Time	10 mins
	Chill time	At least 30 mins

INGREDIENTS

- 8 ounces sour cream
- 1/2 cup whole berry cranberry sauce
- 1/4 teaspoon nutmeg
- 1/4 teaspoon ground ginger
- 4 medium pears, sliced into 12 slices each
- 4 medium apples, cut into 12 slices each
- 4 cups fresh pineapple, cut into bite-size pieces
- 1 teaspoon lemon juice

DIRECTIONS

1. Put sour cream, cranberry sauce, nutmeg and ground ginger in a food processor. It should be well-mixed, then transfer to a small bowl.

2. Then, cut the fresh fruit into small pieces. To prevent browning, toss apple and pear with lemon juice.

3. For final touches, arrange the fruits on platter with dip bowl then chill until ready.

NUTRIENT FACTS	TOTAL	PER SERVING
Calories (kCal):	70	**2.92**
Proteins (g):	0	**0**
Carbohydrates (g):	13	**0.54**
Fats (g):	2	**0.08**
Potassium (mg):	2791	**116.29**
Phosphorus (mg):	320	**13.33**
Sodium (mg):	129	**5.38**

Snacks

Healthy Snack Options

LEMON, GARLIC, & HERB PASTA

Servings:	3	Preparation Time	20 mins

INGREDIENTS	DIRECTIONS
2 cups brown rice penne (uncooked) 2 cups chickpeas (cooked, drained) 1 tbsp extra virgin olive oil 1 1/2 tbsp lemon juice 2 garlic cloves (minced) 1/2 tsp oregano pinch of sea salt & black pepper (to taste) 2 tbsps. parsley (chopped) 2 tbsps. basil leaves (chopped) 2 tbsps. fresh dill (chopped) Note: Pinch = 1/16 teaspoon	1. Cook pasta according to the package. 2. While the pasta is cooking, in a bowl, add the chickpeas, olive oil, lemon juice, garlic, oregano, salt and pepper. Mix to combine and set aside to marinate. 3. Add the pasta to a serving bowl followed by the chickpea mix (including the liquid). 4. Toss to combine. Add the parsley, basil, dill and toss again. Divide into bowls and enjoy!

NUTRIENT FACTS	TOTAL	PER SERVING
Calories (kCal):	*506*	**168.67**
Proteins (g):	*15*	**5**
Carbohydrates (g):	*89*	**29.67**
Fats (g):	*10*	**3.33**
Potassium (mg):	*1087*	**362.33**
Phosphorus (mg):	*622*	**207.33**
Sodium (mg):	*182*	**60.67**

CHOCOLATE PEANUT BUTTER MUFFIN

Servings:	9	Preparation Time	40 mins

INGREDIENTS	DIRECTIONS
3 bananas (medium, ripe, mashed) 3 eggs 1/3 cup maple syrup 1/2 tsp vanilla extract 3 tbsps. Coconut oil 1/2 tsp sea salt 1 cup all natural peanut butter (divided) 1/2 tsp baking soda 1 tsp baking powder 1/2 cup cacao powder	1. Preheat the oven to 375°F (190°C). Line a muffin tray with liners or use a silicone muffin tray. 2. Mix the mashed banana and egg together. Using a hand mixer or stand mixer is best, but a whisk will also work. 3. Slowly add the maple syrup and vanilla and continue mixing. Next, add the oil until an even consistency is achieved. 4. Add the salt and 3/4 of the peanut butter. Continue to mix, then add the baking soda and baking powder. Slowly add the cacao powder. Continue to mix until a pancake batter-like consistency is achieved. 5. Fill each muffin liner with the batter, approximately 1/3 cup each. Add the remaining peanut butter onto the top of each muffin and if desired, swirl with a toothpick. 6. Bake in the oven for 25 minutes or until muffin tops are firm. Remove from the oven, allow to cool in the muffin tin for 10 minutes before removing. Enjoy!

NUTRIENT FACTS	TOTAL	PER SERVING
Calories (kCal):	334	**37.11**
Proteins (g):	10	**1.11**
Carbohydrates (g):	26	**2.89**
Fats (g):	23	**2.56**
Potassium (mg):	3398	**377.56**
Phosphorus (mg):	860	**95.56**
Sodium (mg):	3002	**333.67**

CHEESY TORTILLA ROLLUPS

Servings:	4	Preparation Time	10 mins

INGREDIENTS

½ cup whipped cream cheese

2 flour tortillas, burrito size

½ cup raw spinach leaves, chopped

2 tablespoons onion, diced

2 tablespoons pimento, diced

½ cup crushed pineapple, drained

3 ounces unprocessed cooked turkey breast, diced small

1 teaspoon Mrs. Dash® original blend herb seasoning

DIRECTIONS

1. First, place cream cheese over each tortilla to cover and sprinkle with Mrs. Dash® herb seasoning.

2. In a bowl, put remaining ingredients and mix.

3. Divide mixed ingredients into 2 portions and place half on each tortillas.

4. Roll it up and slice each roll into 4 pieces.

NUTRIENT FACTS	TOTAL	PER SERVING
Calories (kCal):	956	**239**
Proteins (g):	41.3	**10.33**
Carbohydrates (g):	99.5	**24.88**
Fats (g):	45.67	**11.42**
Potassium (mg):	1080	**270**
Phosphorus (mg):	415	**103.75**
Sodium (mg):	916	**229**

Hydration Tips and Safe Beverages

Hydration is essential for everyone, including individuals with chronic kidney disease (CKD). However, those with CKD may need to monitor and potentially limit their fluid intake, particularly as the disease progresses. Here are some key hydration tips and safe beverage suggestions to consider:

Monitor Your Fluid Intake

Depending on the stage of your CKD and whether you're on dialysis, your healthcare provider or dietitian may recommend limiting your fluid intake. This includes not only drinks but also foods that are liquid at room temperature, such as ice cream or gelatin.

Choose Water

Water is typically the best choice for hydration. It is calorie-free and free from sodium, potassium, and phosphorus, making it an ideal option for maintaining hydration without adding unnecessary nutrients that could affect kidney health.

Limit High-Potassium Drinks

Avoid beverages that are high in potassium, such as:

- Orange juice
- Tomato juice
- Prune juice
- Certain sports drinks

Limit High-Phosphorus Drinks

Stay away from drinks that are high in phosphorus, including:

- Beer
- Cola drinks

Many dark-colored sodas contain phosphorus additives that can contribute to elevated phosphorus levels in the body.

Limit Sodium-Rich Drinks

Be cautious with beverages that may be high in sodium, such as:

- Canned soups and broths
- Bottled sauces
- Sports drinks
- Any drinks labeled as "high in sodium"

Limit Alcohol

Alcohol can lead to dehydration and place additional stress on your kidneys. It's best to limit or avoid alcohol consumption altogether.

Beware of Coffee and Tea

Both coffee and tea can be high in potassium. If you choose to drink them, limit your intake to small amounts and consider counting them towards your daily fluid allowance.

Avoid Energy Drinks

Energy drinks often contain high levels of sodium, sugar, and caffeine, which can be detrimental to your kidney health.

Herbal Infusions

Some herbal teas may be a suitable option, but it's crucial to check with your healthcare provider or dietitian first, as certain herbs can affect kidney function.

Stay Cool

Try to avoid overheating, as sweating leads to increased water loss. Staying cool can help you maintain proper hydration levels.

Final Reminder

These guidelines are general in nature, and individual hydration needs can vary significantly. Always consult with your healthcare provider or dietitian to determine the best hydration plan tailored to your specific situation.

Part IV: Thriving with Kidney Disease

Chapter 7: Living with Kidney Disease

Myths and Facts about CKD

Despite the abundance of information available about kidney disease, many people still rely on hearsay, leading to confusion and misinformation. Here are some common myths and facts about Chronic Kidney Disease (CKD) to help clarify misunderstandings and allow you to focus on what truly matters.

Myth 1: CKD is Rare

Fact: CKD is not rare. It affects millions of people worldwide. According to the National Kidney Foundation, approximately 37 million American adults have CKD, and many are unaware of their condition.

Myth 2: There Are Clear Symptoms of CKD in the Early Stages

Fact: Most people with early-stage CKD do not exhibit clear symptoms. CKD is often referred to as a "silent" disease because it can progress without noticeable signs. This highlights the importance of regular check-ups, especially for individuals with risk factors such as diabetes, high blood pressure, or a family history of kidney disease.

Myth 3: If You Have CKD, You Will Definitely Need Dialysis or a Transplant

Fact: Not everyone with CKD progresses to kidney failure requiring dialysis or a transplant. With proper management, including lifestyle changes and medications, the progression of CKD can often be slowed or halted.

Myth 4: A High-Protein Diet is Good for Your Kidneys

Fact: A high-protein diet can actually strain your kidneys and may accelerate kidney damage in individuals with CKD. A balanced diet that includes an appropriate amount of protein is recommended.

Myth 5: Drinking More Water Will Keep Your Kidneys Healthy and Can Cure CKD

Fact: While staying hydrated is important, drinking more water than your body needs won't necessarily improve kidney function or cure CKD. In later stages of CKD, patients may need to limit fluid intake.

Myth 6: Only Adults Can Get CKD

Fact: While CKD is more common in adults, particularly older adults, children can also develop kidney disease.

Myth 7: CKD Only Happens if You Have a Pre-existing Health Condition

Fact: Although conditions like diabetes and high blood pressure significantly increase the risk of developing CKD, it can also be caused by other factors, such as certain medications, urinary tract obstructions, or inherited conditions.

Remember, if you have any questions or concerns about CKD, it's always best to consult with a healthcare provider for accurate information.

Coping Strategies

Living with Chronic Kidney Disease (CKD) presents challenges, but several strategies can help you manage the condition and maintain a good quality of life:

1. Follow Your Treatment Plan: Adhere to the treatment plan laid out by your healthcare team. This often includes managing underlying conditions like diabetes or hypertension, taking prescribed medications, following dietary guidelines, and maintaining a healthy lifestyle with regular exercise and, if applicable, smoking cessation.

2. Focus on Nutrition: Nutrition plays a vital role in managing CKD. Collaborating with a dietitian who specializes in kidney disease can be immensely beneficial. They can provide personalized advice based on your specific needs and help you navigate dietary restrictions while ensuring you receive essential nutrients.

3. Schedule Regular Check-Ups: Regular check-ups are crucial for monitoring kidney function and adjusting treatment as needed. Blood tests can help track the progression of the disease and guide necessary changes in medication or diet.

4. Manage Emotional Health: CKD can impact mental well-being, leading to feelings of anxiety, depression, or fear. Mental health professionals, such as psychologists or counselors, can provide support and teach coping strategies to manage these feelings.

5. Join a Support Group: Connecting with others who share similar experiences can provide comfort, reduce feelings of isolation, and allow for the sharing of practical advice. Organizations like the National Kidney Foundation (NKF) offer resources for finding local support groups.

6. Educate Yourself: Understanding CKD can empower you to manage your condition effectively. Reliable sources of information include your healthcare team and reputable health websites. The NKF and the American Kidney Fund offer extensive resources for patients and their families.

7. Lean on Your Support Network: Friends and family can provide emotional support, assist with practical tasks, and accompany you to medical appointments. Sharing your experiences with them can help them understand what you're going through and how they can support you.

Living with CKD requires adjustments, but with the right resources and support, patients can lead fulfilling lives while managing their condition. Always remember, you are not alone in this journey, and numerous resources are available to help.

Working with Your Healthcare Providers

Effectively collaborating with your healthcare team is crucial for managing Chronic Kidney Disease (CKD). Here are some strategies to help you maximize this relationship:

1. Open Communication: Be honest with your healthcare providers. Share all your symptoms, even those you think might not be related to your kidney disease. The more information they have, the better they can tailor your treatment plan.

2. Prepare for Appointments: Before each appointment, make a list of any questions or concerns you have. This may include new symptoms, side effects from medications, or worries about diet and lifestyle changes.

3. Understand Your Treatment Plan: Ensure you fully understand your treatment plan and the rationale behind each component. If something is unclear, don't hesitate to ask your doctor to explain it in simpler terms.

4. Role of the Dietitian: A dietitian specializing in kidney disease is an essential part of your healthcare team. They can provide personalized dietary advice based on your specific needs while helping you navigate dietary restrictions. Regularly consult with your dietitian and keep them informed about any changes in your health status.

5. Regular Monitoring: Consistent blood tests and other diagnostic evaluations are vital for tracking CKD's progression and adjusting treatment as necessary. Always attend scheduled appointments and follow through with recommended tests.

6. Follow Through: Stick to the prescribed medication regimen and dietary advice, even when you're feeling well. Consistency is key in managing CKD.

7. Share Your Feelings: Don't forget to discuss your emotional health with your healthcare team. CKD can significantly impact mental well-being, leading to anxiety or depression. There are resources available to help manage these aspects of living with a chronic illness.

8. Involve Your Family: If comfortable, consider including family members in discussions with your healthcare team. They can

provide additional support, help remember information or instructions, and gain a better understanding of your experiences.

Remember, your healthcare team is there to support you in managing CKD. Reach out to them with any concerns or questions you may have; they can provide valuable guidance and resources to help you navigate this journey.

Conclusion

Living with Chronic Kidney Disease (CKD) is a journey that requires strength, resilience, and, most importantly, knowledge. This guide has been crafted to equip you with comprehensive information and resources to help you effectively manage your condition. As we conclude this book, it's essential to revisit the key insights and takeaways that can empower you on your path toward better kidney health.

Understanding CKD, including its causes, diagnosis, and symptoms, is the first step in managing this condition. Regular monitoring of your kidney health is vital for tracking your progress and making necessary adjustments to your treatment plan.

The cornerstone of effective CKD management lies in adhering to a kidney-friendly diet. This involves careful monitoring of key nutrients such as potassium, phosphorus, sodium, and protein. Additionally, hydration and fluid management play a crucial role in maintaining kidney health.

The renal diet food list provided in this guide serves as a valuable resource for making informed dietary choices. Remember, it's not just about avoiding certain foods but also about incorporating kidney-friendly options into your meals.

Meal Planning

Meal planning is a significant aspect of managing your diet. The importance of a well-researched food list cannot be overstated; it acts as a roadmap to navigate the often complex dietary needs associated with CKD. By understanding which foods are high in potassium, phosphorus, sodium, and protein, you can effectively control your intake of these key nutrients, which is essential for managing your kidney health.

The guidelines and sample meal plans provided for different stages of CKD offer practical roadmaps for creating balanced meals that cater to your nutritional needs without compromising flavor.

Portion Control and Nutrition Labels

Mastering portion control and understanding nutrition labels are essential skills that can help you manage your dietary intake more effectively. The grocery shopping tips included in this guide provide practical advice for selecting the right foods during your shopping trips.

The recipe sections for breakfast, lunch, dinner, snacks, and beverages offer a variety of options to keep your meals interesting and enjoyable while remaining kidney-friendly.

Knowledge is Power

Living with CKD also involves dispelling myths and understanding the facts about the condition. Knowledge is empowering and can help you take control of your health.

Coping strategies and effective collaboration with your healthcare providers are integral to managing CKD. Open communication with your healthcare team can significantly enhance the effectiveness of your care.

Final Thoughts

In conclusion, while CKD may necessitate specific lifestyle adjustments, having a well-researched food list at your disposal empowers you to take charge of your health. Alongside regular consultations with your healthcare team and the utilization of available resources, you can continue to lead a fulfilling life.

Remember, every step you take toward better management of your condition is a step toward improved health and well-being. You are not alone on this journey; with the right knowledge and support, you can successfully manage CKD.

Appendix A: Glossary

A

- Albumin: A protein in the blood that can indicate kidney function when found in urine.
- Albuminuria: A condition characterized by an excessive amount of the protein albumin in the urine, often indicating kidney damage.

B

- Blood Levels: A term referring to the amount of a particular substance, such as potassium or phosphorus, present in the blood.
- Body Weight: A person's mass or weight, typically measured in kilograms.

C

- Caloric Intake: The total amount of calories consumed in a day, which can vary based on factors like age, sex, weight, and physical activity level.
- Calories: A unit used to measure the amount of energy that food provides when eaten and digested.
- Carbohydrates: One of the three macronutrients, along with protein and fat; carbohydrates are important sources of energy for the body.
- Chronic Kidney Disease (CKD): A long-term condition where the kidneys do not work as well as normal, leading to progressive loss of kidney function.
- Dietary Fiber: Nutrient in our diet that is not digested by gastrointestinal enzymes but fulfills an important role for digestive health.
- Dietitian: A healthcare professional who specializes in diet and nutrition, providing personalized dietary advice based on specific needs and health conditions.

- Dietary Guidelines: Recommendations provided by reputable scientific organizations pertaining to health and nutrition.

D

- Dialysis: A treatment that filters and purifies the blood using a machine to maintain balance in the body when the kidneys cannot perform these functions.

- Diabetes: A chronic disease affecting the body's ability to use sugar for energy, potentially leading to high blood sugar levels and kidney damage.

- Dietary Requirements: The levels of intake of essential nutrients considered adequate to meet the known nutritional needs
of practically all healthy people.

E

- End-Stage Renal Disease (ESRD): A term used when kidney failure reaches an advanced stage, necessitating dialysis or kidney transplantation.

F

- Fats: One of the three main macronutrients, along with carbohydrates and protein; fats are a concentrated source of energy.

- Glomerular Filtration Rate (GFR): A test used to assess how well the kidneys are functioning, specifically estimating how much blood passes through the glomeruli each minute.

H

- Hemodialysis: A treatment for kidney failure that uses a machine to filter the patient's blood outside the body and return it back to circulation.

- Healthcare Provider: A person who helps prevent or treat illness or injury, including doctors, nurses, and allied health professionals.

- Hypertension: Also known as high blood pressure, a condition that can damage blood vessels and organs, including the kidneys.

K

- Kidney Failure: A condition in which the kidneys lose their ability to function properly, often requiring dialysis or transplantation.
- Kidney Function: The ability of the kidneys to filter waste products from the blood and regulate fluid and electrolyte balance.
- Kilogram: The basic unit of mass in the metric system, commonly used to measure body weight.
- Potassium: An essential nutrient that helps nerves and muscles communicate and assists in moving nutrients into cells and waste products out of cells. Excess potassium can be harmful in CKD.

M

- Management: The process of dealing with or controlling health conditions, particularly in the context of chronic illnesses like CKD.
- Myths: Common misconceptions or false beliefs about a subject, such as chronic kidney disease.

N

- Nephrologist: A doctor who specializes in diagnosing and treating diseases of the kidneys.
- Nutrient Requirements: The levels of intake of essential nutrients considered adequate to meet the known nutritional needs of practically all healthy people.
- Peritoneal Dialysis: A treatment for patients with severe chronic kidney disease where sterile fluid containing glucose is introduced into the abdomen, absorbs waste products, and is then drained out.

P

- Phosphorus: A mineral crucial for healthy bones and teeth; excess phosphorus levels can indicate impaired kidney function.

- Physical Activity Level: A measure of a person's daily physical activity, used to estimate total energy expenditure.
- Portion Control: The practice of managing the amount of food consumed in one sitting, which can help control calorie intake.
- Protein: A macronutrient essential for building muscle mass and overall health; its intake may need to be monitored in CKD.
- Proteinuria: The presence of excess proteins in the urine, often indicative of kidney damage.
- Renal Dietitian: A dietitian who specializes in the dietary management of diseases affecting the kidneys, providing personalized advice to patients with CKD.

S

- Serving Size: The amount of food or drink that is generally served, used to quantify recommended amounts, nutrient content, and caloric values in dietary guidelines and food labels.
- Sodium: A mineral crucial for maintaining blood pressure and fluid balance; CKD patients may have difficulty regulating sodium levels.
- Trans Fat: A type of dietary fat associated with an increased risk of heart disease.
- Unsaturated Fats: Healthy fats that are liquid at room temperature, such as olive oil and canola oil, which can help improve cholesterol levels.

U

- Uremia: A high level of waste products in the blood due to poor kidney function or kidney failure.
- Urine: Liquid waste produced by the kidneys and excreted by the body; in CKD, the kidneys may not effectively produce urine.

V

- Vitamins: Organic compounds required by the body in small amounts to sustain life; essential for various bodily functions.
- World Health Organization (WHO): A specialized agency of the United Nations responsible for international public health.

Appendix B: Resources

BIDMC Food Prioritization Project by https://www.renaltracker.com
Food List Reference: USDA FoodData Central – https://www.fdc.nal.usda.gov

The Basics of a Kidney-Friendly Diet:
1. National Kidney Foundation. (2015). A to Z Health Guide. https://www.kidney.org/atoz/content/diet
2. Kidney Care UK. (2021). Fluid control for kidney patients. https://www.kidneycareuk.org/about-kidney-health/living-kidney-disease/kidney-kitchen/factsheets/fluid-control-kidney-patients/
3. National Institute of Diabetes and Digestive and Kidney Diseases. (2017). Eating & Nutrition for Hemodialysis. https://www.niddk.nih.gov/health-information/kidney-disease/kidney-failure/hemodialysis/eating-nutrition

Meal Planning for Kidney Health
1. National Kidney Foundation: Nutrition and Chronic Kidney Disease (Stages 1–4) https://www.kidney.org/atoz/content/nutrichronic
2. National Kidney Foundation: Nutrition and Early Kidney Disease (Stages 1–4)
   https://www.kidney.org/sites/default/files/11-50-0113_patbro_nutrition.pdf
3. National Kidney Foundation: Potassium and Your CKD Diet
   https://www.kidney.org/atoz/content/potassium
4. National Kidney Foundation: Phosphorus and Your CKD Diet
   https://www.kidney.org/atoz/content/phosphorus
5. American Dietetic Association: Chronic Kidney Disease (CKD) and Diet: Assessment, Management, and Treatment
   https://www.eatrightpro.org/-/media/eatrightpro-files/practice/position-and-practice-papers/position-papers/kidneydisease.pdf
6. World Health Organization: Protein and Amino Acid Requirements in Human Nutrition
   https://www.who.int/nutrition/publications/nutrientrequirements/WHO_TRS_935/en/
7. Dietary Guidelines for Americans
   https://www.dietaryguidelines.gov/sites/default/files/2019-05/2015-2020_Dietary_Guidelines.pdf

Portion Control and Serving Sizes
1. https://www.niddk.nih.gov/health-information/weight-management/just-enough-food-portions
2. Food Portioning: www.covenanthome.care

Myths and Facts about CKD
1. National Kidney Foundation: 10 Common Myths About Chronic Kidney Disease
   https://www.kidney.org/news/ekidney/march_2013/myths
2. American Kidney Fund: Kidney disease facts
   https://www.kidneyfund.org/kidney-disease/kidney-disease-facts/
3. National Institute of Diabetes and Digestive and Kidney Diseases: Eating & Nutrition for Hemodialysis
   https://www.niddk.nih.gov/health-information/kidney-disease/kidney-failure/hemodialysis/eating-nutrition
4. Mayo Clinic: Chronic kidney disease
   https://www.mayoclinic.org/diseases-conditions/chronic-kidney-disease/symptoms-causes/syc-20354521

Appendix C: Index

	Page		Page
CARBOHYDRATES	**271**	**FATS (NUTS AND OILS)**	**215**
Amaranth	275	Olive	225
Barley	275	Peanut	219
Breads	278	Pecans	221
Cereals	276	Pine	218
Couscous	275	Pistachios	221
Crackers	282	Poppyseed	223
Grits	280	Pumpkin	223
Oats	237	Safflower	226
Pancake	277	Sesame	222
Pasta	281	Soybean	226
Polenta (cornmeal)	275	Sunflower	222
Quinoa	275	Walnut	217
Rice	272	**FRUITS**	**245**
Waffle	277	Apple	246
Wheat	274	Apricot	258
FATS (NUTS AND OILS)	**215**	Avocado	260
Acorn	223	Banana	254
Almond	216	Blackberries	246
Butter	226	Blueberries	248
Canola	226	Canteloupe/ Melon	254
Cashew	220	Cherries	252
Chestnut	218	Coconut	225
Chia	223	Cranberry	247

Coconut	225	Dates	263
Flaxseed	223	Durian	263
Ghee	226	Elderberries	251
Hazelnut	220	Fig	262
Hemp	223	Gooseberries	251
Macadamia	221	Grapefruit	251
Margarine	226	Grapes	250

	Page		Page
FRUITS	*245*	**HERBS AND SPICES**	*265*
Guava	262	Anise	268
Jackfruit	263	Basil	267
Kiwi	251	Cardamom	268
Lemon	256	Cayenne	268
Lime	257	Celery	268
Loganberries	251	Chives	267
Lychee	257	Cinnamon	266
Mango	257	Cloves	266
Mangosteen	263	Coriander	266
Nectarine	261	Cumin	266
Orange	255	Curry Powder	268
Papaya	261	Dill	268
Peaches	253	Fennel	268
Pears	247	Fennel Seeds	268
Persimmon	261	Garlic	267
Pineapple	249	Ginger	267
Plantain	260	Horseradish	269
Plum	258	Lemon grass	266
Pomegranate	259	Marjoram	267
Pomelo	263	Nutmeg	266
Prune	259	Onion	267
PurplePassionFruit/Granadilla	261	Oregano	267
Raspberries	247	Paprika	268
Rhubarb	259	Parsley	266
Sapodilla	264	Pepper, black	269
Soursop	263	Pepper, white	269

Starfruit (Carambola)	264	Rosemary	267
Strawberries	248	Saffron	269
Sugar apple (sweetsop)	264	Sage	266
Tamarind	264	Spring Onions	267
Watermelon	262	Tarragon	269
		Thyme	266

		Page			*Page*
ANIMAL PROTEIN		**183**	**MILKS AND CHEESE**		**205**
Anchovies		199	Cheeses		211
Beef		191	Cream		214
Carp		197	Milk		206
Catfish		200	Milk Sub		207
Chicken		184	Yogurt		208
Clams		202	**VEGETABLES**		**227**
Cod		199	Alfalfa		237
Crab		200	Artichokes		237
Crayfish/Crawfish		201	Arugula		239
Eggs		187	Asparagus		229
Flatfish		198	Beans		229
Halibut		198	Beets		234
Herring		203	Broccoli		234
Lamb		192	Brussel Sprouts		242
Lobster		198	Cabbage		232
Mackerel		196	Carrots		229
Mahi-Mahi		197	Cassava/ Yucca/Manioc		240
Mussels		196	Cauliflower		234
Oysters		202	Celery		237
Pangasius (Cream Dory) (Swai)		195	Collards		238
Pollock		195	Corn		230
Pork		188	Cucumber		234
Salmon		194	Eggplant (aubergine)		238
Sardines		195	Endive or Escarole		239
Scallops		203	Jicama (Yambean)		238
Shrimp		199	Kale		244
Squid (Calamari)		201	Kohlrabi		240

Tilapia	195	Leeks	240
Trout	197	Lettuce	231
Tuna	194	Mixed Vegetables	242
Turkey	186	Mushroom	231
Veal	192	Mustard Greens	244

	Page
VEGETABLES	**227**
Okra	239
Parsnips	241
Peas	236
Pepper	233
Potatoes	235
Pumpkin	239
Radish	240
Rutabaga	241
Spinach	243
Squash	240
Swiss Chard	243
Tomatillos	243
Tomato	228
Turnip Greens	241
Turnips	243
Waterchestnuts	242
Watercress	242
Yam	242
VEGETABLES PROTEIN	*179-182*
Beans	180
Chickpeas	181
Edamame	182
Spirulina	182
Tempeh	182
Tofu	182

Low Potassium Food List for Kidney Disease Patients

A Comprehensive Printable

Low Potassium Diet Book

with Thousands of Validated Low Potassium Foods for CKD Cookbooks and Recipes

by Janeth Kingston BSN, RN

A Comprehensive Printable

Low Potassium Diet Book

Low Potassium Food List
for Kidney Disease Patients

by Janeth Kingston, BSN RN

INTRODUCTION

About this Book

Welcome to this comprehensive guide to a low-potassium diet for Chronic Kidney Disease (CKD) patients. This book is designed as a valuable resource for those navigating the complexities of dietary restrictions associated with CKD. It is our goal to provide you with the knowledge and tools necessary to manage your potassium intake effectively, thereby improving your overall health and quality of life.

Purpose

The purpose of this book is twofold:

1. Educational: To provide clear, accurate, and comprehensive information about the role of potassium in the body, why its regulation is crucial in CKD, and how a low-potassium diet can help manage this condition.

2. Practical: To offer an extensive food list comprising over 1000 items, categorized by their potassium content. This list will serve as a handy reference when planning meals, shopping for groceries, or eating out.

Scope

The scope of this book extends beyond merely listing foods and their potassium content. It aims to provide an understanding of the science behind the dietary recommendations, equipping you with the knowledge to make informed decisions about your diet.

We delve into the nuances of meal planning, portion control, reading food labels, and even tips for dining out or traveling. The book also includes sample meal plans tailored to different stages of CKD, providing practical examples of how to implement a low-potassium diet in daily life.

A Comprehensive Food List

One of the key features of this book is the extensive food list containing over 1000 foods, categorized by their food groups. The potassium content in each food are specifically highlighted so that this list can serve as a handy tool for those seeking to limit their potassium intake.

The list covers various food groups including fruits, vegetables, grains, meats, dairy products, beverages, and snacks, making it a comprehensive resource for meal planning.

A Word of Caution

While this book is a comprehensive guide to low-potassium dieting for CKD patients, it is crucial to remember that it does not replace professional medical advice. Each person's health situation is unique, and dietary needs can vary widely depending on the stage of CKD, presence of other health conditions, and overall nutritional status.

Always consult with your healthcare provider or a registered dietitian before making any significant changes to your diet. Regular blood tests are necessary to monitor your potassium levels and other important parameters. Your healthcare team will provide personalized advice based on these results and your specific health needs.

Remember, managing CKD is a team effort. This book is intended to be part of your toolkit, working in conjunction with the guidance from your healthcare team. With the right knowledge and resources, you can take proactive steps towards managing your CKD effectively and living a healthier life.

Chapter 1: Understanding Potassium and Kidney Health

Potassium is a fairly common nutrient that can be found in almost any food. It is responsible for the following:

- Keeping nerves and muscles healthy
- Maintaining your body's pH level
- Regulating fluid and electrolyte balance, and;
- Maintaining the normal rhythm of your heart beats.

So, what happens if I have too much potassium in the body?

It can cause significant heart problems, such as:

- Irregular heartbeats or a slow pulse,
- A heart attack, or;
- Your heart could just stop beating altogether

Other, less severe, symptoms include:

- Weakness,
- Numbness, and
- Nausea

To avoid these complications, you need to keep your blood potassium level in the normal range.

The secret to maintaining potassium levels? *Moderation.*

According to The National Kidney Foundation, the normal amount in a typical healthy American is **3,500 to 4,500 milligrams per day.** For patients with a potassium-restricted diet, they can go low as **2,000 mg per day**. However, it depends on what your physician or dietitian advises you to take based on your health.

You'll need a blood test to confirm whether your current potassium levels are high or not and you can use these values as a general reference:

Blood Potassium Level (mmol/L)	Description
3.5 - 5.0	Your blood potassium is **normal**
5.1 - 6.0	Your blood potassium is **elevated**
6.0 and above	Your blood potassium is **exceedingly high**

But don't worry, with the right strategies and tips, you can do it!

Speaking of... here's two:

1. Be picky with your produce (the food list chart will really come in handy for this). You have to be careful with what you eat, as well as how much, is the most important point in a low-potassium diet.

In general, any food that contains more than 200mg potassium per serving is high in potassium. So, you'll have to start watching out for high-potassium foods, such as:

Item	Sodium (mg)	Protein (g)	Potassium (mg)	Phosphorus (mg)
Potatoes	6	2.05	425	57
Banana	1	1.09	358	22
Spinach, Raw	79	2.86	558	49
Avocados, Raw	7	2.00	485	52
Brussels Sprouts	25	3.38	389	69

USDA values per 100g

You need to avoid high potassium food items and find lower potassium foods. Such as:

Item	Sodium (mg)	Protein (g)	Potassium (mg)	Phosphorus (mg)
Cabbage	18	1.28	170	26
Apple	1	0.27	104	12
Cucumber	2	0.65	147	24
Blueberries	1	0.74	77	12
Onions, Raw	4	1.10	146	29

USDA values per 100g

2. Practice Leaching

Leaching is a process that helps reduce the potassium content of food. It means that you don't have to give up high-potassium vegetables, you just need more time to prepare them. Here's how you can do it:

1. For beets, carrots, potatoes, sweet potatoes, rutabagas, and winter squash:
2. Peel and place vegetables in cold water (to avoid darkening)
3. Slice into ⅛ inch-thick pieces
4. Briefly rinse in warm water
5. Soak in warm water for a minimum of 2 hours. Use ten times the amount of water to the amount of vegetables. For example, 10 cups of water for 1 cup of vegetables.

Now remember, although leaching is an effective process, it only **reduces potassium but DOES NOT eliminate it entirely.**

For this reason, it's always better and safe to take in foods that are low in potassium.

Part 1.
The Comprehensive Food List

Now, we dive right away to the core of this book. The food list chart contained in the next few chapters are a result of meticulous efforts by renal nurses and dietitians who helped in coming up with this guide. Unlike any other books, we have arranged the food items in food groups and in chart forms so you can easily navigate the charts and find what you are looking for.

The Food List in this book specifically focuses on highlighting the Potassium content of each food item acknowledging the need to emphasize these values and eliminate mistakes in picking and portioning your food.

Why do I see food items that are high-potassium in the list?

While I initially debated whether to only list down foods that are specifically Low in Potassium or not, I've come to the conclusion that with every recipe comes at least an ingredient or two with varying amounts of potassium in them. So instead of leaving those ingredients out which will in turn leave you with more guess work, you will now have the opportunity to add the ingredients while applying the proper portioning according to your daily potassium limits. Or, skip right through the ingredient, because you now know that a pinch obviously screams "high potassium."

Navigating Through The Charts

1. The charts are systematically arranged according to broad food classifications: Carbohydrates, Fats (inclusive of oils, nuts, and seeds), Dairy Products, Fruits & Vegetables, Plant-Based Proteins, Meats, Poultry, & Seafoods, and Herbs & Spices.

2. Identify your particular food item within these categories or alternatively, use the Low Potassium Food List Index provided at Page 479.

3. Each broad food group is further divided into specific preparations standardized to a quantity of 100 grams. Additional measurements such as slices or cups are also provided, but these may vary based on the nature of the food item.

4. For every 100 grams of a specific food category, you will discover its corresponding nutritional values: Calories, Carbs, Proteins, Fats, Sodium, Phosphorus, and Potassium.

5. You can then adjust these values by dividing or multiplying them based on the quantity of food you are using in your recipe to ascertain the precise nutritional content.

Example:

The recipe calls for 1 cup of boiled asparagus. Based on the food list chart, you will need to multiply the amount of nutrients by 2, since 100 grams of boiled asparagus is only ½ of a cup (or 0.50 cup).

ASPARAGUS	SERVING QUANTITY	SERVING UNIT	CALORIES (kcal)	PROTEIN (g)	TOTAL CARBOHYDRATES (g)	POTASSIUM (mg)	TOTAL FAT (g)
boiled, drained	100.00	g	22	2.4	4.1	224.00	0.22
	90.00	g	20	2.2	3.7	201.60	0.20
	0.50	c					

For this specific example, the nutrient content of 1 cup of asparagus will now be:

    Calories: *44 kCal*
    Protein: *4.8 g*
    Carbs: *8.2 g*
    Fats: *0.44g*
    Potassium: *448 g* ↑

You may then conclude that a cup of Asparagus may contain too much potassium for you and decide to cut back on what the actual recipe calls for.

As much as I love for you to flip through every page of this food chart, that might not make any sense if you really are looking to make good use of it.

Thus, you might find value in the Food Item Index that I have created for you at Page 479 of this book.

Chapter 2: Carbohydrates

Do you want to print the charts in letter-size (8.5x11")?

I have created downloadable printables of this chart. You can scan the QR code below or copy the link to your computer browser to be able to get your printable copies of the food charts

https://go.renaltracker.com/lowpotassiumprint

Grains and Cereals

RICE	SERVING QUANTITY	SERVING UNIT	CALORIES (kcal)	PROTEIN (g)	TOTAL CARBOHYDRATES (g)	POTASSIUM (mg)	TOTAL FAT (g)
white, unenriched	100.00	g	359	6.9	79.8	75.00	1.30
white, cooked, glutinous	100.00	g	96	2.0	21.0	20.00	0.27
	174.00	g	167	3.5	36.5	26.40	0.36
	1.00	c					
white, long-grain, parboiled enriched, cooked	100.00	g	123	2.9	26.1	29.00	0.21
	158.00	g	194	4.6	41.2	53.90	0.39
	1.00	c					
flour, white, unenriched	100.00	g	359	6.9	79.8	26.00	0.19
						53.30	0.39
white, steamed, Chinese restaurant	100.00	g	151	3.2	33.9		
	132.00	g	199	4.2	44.7	265.00	3.85
cup, loosely packed	1.00	c					
white, medium-grain, cooked unenriched	100.00	g	130	2.4	28.6	86.00	0.96
	186.00	g	242	4.4	53.2	169.00	1.88
	1.00	c					
white, short-grain, cooked unenriched	100.00	g	130	2.4	28.7	101.00	0.34
	205.00	g	266	4.8	58.8	166.00	0.56
	1.00	c					
flour, brown,	100.00	g	365	7.2	75.5	427.00	1.08
						683.00	1.73
brown, cooked, no salt, no fat	100.00	g	122	2.7	25.5		
	196.00	g	239	5.4	49.9	75.00	1.30
	1.00	c					
wild, cooked	100.00	g	101	4.0	21.3	20.00	0.27
	164.00	g	166	6.5	35.0	26.40	0.36
	1.00	c					
wild, raw	100.00	g	357	14.7	74.9	29.00	0.21
	160.00	g	571	23.6	120.0	53.90	0.39
	1.00	c					

OATS

	SERVING QUANTITY	SERVING UNIT	CALORIES (kcal)	PROTEIN (g)	TOTAL CARBOHYDRATES (g)	POTASSIUM (mg)	TOTAL FAT (g)
raw	100.00	g	379	12.2	67.7	362.00	6.52
	81.00	g	307	10.7	54.8	293.00	5.28
	1.00	c					
cereal, oat,	100.00	g	372	12.4	73.2	633.00	6.60
	33.00	g	123	4.1	24.2	209.00	2.18
	1.00	c					
steel cut	100.00	g	378	13.3	66.7	356.00	6.67
Brand: ARROWHEAD MILLS	45.00	g	170	6.0	30.0	160.00	3.00
	1.00	svg					
rolled	100.00	g	350	12.5	67.5	350.00	6.25
Brand: MILLVILLE by Aldi	40.00	g	140	5.0	27.0	140.00	2.50
	1.00	svg					
bran, cooked	100.00	g	40	3.2	11.4	92.00	0.86
	219.00	g	88	7.0	25.1	201.00	1.88
	1.00	c					
bran, uncooked (raw)	100.00	g	246	17.3	66.2	566.00	7.03
	94.00	g	231	16.3	62.2	532.00	6.61
	1.00	c					
flour, partially debranned	100.00	g	404	14.7	65.7	371.00	9.12
	104.00	g	420	15.2	68.3	386.00	9.48
	1.00	c					
regular, rolled, not fortified, dry	100.00	g	379	13.2	67.7	362.00	6.52
	81.00	g	307	10.7	54.8	293.00	5.28
	1.00	c					
AMARANTH							
Grain	100.00	g	102	3.8	18.7	135.00	1.58
cooked	246.00	g	251	9.4	46.0	332.00	3.89
	1.00	c					

WHEAT

	SERVING QUANTITY	SERVING UNIT	CALORIES (kcal)	PROTEIN (g)	TOTAL CARBOHYDRATES (g)	POTASSIUM (mg)	TOTAL FAT (g)
durum	100.00	g	399	13.7	71.1	431.00	2.47
	192.00	g	651	26.3	137.0	828.00	4.74
	1.00	c					
sprouted	100.00	g	198	7.5	42.5	169.00	1.27
	108.00	g	214	8.1	45.9	183.00	1.37
	1.00	c					
germ	100.00	g	360	23.2	51.8	892.00	9.72
	115.00	g	414	26.7	59.6	1,030.00	11.20
	1.00	c					
bran	100.00	g	216	15.6	64.5	1,180.00	4.25
	58.00	g	125	9.1	37.4	684.00	2.46
	1.00	c					
cream of wheat, instant, dry	100.00	g	366	10.6	75.5	115.00	1.40
	11.50	g	42	1.2	8.7	13.20	0.16
	1.00	tbsp					
flour, whole wheat, unenriched	100.00	g	370	15.1	71.2	376.00	2.73
whole grain, soft wheat	100.00	g	332	9.6	74.5	394.00	1.95
bread flour, unenriched	100.00	g	361	12.0	72.5	100.00	1.66
unsifted	137.00	g	495	16.4	99.4	137.00	2.27
	1.00	c					
flour, bread, white, enriched	100.00	g	361	12.0	72.5	100.00	1.66
	137.00	g	495	16.4	99.4	137.00	2.27
	1.00	c					
flour, cake, enriched	100.00	g	362	8.2	78.0	105.00	0.86
unsifted	137.00	g	496	11.2	107.0	144.00	1.18
	1.00	c					

CUOSCUOS	SERVING QUANTITY	SERVING UNIT	CALORIES (kcal)	PROTEIN (g)	TOTAL CARBOHYDRATES (g)	POTASSIUM (mg)	TOTAL FAT (g)
dry	100.00	g	376	12.8	77.4	166.00	0.64
	173.00	g	680	22.1	134.0	287.00	1.11
	1.00	c					
cooked	100.00	g	112	3.8	23.2	58.00	0.16
	157.00	g	176	6.0	36.4	91.10	0.25
	1.00	c					

BARLEY

pearled, cooked	100.00	g	123	2.3	28.2	93.00	0.44
	157.00	g	193	3.6	44.3	146.00	0.69
	1.00	c					
flour or meal	100.00	g	345	10.5	74.5	309.00	1.60
	148.00	g	511	15.5	110.0	457.00	2.37
	1.00	c					

QUINOA

cooked	100.00	g	120	4.4	21.3	172.00	1.92
	185.00	g	222	8.1	39.4	318.00	3.55
	1.00	c					
uncooked	100.00	g	368	14.1	64.2	563.00	6.07
	170.00	g	626	24.0	109.0	957.00	10.30
	1.00	c					
pasta from quinoa flour (gluten-free)	100.00	g	152	3.2	31.1	63.00	2.07
	132.00	g	201	4.3	41.1	83.20	2.73
not packed	1.00	c					

GRITS

corn, yellow, quick, unenriched cooked with water, no salt	100.00	g	59	1.4	12.9	21.00	0.19
	242.00	g	143	3.4	31.2	50.82	0.46
	1.00	c					
corn, white, quick, unenriched cooked with water	100.00	g	59	1.4	12.9	21.00	0.19
	242.00	g	143	3.4	31.2	50.82	0.46
	1.00	c					
POLENTA (cornmeal)	100.00	g					
	240.00	g	139	2.7	30.0	50.40	0.67
	1	c					
corn, yellow, quick, unenriched cooked with water, no salt	100.00	g	59	1.4	12.9	21.00	0.19
	242.00	g	143	3.4	31.2	50.82	0.46
	1.00	c					

CEREALS

	SERVING QUANTITY	SERVING UNIT	CALORIES (kcal)	PROTEIN (g)	TOTAL CARBOHYDRATES (g)	POTASSIUM (mg)	TOTAL FAT (g)
corn flakes, plain (store brands)	100.00	g	357	7.5	84.1	168.00	0.40
	25.00	g	89	1.9	21.0	42.00	0.10
	1.00	c					
corn flakes, frosted (store brands)	100.00	g	389	4.3	90.2	82.00	0.87
	40.00	g	156	1.7	36.1	32.80	0.35
	1.00	c					
crsipy rice	100.00	g	383	6.7	86.2	106.00	1.26
	26.00	g	100	1.7	22.4	27.60	0.33
	1.00	c					
cocoa puffs (General Mills)	100.00	g	383	5.6	83.7	272.00	5.20
	36.00	g	138	2.0	30.1	97.90	1.87
	1.00	c					
muesli, with fruits & nuts	100.00	g	335	8.6	74.9	324.00	5.40
	85.00	g	302	7.3	63.7	275.00	4.59
	1.00	c					
muesli Brand: Safeway	100.00	g	386	8.8	73.7	474.00	5.26
	57.00	g	220	5.0	42.0	270.00	3.00
	1.00	svg					
granola, homemade, ready-to-eat	100.00	g	489	13.7	53.9	539.00	24.30
	122.00	g	597	16.7	65.8	658.00	29.60
	1.00	c					
granola bars, plain	100.00	g	471	10.1	64.4	336.00	19.80
	28.00	g	132	2.8	18.0	94.10	5.54
	1.00	bar/ oz					
granola bars, almond	100.00	g	495	7.7	62.0	273.00	25.50
	28.35	g	140	2.2	17.6	77.40	7.23
	1.00	oz					

Breads and Pastries

BREADS	SERVING QUANTITY	SERVING UNIT	CALORIES (kcal)	PROTEIN (g)	TOTAL CARBOHYDRATES (g)	POTASSIUM (mg)	TOTAL FAT (g)
muffins, english, mixed-grain includes granola	100.00	g	235	9.1	46.3	156.00	1.80
	66.00	g	155	6.0	30.6	103.00	1.19
	1.00	pc					
pumpernickle, med or regular slice	100.00	g	250	8.7	47.5	208.00	3.10
	32.00	g	80	2.8	15.2	66.60	0.99
	1.00	pc					
cinammon, medium or regular slice	100.00	g	253	7.1	44.4	74.00	5.29
	28.00	g	71	2.0	12.4	20.70	1.48
	1.00	pc					
raisin, med or regular slice	100.00	g	273	8.8	52.2	180.00	3.26
	28.00	g	76	2.5	14.6	50.40	0.91
	1.00	pc					
roll, multigrain med, reg, sandwich size	100.00	g	263	9.6	44.6	160.00	6.00
	43.00	g	113	4.1	19.2	68.80	2.58
	1.00	pc					
bread stuffing, homemade	100.00	g	177	3.1	21.7	72.00	8.51
dry mix, prepared	228.00	g	404	7.2	49.5	164.00	19.40
	1.00	pc					

BREADS

	SERVING QUANTITY	SERVING UNIT	CALORIES (kcal)	PROTEIN (g)	TOTAL CARBOHYDRATES (g)	POTASSIUM (mg)	TOTAL FAT (g)
whole wheat	100.00	g	252	12.5	42.7	254.00	3.50
	50.00	g	126	6.2	21.4	127.00	1.75
	2.00	slices					
white	100.00	g	266	8.9	49.4	126.00	490.00
	50.00	g	133	4.4	24.7	63.00	245.00
	2.00	slices					
french, small (2"x2.5"x1.75")	100.00	g	272	10.8	51.9	117.00	2.42
	32.00	g	87	3.4	16.6	37.44	0.77
	1.00	slice					
pita, 6.5"	100.00	g	275	9.1	55.7	120.00	1.20
	60.00	g	165	5.5	33.4	72.00	0.72
	1.00	pc					
sourdough	100.00	g	272	10.8	51.9	117.00	2.42
	50.00	g	136	5.4	25.9	58.50	1.21
	2.00	slices					
rye	100.00	g	259	8.5	48.3	166.00	33.00
	32.00	g	83	2.7	15.5	53.12	1.06
	1.00	slice					
bagels, wheat	100.00	g	250	10.2	48.9	165.00	1.53
	105.00	g	262	10.7	51.3	173.00	1.61
	1.00	reg pc					
biscuits	100.00	g	362	7.5	43.9	184.00	18.19
	45.00	g	163	3.4	19.8	82.80	8.19
	1.00	pc					
sprouted, wheat	100.00	g	188	13.2	33.9	198.00	0.00
	26.00	g	49	3.4	8.8	51.50	0.00
	1.00	slice					
cracked, wheat	100.00	g	274	10.7	47.5	141.00	4.53
	28.00	g	77	3.0	13.3	39.50	1.27
	1.00	reg slice					
tortillas, corn ready-to-bake or fry	100.00	g	218	5.7	44.6	186.00	2.85
	24.00	g	52	1.4	10.7	44.60	0.68
	1.00	Pc					
tortillas, flour approx. 6" diameter ready-to-bake or fry, refrigerated	100.00	g	306	8.2	49.4	125.00	7.99
	30.00	g	92	2.5	14.8	37.50	2.40
	1.00	pc					

BREADS

	SERVING QUANTITY	SERVING UNIT	CALORIES (kcal)	PROTEIN (g)	TOTAL CARBOHYDRATES (g)	POTASSIUM (mg)	TOTAL FAT (g)
tortilla, whole wheat	100.00	g	310	9.8	45.9	262.00	9.76
ready-to-bake or fry	41.00	g	127	4.0	18.8	107.00	4.00
	1.00	pc					
ciabatta (yeast bread) italian, grecian, aarmenian thick slice	100.00	g	259	9.5	48.1	124.00	2.73
	43.00	g	111	4.1	20.7	53.30	1.17
	1.00	pc					
focaccia, plain (italian flatbread)	100.00	g	249	8.8	35.8	114.00	7.89
	57.00	g	142	5.0	20.4	65.00	4.50
	1.00	pc					
Pita, medium	100.00	g	275	9.1	55.7	120.00	1.20
	57.00	g	157	5.2	31.7	68.40	0.68
	1.00	pc					
Naan, plain	100.00	g	291	9.6	50.4	125.00	5.65
	90.00	g	262	8.7	45.4	112.00	5.08
	1.00	pc					
Paratha, whole wheat, frozen	100.00	g	326	6.4	45.4	185.00	6.70
	79.00	g	258	5.0	35.9	196.00	7.10
	1.00	pc					
brioche	100.00	g	418	8.8	35.8	139.00	13.20
	77.00	g	322	6.7	27.6	110.00	10.40
	1.00	pc					
croissants, plain	100.00	g	406	8.2	45.8	120.00	26.80
medium	57.00	g	231	4.7	26.1	92.40	20.60
	1.00	pc					
croissants, chocolate	100.00	g	421	7.4	49.4	118.00	21.00
	57.00	g	240	4.2	28.2	67.30	12.00
	1.00	pc					
croissants, cheese	100.00	g	414	9.2	47.0	132.00	20.90
	57.00	g	236	5.2	26.8	75.22	11.90
	1.00	pc					
muffins, english, whole grain white	100.00	g	245	7.0	50.2	130.00	1.75
	57.00	g	140	4.0	28.6	74.10	1.00
	1.00	pc					
muffins, english, whole wheat	100.00	g	203	8.8	40.4	210.00	2.10
	66.00	g	134	5.8	26.7	139.00	1.39
	1.00	pc					

CRACKERS

	SERVING QUANTITY	SERVING UNIT	CALORIES (kcal)	PROTEIN (g)	TOTAL CARBOHYDRATES (g)	POTASSIUM (mg)	TOTAL FAT (g)
melba toast, rye	100.00	g	389	11.6	77.3	193.00	3.40
3 3/4" x 1 3/4" x 1/8"	15.00	g	58	1.7	11.6	28.95	0.51
	3.00	pcs					
melba toast, wheat	100.00	g	374	12.9	76.4	148.00	2.30
	15.00	g	56	1.9	11.5	22.20	0.35
	3.00	pcs					
saltine, low salt (square)	100.00	g	421	9.5	74.3	724.00	8.85
	15.00	g	63	1.4	11.2	108.60	1.33
	5.00	pcs					
saltine, fat-free, low sodium	100.00	g	393	10.5	82.3	115.00	1.60
	15.00	g	59	1.6	12.4	17.25	0.24
	3.00	pcs					
saltines, whole wheat/multi-grain	100.00	g	398	7.1	68.3	221.00	10.71
	14.00	g	56	1.0	9.6	30.94	1.50
	1.00	svg					
whole wheat, low salt	100.00	g	443	8.8	68.6	297.00	17.20
	28.00	g	124	2.5	19.2	83.16	4.82
	7.00	pcs					
whole wheat, reduced fat	100.00	g	416	11.3	75.5	373.00	7.59
1 svg = 29g	4.20	g	17	0.5	3.2	15.67	0.32
	1.00	pcs					
graham, plain or honey, low fat	100.00	g	386	5.7	78.0	171.00	5.71
	35.00	g	135	2.0	27.3	59.85	2.00
	1.00	svg					
goldfish (fish-shaped), flavored	100.00	g	463	10.2	65.7	224.00	17.71
	5.20	g	24	0.5	3.4	11.65	0.92
	10.00	pcs					
toast thins, low sodium	100.00	g	442	6.5	67.7	306.00	16.13
	31.00	g	137	2.0	21.0	94.86	5.00
	1.00	svg					

PANCAKE

	SERVING QUANTITY	SERVING UNIT	CALORIES (kcal)	PROTEIN (g)	TOTAL CARBOHYDRATES (g)	POTASSIUM (mg)	TOTAL FAT (g)
buttermilk (from recipe)	100.00	1	227	6.8	28.7	145.00	9.30
	38.00	1	86	2.6	10.9	55.10	3.53
	1-4" diameter	pc					
plain, (prepared from recipe)	100.00	1	227	6.4	28.3	132.00	9.70
	38.00	1	86	2.4	10.8	50.20	3.69
	1-4" diameter	pc					
plain, reduced fat	100.00	g	269	5.7	57.3	97.00	1.90
	105.00	g	282	6.0	60.2	102.00	2.00
	3.00	pcs					
plain, frozen, ready to heat includes buttermilk	100.00	g	233	5.2	37.8	90.00	6.83
	40.00	g	93	2.1	15.1	36.00	2.73
	1 (4")	pc					
gluten-free, frozen, ready to heat	100.00	g	215	3.3	40.3	127.00	4.55
	48.00	g	103	1.6	19.3	61.00	2.18
	1.00	pc					

WAFFLE

	SERVING QUANTITY	SERVING UNIT	CALORIES (kcal)	PROTEIN (g)	TOTAL CARBOHYDRATES (g)	POTASSIUM (mg)	TOTAL FAT (g)
plain, prepared from recipe	100.00	g	291	7.9	32.9	159.00	14.10
	75.00	g	218	5.9	24.7	119.00	10.60
	1 (7")	pc					

Pasta

PASTA	SERVING QUANTITY	SERVING UNIT	CALORIES (kcal)	PROTEIN (g)	TOTAL CARBOHYDRATES (g)	POTASSIUM (mg)	TOTAL FAT (g)
spaghetti, unenriched, cooked	100.00	g	158	5.8	30.9	44.00	0.93
	70.00	g	111	4.1	21.6	30.80	0.65
	0.50	c					
spaghetti, enriched, cooked	100.00	g	158	5.8	30.9	44.00	0.93
	140.00	g	221	8.1	43.2	61.60	1.30
	1.00	c					
spaghetti, whole wheat, cooked	100.00	g	149	6.0	30.1	96.00	1.71
	140.00	g	209	8.4	42.1	134.40	2.39
	1.00	c					
bowtie/farfalle, enriched, cooked	100.00	g	136	4.8	27.4	24.51	0.55
	154.79	g	210	7.4	42.3	37.93	0.86
	1.00	c					
fusilli, enriched, cooked	100.00	g	161	5.7	32.5	29.09	0.66
	130.41	g	210	7.4	42.3	37.93	0.86
	1.00	c					
penne, enriched, cooked	100.00	g	169	6.0	34.1	30.55	0.69
	124.17	g	210	7.4	42.3	37.93	0.86
	1.00	c					
macaroni, enriched, cooked	100.00	g	133	4.7	26.8	24.04	0.54
	157.79	g	210	7.4	42.3	37.93	0.86
	1.00	c					
lasagna, enriched, boiled/drained	100.00	g	150	5.3	30.1	26.98	0.61
	140.62	g	210	7.4	42.3	37.93	0.86
	1.00	c					
whole grain, 51% whole wheat rest enriched semolina, cooked spaghetti, unenriched, cooked	100.00	g	156	5.7	30.9	71.00	1.48

Chapter 3: Proteins

Do you want to print the charts in letter-size (8.5x11")?

I have created downloadable printables of this chart. You can scan the QR code below or copy the link to your computer browser to be able to get your printable copies of the food charts

https://go.renaltracker.com/lowpotassiumprint

Vegetable Proteins

TOFU	SERVING QUANTITY	SERVING UNIT	CALORIES (kcal)	PROTEIN (g)	TOTAL CARBOHYDRATES (g)	POTASSIUM (mg)	TOTAL FAT (g)
soft with calcium	100.00	g	61	7.2	1.2	120.00	3.69
sulfate and magnesium chloride (Nigari)	85.05	g	52	6.1	1.0	102.06	3.14
	3.00	oz					
firm with calcium	100.00	g	78	9.0	2.9	148.00	4.17
sulfate and magnesium chloride (Nigari)	85.05	g	66	7.7	2.4	125.87	3.55
	3.00	oz					
silken tofu (Vitasoy USA)	100.00	g	43	4.8	0.6	na	2.40
	91.00	g	39	4.4	0.5	na	2.18
	0.20	package					
TEMPEH							
raw	100.00	g	192	20.3	7.6	412.00	10.80
	83.00	g	159	16.8	6.3	341.96	8.96
	0.50	c					
cooked	100.00	g	185	19.9	7.6	401.00	11.38
EDAMAME							
frozen, unprepared	100.00	g	109	11.2	7.6	482.00	4.73
	118.00	g	129	13.2	9.0	568.76	5.58
	1.00	c					
frozen, prepared	100.00	g	121	11.9	8.9	436.00	5.20
	155.00	g	188	18.5	13.8	675.80	8.06
	1	c					
SPIRULINA							
seaweed, fresh/raw	100.00	g	26	5.9	2.4	127.00	0.39
	28.35	g	7	1.7	0.7	36.00	0.11
	1.00	oz					
seaweed, dried	100.00	g	290	57.5	23.9	1363.00	7.72
	112.00	g	325	64.4	26.8	1526.56	8.65
	1.00	c					

BEANS

	SERVING QUANTITY	SERVING UNIT	CALORIES (kcal)	PROTEIN (g)	TOTAL CARBOHYDRATES (g)	POTASSIUM (mg)	TOTAL FAT (g)
Lentils/Pinto/	100.00	g	131	8.6	23.9	398.91	0.49
Navy	92.00	g	121	8.0	22.0	367.00	0.45
	0.50	c					
Lima	100.00	g	113	6.8	20.2	467.00	0.86
	78.00	g	88	5.3	15.7	364.26	0.67
	0.50	c					
Broad or	100.00	g	72	5.6	11.7	250.00	0.60
Fava	81.75	g	59	4.6	9.6	204.38	0.49
	0.75	c					
Black beans,	100.00	g	132	8.9	23.7	355.00	0.54
boiled	86.00	g	114	7.6	20.4	305.30	0.46
	0.50	c					
Mungo,	100.00	g	105	7.5	18.3	231.00	0.55
boiled	90.00	g	95	6.8	16.5	207.90	0.50
	0.50	c					
sprouts,	100.00	g	30	3.0	5.9	149.00	0.18
Mung	78.00	g	23	2.4	4.6	116.22	0.14
	0.75	c					
Kidney,	100.00	g	127	8.7	22.8	405.00	0.50
boiled	88.50	g	112	7.7	20.2	358.43	0.44
	0.50	c					
Navy, boiled	100.00	g	140	8.2	26.1	389.00	0.62
	91.00	g	127	7.5	23.7	353.99	0.56
	0.50	c					
Lupin, boiled	100.00	g	119	15.6	9.9	245.00	2.92
	83.00	g	99	12.9	8.2	203.35	2.42
	0.50	c					
Pinto, frozen	100.00	g	170	9.8	32.5	755.98	0.50
	94.49	g	161	9.3	31.0	714.34	0.47
	3.33	oz					
Pinto, boiled	100.00	g	143	9.0	26.2	436.00	0.65
	85.50	g	122	7.7	22.4	372.78	0.56
	0.50	c					
White (Cannellini), boiled no salt	100.00	g	139	9.7	25.1	561.00	0.35
	89.50	g	124	8.7	22.5	502.10	0.31
	0.50	c					

BEANS

	SERVING QUANTITY	SERVING UNIT	CALORIES (kcal)	PROTEIN (g)	TOTAL CARBOHYDRATES (g)	POTASSIUM (mg)	TOTAL FAT (g)
White, small,	100.00	g	142	9.0	25.8	463.00	0.64
boiled, no salt	89.50	g	127	8.0	23.1	414.39	0.57
	0.50	c					
sprouts,	100.00	g	29	4.2	4.1	187.00	0.50
Kidney	92.00	g	27	3.9	3.8	172.04	0.46
	0.50	c					
sprouts, Navy	100.00	g	67	6.2	13.1	307.00	0.70
	78.00	g	52	4.8	10.2	239.46	0.55
	0.75	c					
sprouts, Pinto	100.00	g	62	5.3	11.6	307.00	0.90
	85.05	g	53	4.5	9.9	262.10	0.77
	3.00	oz					
French, boiled	100.00	g	129	7.1	24.0	370.00	0.76
	88.50	g	114	6.2	21.3	327.45	0.67
	0.50	c					
baked,	100.00	g	155	5.5	21.6	358.00	5.15
prepared	126.50	g	196	7.0	27.4	452.87	6.51
	0.50	c					
Refried,	100.00	g	90	5.0	13.6	319.00	2.01
canned	119.00	g	107	5.9	16.1	379.61	2.39
	0.50	c					

CHICKPEAS

	SERVING QUANTITY	SERVING UNIT	CALORIES (kcal)	PROTEIN (g)	TOTAL CARBOHYDRATES (g)	POTASSIUM (mg)	TOTAL FAT (g)
garbanzos/	100.00	g	88	4.9	13.5	144.00	1.95
bengal gram, canned	120.00	g	106	5.9	16.2	172.80	2.34
	0.50	c					
garbanzos/	100.00	g	164	8.9	27.4	291.00	2.59
bengal gram, boiled	82.00	g	134	7.3	22.5	238.62	2.12
	0.50	c					
garbanzos/	100.00	g	138	7.0	22.9	109.00	2.47
bengal gram,	152.00	g	210	10.7	34.8	165.68	3.75
canned drained, rinsed in tap water	1.00	c					
garbanzos/	100	g	88	4.9	13.5	144.00	1.95
bengal gram,	240	g	211	11.8	32.4	345.60	4.68
canned low sodium	1	c					
flour	100.00	g	387	22.4	57.8	846.00	6.69
	92.00	g	110	6.4	16.4	239.84	1.90
	1.00	c					

Poultry

EGG	SERVING QUANTITY	SERVING UNIT	CALORIES (kcal)	PROTEIN (g)	TOTAL CARBOHYDRATES (g)	POTASSIUM (mg)	TOTAL FAT (g)
chicken, raw, large	100.00	g	143	12.6	0.7	138.00	9.51
	50.00	g	72	6.3	0.4	69.00	4.76
	1.00	pc					
chicken, fried, large	100.00	g	196	13.6	0.8	152.00	14.84
	46.00	g	90	6.3	0.4	69.92	6.83
	1.00	pc					
chicken, poached, large	100.00	g	143	12.5	0.7	138.00	9.47
	50.00	g	72	6.3	0.4	69.00	4.74
	1.00	pc					
chicken, hard boiled, large	100.00	g	155	12.6	1.1	126.00	10.61
	50.00	g	78	6.3	0.6	63.00	5.31
	1.00	pc					
scrambled, fast food	100.00	g	212	13.8	2.1	147.00	16.18
	94.00	g	199	13.0	2.0	138.18	15.21
	2.00	pc					
substitute, liquid	100.00	g	84	12.0	0.6	330.00	3.31
	251.00	g	211	30.1	1.6	828.30	8.31
	1.00	c					
substitute, powder	100.00	g	443	55.8	21.8	742.31	12.97
	9.92	g	44	5.5	2.2	73.66	1.29
	0.35	oz					
substitute, frozen	100.00	g	160	11.3	3.2	213.00	11.11
	60.00	g	96	6.8	1.9	127.80	6.67
	0.25	c					
chicken, egg whites only, raw large egg	100.00	g	52	10.9	0.7	163.00	0.17
	33.00	g	17	3.6	0.2	53.79	0.06
	1.00	pc					
chicken, yolk only, raw large egg	100.00	g	322	15.9	3.6	109.00	26.54
	17.00	g	55	2.7	0.6	18.53	4.51
	1.00	pc					
chicken, whole, raw, frozen	100.00	g	147	12.3	1.0	135.00	9.95
	56.70	g	83	7.0	0.6	76.54	5.64
	2.00	oz					
yolk only, frozen, raw	100.00	g	296	15.5	0.8	121.00	25.60
	56.70	g	168	8.8	0.5	68.61	14.51
	2.00	oz					
whites, frozen, raw	100.00	g	48	10.2	1.0	169.00	0.00
	56.70	g	27	5.8	0.6	95.82	0.00
	2.00	oz					
duck, raw	100.00	g	185	12.8	1.5	222.00	13.77
	70.00	g	130	9.0	1.0	155.40	9.64
	1.00	pc					
quail, raw	100.00	g	158	13.1	0.4	132.00	11.09
	9.00	g	14	1.2	0.0	11.88	1.00
	1.00	pc					

CHICKEN	SERVING QUANTITY	SERVING UNIT	CALORIES (kcal)	PROTEIN (g)	TOTAL CARBOHYDRATES (g)	POTASSIUM (mg)	TOTAL FAT (g)
ground, raw	100.00	g	143	17.4	0.0	522.00	8.10
meat and skin, raw	100.00	g	215	18.6	0.0	189.00	15.06
	113.40	g	244	21.1	0.0	214.33	17.08
	4.00	oz					
meat and skin, roasted	100.00	g	239	27.3	0.0	223.00	13.60
	85.05	g	203	23.2	0.0	189.66	11.57
	3.00	oz					
thigh meat only, fried	100.00	g	218	28.2	1.2	259.00	10.30
	85.05	g	185	24.0	1.0	220.28	8.76
	3.00	oz					
thigh meat only, roasted	100.00	g	179	24.8	0.0	269.00	8.15
	85.05	g	152	21.1	0.0	228.78	6.93
	3.00	oz					
wing meat only, fried	100.00	g	211	30.2	0.0	208.00	9.15
	85.05	g	179	25.6	0.0	176.90	7.78
	3.00	oz					
wing meat only, roasted	100.00	g	203	30.5	0.0	210.00	8.13
	85.05	g	173	26.0	0.0	178.60	6.91
	3.00	oz					
wing meat only, stewed	100.00	g	181	27.2	0.0	153.00	7.18
	85.05	g	154	23.1	0.0	130.12	6.11
	3.00	oz					
back meat only, fried	100.00	g	288	30.0	5.7	251.00	4.12
	85.05	g	245	25.5	4.8	213.47	3.50
	3.00	oz					
back meat only, roasted	100.00	g	239	28.2	0.0	237.00	13.16
	85.05	g	203	24.0	0.0	201.57	11.19
	3.00	oz					
back meat only, stewed	100.00	g	209	25.3	0.0	158.00	11.19
	85.05	g	178	21.5	0.0	134.38	9.52
	3.00	oz					
drumstick meat only, fried	100.00	g	195	28.6	0.0	249.00	8.08
	85.05	g	166	24.3	0.0	211.77	6.87
	3.00	oz					
drumstick meat only, roasted	100.00	g	155	24.2	0.0	256.00	5.70
	85.05	g	132	20.6	0.0	217.73	4.85
	3	oz					

CHICKEN	SERVING QUANTITY	SERVING UNIT	CALORIES (kcal)	PROTEIN (g)	TOTAL CARBOHYDRATES (g)	POTASSIUM (mg)	TOTAL FAT (g)
drumstick meat only, stewed	100.00	g	169	27.5	0.0	199.00	5.71
	85.05	g	144	23.4	0.0	169.25	4.86
	3.00	oz					
leg meat only, fried	100.00	g	208	28.4	0.7	254.00	9.32
	85.05	g	177	24.1	0.6	216.02	7.93
	3.00	oz					
leg meat only, roasted	100.00	g	174	24.2	0.0	269.00	7.80
	85.05	g	148	20.6	0.0	228.78	6.63
	3.00	oz					
leg meat only, stewed	100.00	g	185	26.3	0.0	190.00	8.06
	85.05	g	157	22.3	0.0	161.59	6.85
	3.00	oz					
pate, chicken liver, canned	100.00	g	201	13.5	6.6	95.00	13.10
	52.00	g	105	7.0	3.4	49.40	6.81
	4.00	tbsp					
chicken tenders, fast food	100.00	g	271	19.2	17.3	373.00	13.95
	62.00	g	168	11.9	10.7	231.26	8.65
	4.00	pcs					
chicken patty, frozen, cooked	100.00	g	287	14.9	12.8	261.00	19.58
bratwurst, chicken, cooked	100.00	g	176	19.4	0.0	211.00	10.30
	83.92	g	148	16.3	0.0	177.06	8.69
	2.96	oz					
sausage, chicken/beef, smoked	100.00	g	295	18.5	0.0	139.00	244.00
	138.00	g	251	15.7	0.0	118.22	20.41
	1.00	c					

TURKEY

	SERVING QUANTITY	SERVING UNIT	CALORIES (kcal)	PROTEIN (g)	TOTAL CARBOHYDRATES (g)	POTASSIUM (mg)	TOTAL FAT (g)
breast, meat &	100.00	g	144	21.6	0.1	224.00	5.64
skin, raw	113.40	g	163	24.5	0.2	254.02	6.40
	4.00	oz					
breast, meat &	100.00	g	189	28.6	0.1	239.00	7.39
skin, roasted	85.05	g	161	24.3	0.1	203.27	6.29
	3.00	oz					
breast, meat	100.00	g	114	23.3	0.0	267.00	2.33
only, raw	85.05	g	97	19.9	0.0	227.08	1.98
	3.00	oz					
breast, meat	100.00	g	136	29.5	0.0	297.00	1.97
only, roasted	85.05	g	116	25.1	0.0	252.60	1.68
	3.00	oz					
ground, raw	100.00	g	148	20.0	0.0	237.00	7.66
	113.40	g	168	22.3	0.0	268.76	8.69
	4.00	oz					
ground,	100.00	g	203	27.4	0.0	294.00	10.40
cooked	85.05	g	173	23.3	0.0	250.04	8.85
	3.00	oz					
white rotisserie, deli cut	100.00	g	112	13.5	7.7	349.00	3.00
	56.70	g	64	7.7	4.4	197.88	1.70
	2.00	oz					
ham, extra	100.00	g	134	19.6	0.9	299.00	5.80
lean, sliced	20.00	g	27	3.9	0.2	59.80	1.16
	1.00	pc					
pastrami,	100.00	g	139	16.3	3.3	345.00	6.21
sliced	56.70	g	79	9.2	1.9	195.62	3.52
	2.00	slices					
bologna	100.00	g	209	11.4	4.7	135.00	16.05
	56.70	g	119	6.5	2.7	76.55	9.10
	2.00	slices					
salami	100.00	g	172	19.2	1.6	216.00	9.21
	56.70	g	98	10.9	0.9	122.47	5.22
	2.00	slices					
bacon, turkey,	100.00	g	382	29.6	3.1	395.00	27.90
cooked	28.35	g	108	8.4	0.9	111.98	7.91
	1.00	oz					
bacon, turkey,	100.00	g	253	13.3	4.8	156.00	20.00
low sodium	15.00	g	38	2.0	0.7	23.40	3.00
	1.00	svg					
sausage,	100.00	g	196	23.9	0.0	298.00	10.44
turkey, cooked	56.70	g	111	13.6	0.0	168.97	5.92
	2.00	oz					

Meats

PORK	SERVING QUANTITY	SERVING UNIT	CALORIES (kcal)	PROTEIN (g)	TOTAL CARBOHYDRATES (g)	POTASSIUM (mg)	TOTAL FAT (g)
ground, cooked	100.00	g	297	25.7	0.0	362.00	20.77
	85.05	g	253	21.9	0.0	307.88	17.66
	3.00	oz					
ground, raw	100.00	g	263	16.9	0.0	287.00	21.19
	113.40	g	298	19.1	0.0	325.46	24.03
	4.00	oz					
loin, sirloin, roasts, separable lean roasted	100.00	g	204	27.8	0.0	352.00	9.44
	85.05	g	174	23.6	0.0	299.37	8.03
	3.00	oz					
loin, center rib, separable lean, roasted	100.00	g	206	28.8	0.0	287.00	9.21
	85.05	g	175	24.5	0.0	244.09	7.83
	3.00	oz					
loin, sirloin, boneless, separable lean roasted	100.00	g	178	30.4	0.0	408.00	5.31
	85.05	g	151	25.9	0.0	347.00	4.52
	3.00	oz					
loin, center rib, boneless roasted	100.00	g	214	28.8	0.0	363.00	10.13
	85.05	g	182	24.5	0.0	308.73	8.62
	3.00	oz					
shoulder, blade, boston roasts roasted turkey, salt.	100.00	g	232	24.2	0.0	427.00	14.30
	85.05	g	197	20.6	0.0	363.16	12.16
	3.00	oz					
shoulder, whole, roasted	100.00	g	230	25.3	0.0	345.80	13.53
	85.05	g	196	21.5	0.0	294.10	11.51
	3.00	oz					
loin, whole, roasted	100.00	g	209	28.6	0.0	425.00	9.63
	85.05	g	178	24.3	0.0	361.46	8.19
	3.00	oz					
leg or ham, whole, roasted	100.00	g	211	29.4	0.0	373.00	9.44
	85.05	g	179	25.0	0.0	317.23	8.03
	3.00	oz					
loin, tenderloin, separable lean & fat roasted	100.00	g	147	26.0	0.0	419.00	3.96
	85.05	g	125	22.2	0.0	356.36	3.37
	3.00	oz					
ground, cooked	100.00	g	297	25.7	0.0	362.00	20.77
	85.05	g	253	21.9	0.0	307.88	17.66
	3.00	oz					

PORK

	SERVING QUANTITY	SERVING UNIT	CALORIES kcal	PROTEIN (g)	TOTAL CARBOHYDRATES (g)	POTASSIUM (mg)	TOTAL FAT (g)
bacon, cured, broiled, panfried or roasted	100.00	g	541	37.0	1.4	565.00	41.78
	8.00	g	43	3.0	0.1	45.20	3.34
	1.00	slice					
bacon, reduced sodium, cured broiled, panfried or roasted	100.00	g	541	37.0	1.4	565.00	41.78
	56.70	g	307	21.0	0.8	320.36	23.69
	2.00	oz					
country style ribs, separable lean & fat roasted	100.00	g	359	21.8	0.0	322.00	29.46
	85.05	g	305	18.5	0.0	273.86	25.06
	3.00	oz					
sirloin, chops or roasts, boneless, raw	100.00	g	121	22.8	0.0	354.00	2.59
	113.40	g	137	25.9	0.0	401.44	2.94
	4.00	oz					
kidney, braised	100.00	g	151	25.4	0.0	143.00	4.70
	85.05	g	128	21.6	0.0	121.62	4.00
	3.00	oz					
liver, braised	100.00	g	165	26.0	3.8	150.00	4.40
	85.05	g	140	22.1	3.2	127.57	3.74
	3.00	oz					
ham, minced, sliced	100.00	g	263	16.3	1.8	311.00	20.68
	21.00	g	55	3.4	0.4	65.31	4.34
	1.00	slice					
ham, extra lean, 5% fat	100.00	g	107	16.9	0.7	463.00	4.04
	85.05	g	91	14.3	0.6	393.78	3.44
	3.00	oz					
ham, low sodium, cured, cooked	100.00	g	165	22.0	0.5	362.00	7.70
	85.05	g	140	18.7	0.4	307.88	6.55
	3.00	oz					
sausages, Kielbasa, grilled	100.00	g	337	12.5	5.0	306.00	29.68
	85.05	g	287	10.6	4.3	260.25	25.24
	3.00	oz					
Kielbasa, panfried	100.00	g	333	12.4	4.8	304.00	29.43
	85.05	g	283	10.5	4.1	258.55	25.03
	3.00	oz					
Beerwurst, pork/beef	100.00	g	276	14.0	4.3	244.00	22.53
	56.70	g	156	7.9	2.4	138.35	12.77
	2.00	oz					

PORK	SERVING QUANTITY	SERVING UNIT	CALORIES (kcal)	PROTEIN (g)	TOTAL CARBOHYDRATES (g)	POTASSIUM (mg)	TOTAL FAT (g)
Italian Sweet, links	100.00	g	149	16.1	2.1	194.00	8.42
	85.05	g	127	13.7	1.8	165.00	7.16
	3.00	oz					
Polish, pork, cooked	100.00	g	326	14.1	1.6	237.00	28.72
	56.70	g	185	8.0	0.9	134.38	16.28
	2.00	oz					
Bratwurst, pork, cooked	100.00	g	333	13.7	2.9	347.99	29.18
	56.70	g	189	7.8	1.6	197.31	16.54
	2.00	oz					
meatloaf/ luncheon meat pork/beef	100.00	g	260	15.4	1.6	245.00	20.90
	23.00	g	60	3.5	0.4	56.35	4.81
	1.00	slice					
peperoni, beef/pork	100.00	g	504	19.3	1.2	274.00	46.28
	56.70	g	286	11.0	0.7	155.36	26.24
	2.00	oz					
salami, italian, pork	100.00	g	425	21.7	1.2	340.00	37.00
	28.35	g	120	6.2	0.3	96.39	10.49
	1.00	oz					

BEEF

	SERVING QUANTITY	SERVING UNIT	CALORIES (kcal)	PROTEIN (g)	TOTAL CARBOHYDRATES (g)	POTASSIUM (mg)	TOTAL FAT (g)
chuck eyeroast, boneless, all grades 0" fat, separable lean only, roasted	3	g	183	26.7	0.0	344.00	8.46
	85.05	g	156	22.7	0.0	292.57	7.20
	3.00	oz					
chuck eyeroast, boneless, all grades separable lean only, 0", raw	100.00	g	137	20.6	0.0	357.00	6.01
	85.05	g	117	17.5	0.0	303.63	5.11
	3.00	oz					
Chuck eyeroast, boneless, all grades sep lean & fat, 0" fat, roasted	100.00	g	236	24.6	0.0	308.00	15.29
	85.05	g	201	21.0	0.0	261.95	13.00
	3.00	oz					
chuck eyeroast, boneless, all grades sep lean & fat, 0" fat, raw	100.00	g	173	19.3	0.0	367.00	10.67
	85.05	g	147	16.4	0.0	312.13	9.07
	3.00	oz					
jerky	100.00	g	410	33.2	11.0	597.00	25.60
	28.35	g	116	9.4	3.1	169.25	7.26
	1.00	oz					
corned beef, brisket, raw	100.00	g	198	14.7	0.1	297.00	14.90
	113.40	g	225	16.7	0.2	336.80	16.90
	4.00	oz					
corned beef, brisket, cooked	100.00	g	251	18.2	0.5	145.00	18.98
	85.05	g	213	15.5	0.4	123.32	16.14
	3.00	oz					
broth cube 1 cube, 6 fl. oz prepared	100.00	g	170	17.3	16.1	403.00	4.00
	3.60	g	6	0.6	0.6	14.51	0.14
	1.00	cube					
liver, pan fried	100.00	g	175	26.5	5.2	351.00	4.68
	81.00	g	142	21.5	4.2	284.31	3.79
	1.00	slice					
liver, braised	100.00	g	191	29.1	5.1	352.00	5.26
	85.05	g	162	24.7	4.4	299.37	4.47
	3.00	oz					
tongue, simmered	100.00	g	284	19.3	0.0	184.00	22.30
	85.05	g	242	16.4	0.0	156.49	18.97
	3.00	oz					
kidney simmered	100.00	g	158	27.3	0.0	135.00	4.65
	85.05	g	134	23.2	0.0	114.82	3.95
	3.00	oz					
tripe, simmered	100.00	g	94	11.7	2.0	42.00	4.05
	85.05	g	80	10.0	1.7	35.72	3.44
	3.00	oz					

LAMB	SERVING QUANTITY	SERVING UNIT	CALORIES (kcal)	PROTEIN (g)	TOTAL Carbohydrates (g)	POTASSIUM (mg)	TOTAL FAT (g)
tenderloin, New Zealand, separable lean only, raw	100.00	g	116	20.5	0.0	381.00	3.81
	85.05	g	99	17.5	0.0	324.04	3.24
	3.00	oz					
loin, NZ, separable lean, frozen, broiled	100.00	g	199	29.3	0.0	189.00	8.24
	85.05	g	169	24.9	0.0	160.74	7.01
	3.00	oz					
australian, separable lean, 1/8" fat, cooked	100.00	g	201	26.7	0.0	318.00	9.63
	85.05	g	171	22.7	0.0	270.46	8.19
	3.00	oz					
Australian, separable lean, 1/8" fat, raw	100.00	g	142	20.3	0.0	320.00	6.18
	113.40	g	161	23.0	0.0	362.88	7.01
	4.00	oz					
Australian, ground, 85%Lean/15%fat, raw	100.00	g	255	17.1	0.0	na	20.17
	85.05	g	217	14.6	0.0	na	17.61
	3.00	oz					
NZ, rib, separable lean, frozen, raw	100.00	g	160	20.7	0.0	309.00	8.61
	113.40	g	181	23.4	0.0	350.41	9.76
	4.00	oz					
NZ, rib, separable lean, frozen, roasted	100.00	g	193	24.4	0.0	323.00	10.63
	85.05	g	164	20.8	0.0	274.71	9.04
	3.00	oz					

VEAL							
separable lean, cooked	100.00	g	196	32.0	0.0	338.00	6.58
	85.05	g	167	27.1	0.0	287.47	5.60
	3.00	oz					
liver, pan fried	100.00	g	193	27.4	4.5	353.00	6.51
	85.05	g	164	23.3	3.8	300.22	5.54
	3.00	oz					
sausage, bratwurst, veal, cooked	100.00	g	341	14.0	0.0	231.00	31.70
	83.92	g	286	11.7	0.0	193.85	26.60
	2.96	oz					
ground, pan fried	100.00	g	503	8.9	0.9	107.00	51.60
	85.05	g	428	7.5	0.8	91.00	43.89
	3.00	oz					

VEAL

	SERVING QUANTITY	SERVING UNIT	CALORIES (kcal)	PROTEIN (g)	TOTAL CARBOHYDRATES (g)	POTASSIUM (mg)	TOTAL FAT (g)
sirloin, separable, lean, braised	100.00	g	204	34.0	0.0	339.00	6.51
	85.05	g	174	28.9	0.0	288.32	5.54
	3.00	oz					
sirloin separable lean, roasted	100.00	g	168	26.3	0.0	365.00	6.22
	85.05	g	143	22.4	0.0	310.43	5.29
	3.00	oz					
sirloin, lean, raw	100.00	g	110	20.2	0.0	348.00	2.59
	113.40	g	125	22.9	0.0	394.63	2.94
	4.00	oz					
loin, lean and fat, braised	100.00	g	284	30.2	0.0	280.00	17.21
	85.05	g	242	25.7	0.0	238.14	14.64
	3.00	oz					
loin, lean and fat, roasted	100.00	g	217	25.0	0.0	325.00	12.32
	85.05	g	185	21.1	0.0	276.41	10.48
	3.00	oz					
loin, lean, braised	100.00	g	226	33.6	0.0	297.00	9.15
	85.05	g	192	28.6	0.0	252.60	7.78
	3.00	oz					
loin, lean, roasted	100.00	g	175	26.3	0.0	340.00	6.94
	85.05	g	149	22.4	0.0	289.17	5.90
	3.00	oz					
loin, lean, raw	100.00	g	114	21.9	0.0	260.00	2.90
	113.40	g	129	24.8	0.0	294.84	3.29
	4.00	oz					
loin, chop, lean and fat, grilled	100.00	g	198	28.0	0.2	229.00	9.48
	85.05	g	168	23.9	0.1	194.76	8.06
	3.00	oz					
bratwurst, veal, cooked	100.00	g	341	14.0	0.0	231.00	31.70
	83.92	g	286	11.7	0.0	193.85	26.60
	2.96	oz					

Seafoods

SALMON	SERVING QUANTITY	SERVING UNIT	CALORIES (kcal)	PROTEIN (g)	TOTAL CARBOHYDRATES (g)	POTASSIUM (mg)	TOTAL FAT (g)
pink, raw	100.00	g	127	20.5	0.0	365.96	4.40
	113.40	g	144	23.2	0.0	415.00	4.99
	4.00	oz					
atlantic, wild, raw	100.00	g	142	19.8	0.0	489.95	0.98
	113.40	g	161	22.5	0.0	555.61	1.11
	4.00	oz					
atlantic, farmed, raw	100.00	g	208	20.4	0.0	362.97	13.42
	113.39	g	236	23.2	0.0	411.60	15.22
	4.00	oz					
pink, canned, drained solids, w/ bone	100.00	g	138	23.1	0.0	332.80	5.02
	85.05	g	117	19.6	0.0	283.05	4.27
	3.00	oz					
pink, canned, with bone and liquid no salt	100.00	g	139	19.8	0.0	325.99	6.05
	56.70	g	79	11.2	0.0	184.84	3.43
	2.00	oz					
pink, canned, drained solids without skin and bones	100.00	g	136	24.6	0.0	326.00	4.21
	85.05	g	116	20.9	0.0	277.26	3.58
	3.00	oz					
chum, canned, drained, with bone no salt	100.00	g	141	21.4	0.0	300.00	5.50
	56.70	g	80	12.2	0.0	170.10	3.12
	2.00	oz					
nuggets, breaded, frozen	100.00	g	212	12.7	14.0	165.00	11.72

TUNA

	SERVING QUANTITY	SERVING UNIT	CALORIES	PROTEIN (g)	TOTAL CARBOHYDRATES (g)	POTASSIUM (mg)	TOTAL FAT (g)
bluefin, raw	100.00	g	144	23.3	0.0	251.98	4.90
	113.40	g	163	26.5	0.0	285.74	5.56
	4.00	oz					
yellowfin or Ahi, raw	100.00	g	109	24.4	0.0	440.96	0.49
	113.40	g	124	27.7	0.0	500.05	0.56
	4.00	oz					
canned in oil, drained, light no salt	100.00	g	198	29.1	0.0	207.00	8.21
	56.70	g	112	16.5	0.0	117.37	4.65
	2.00	oz					
white, canned in water, drained no salt	100.00	g	128	23.6	0.0	237.00	2.97
	56.70	g	73	13.4	0.0	134.38	1.68
	2.00	oz					
canned in water, drained, light no salt	100.00	g	116	25.5	0.0	237.00	0.82
	56.70	g	66	14.5	0.0	134.38	0.46
	2.00	oz					
white, canned in oil, drained, no salt	100.00	g	186	26.5	0.0	332.99	8.08
	56.70	g	105	15.0	0.0	188.81	4.58
	2.00	oz					

COD	SERVING QUANTITY	SERVING UNIT	CALORIES (kcal)	PROTEIN (g)	TOTAL CARBOHYDRATES (g)	POTASSIUM (mg)	TOTAL FAT (g)
atlantic, raw	100.00	g	82	17.8	0.0	412.96	0.67
	113.40	g	93	20.2	0.0	468.30	0.76
	4.00	oz					
atlantic, canned	100.00	g	105	22.8	0.0	527.99	0.86
	56.70	g	60	12.9	0.0	299.37	0.49
	2.00	oz					
atlantic, cooked, dry heat	100.00	g	105	22.8	0.0	244.00	0.86
	85.05	g	89	19.4	0.0	207.52	0.73
	3.00	oz					
pacific, raw	100.00	g	69	15.3	0.0	234.98	0.41
	113.40	g	78	17.3	0.0	266.46	0.46
	4.00	oz					
pacific, cooked, dry heat	100.00	g	85	18.7	0.0	289.00	0.50
	85.05	g	72	15.9	0.0	245.79	0.43
	3.00	oz					
ANCHOVIES							
Raw	100.00	g	131	20.4	0.0	382.96	4.84
	113.40	g	149	23.1	0.0	434.28	5.49
	4.00	oz					
canned, in oil, drained	100.00	g	210	28.9	0.0	544.00	9.71
	16.00	g	34	4.6	0.0	87.04	1.55
	4.00	pcs					
SHRIMP							
mixed species, raw	100.00	g	71	13.6	0.9	113.00	1.01
	113.40	g	81	15.4	1.0	128.14	1.15
	4.00	oz					
mixed species, breaded, fried	100.00	g	242	21.4	11.5	224.87	12.27
	85.05	g	206	18.2	9.8	191.25	10.44
	3.00	oz					
mixed species, cooked, moist heat	100.00	g	119	22.8	1.5	170.00	1.70
	85.05	g	101	19.4	1.3	144.58	1.45
	3.00	oz					
cracker	100.00	g	426	7.1	59.1	193.00	17.86

SARDINES	SERVING QUANTITY	SERVING UNIT	CALORIES (kcal)	PROTEIN (g)	TOTAL CARBOHYDRATES (g)	POTASSIUM (mg)	TOTAL FAT (g)
spanish	100.00	g	212	6.2	14.2	0.00	14.16
	113.00	g	240	7.0	16.0	0.00	16.00
	4.00	oz					
atlantic, canned in oil, with bones	100.00	g	208	24.6	0.0	397.00	11.45
	24.00	g	50	5.9	0.0	95.28	2.75
	2.00	oz					
portuguese	100.00	g	236	25.5	0.0	na	12.73
	55.00	g	130	14.0	0.0	na	7.00
	0.50	c					
fillets, canned	100.00	g	338	18.2	7.3	na	26.36
	55.00	g	186	10.0	4.0	na	14.50
	0.25	c					
TILAPIA							
raw	100.00	g	96	20.1	0.0	302.00	1.70
	113.40	g	107	22.8	0.0	342.47	1.93
	4.00	oz					
cooked, dry heat	100.00	g	128	26.2	0.0	379.78	2.65
	85.05	g	109	22.2	0.0	323.00	2.25
	3.00	oz					
POLLOCK							
atlantic, raw	100.00	g	92	19.4	0.0	355.97	0.98
	113.40	g	104	22.0	0.0	403.66	1.11
	4.00	oz					
atlantic, cooked, dry heat	100.00	g	118	24.9	0.0	456.00	1.26
	85.05	g	100	21.2	0.0	387.82	1.07
	3.00	oz					
alaska, untreated, cooked	100.00	g	87	19.4	0.0	364.00	1.00
	85.05	g	74	16.5	0.0	309.58	0.85
	3.00	oz					
PANGASIUS (CREAM DORY/SWAI)							
fillets, boneless	100.00	g	71	14.2	0.0	na	1.77
	113.00	g	80	16.0	0.0	na	2.00
	4.00	oz					
fillets, skinless, boneless	100.00	g	177	20.4	0.0	na	1.77
	113.00	g	200	23.0	0.0	na	2.00
	4.00	oz					

TROUT

	SERVING QUANTITY	SERVING UNIT	CALORIES (kcal)	PROTEIN (g)	TOTAL CARBOHYDRATES (g)	POTASSIUM (mg)	TOTAL FAT (g)
rainbow, wild, raw, fillet	100.00	g	119	20.5	0.0	481.00	3.46
	113.40	g	135	23.2	0.0	545.45	3.92
	4.00	oz					
rainbow, farmed, raw, fillet	100.00	g	141	19.9	0.0	376.96	6.18
	113.40	g	160	22.6	0.0	427.48	7.01
	4.00	oz					
mixed species, raw fillet	100.00	g	148	20.8	0.0	360.97	6.61
	113.40	g	168	23.6	0.0	409.33	7.50
	4.00	oz					
sea trout, mixed species, raw	100.00	g	104	16.7	0.0	340.97	3.61
	113.40	g	118	19.0	0.0	386.66	4.09
	4.00	oz					
rainbow, wild, cooked, dry heat	100.00	g	150	22.9	0.0	448.00	5.82
	85.05	g	128	19.5	0.0	381.02	4.95
	3.00	oz					
rainbow, farmed, cooked, dry heat	100.00	g	168	23.8	0.0	450.00	7.38
	85.05	g	143	20.2	0.0	382.72	6.28
	3.00	oz					
mixed species, cooked, dry heat	100.00	g	190	26.6	0.0	463.00	8.47
	85.05	g	162	22.7	0.0	393.78	7.20
	3.00	oz					
sea trout, mixed species, cooked, dry heat	100.00	g	133	21.5	0.0	437.00	4.63
	85.05	g	113	18.3	0.0	371.66	3.94
	3.00	oz					

CARP

	SERVING QUANTITY	SERVING UNIT	CALORIES	PROTEIN	TOTAL CARBOHYDRATES	POTASSIUM	TOTAL FAT
raw	100.00	g	127	17.8	0.0	332.97	5.60
	113.40	g	144	20.2	0.0	377.59	6.35
	4.00	oz					
cooked, dry heat	100.00	g	162	22.9	0.0	427.00	7.17
	85.05	g	138	19.4	0.0	363.16	6.10
	3.00	oz					

MAHI-MAHI

	SERVING QUANTITY	SERVING UNIT	CALORIES	PROTEIN	TOTAL CARBOHYDRATES	POTASSIUM	TOTAL FAT
Dorado or Dolphinfish, raw	100.00	g	85	18.5	0.0	415.96	0.70
	113.40	g	96	21.0	0.0	471.70	0.79
	4.00	oz					
Doradao or Dolphinfish, cooked, dry heat	100.00	g	109	23.7	0.0	532.99	0.90
	85.05	g	93	20.2	0.0	452.31	0.77
	3.00	oz					

FLATFISH	SERVING QUANTITY	SERVING UNIT	CALORIES (kcal)	PROTEIN (g)	TOTAL CARBOHYDRATES (g)	POTASSIUM (mg)	TOTAL FAT (g)
raw	100.00	g	70	12.4	0.0	159.98	1.93
	113.40	g	79	14.1	0.0	181.42	2.19
	4.00	oz					
cooked, dry	100.00	g	86	15.2	0.0	197.00	2.37
heat	85.05	g	73	13.0	0.0	167.55	2.02
	3.00	oz					

HALIBUT

greenland, raw	100.00	g	186	14.4	0.0	267.97	13.84
	113.40	g	211	16.3	0.0	303.88	15.69
	4.00	oz					
atlantic and	100.00	g	91	18.6	0.0	434.96	1.33
pacific, raw	113.40	g	103	21.0	0.0	493.24	1.51
	4.00	oz					
greenland,	100.00	g	239	18.4	0.0	344.00	17.71
cooked, dry heat	85.05	g	203	15.7	0.0	292.57	15.09
	3.00	oz					
atlantic and pacific, cooked, dry heat	100.00	g	111	22.5	0.0	527.99	1.61
	85.05	g	94	19.2	0.0	449.06	1.37
	3.00	oz					

LOBSTER

Northern, raw (Langoustine)	100.00	g	77	16.5	0.0	200.00	0.75
	113.40	g	87	18.7	0.0	226.80	0.85
	4.00	oz					
Spiny, mixed	100.00	g	112	20.6	2.4	180.00	1.51
species, raw	113.40	g	127	23.4	2.8	104.12	1.71
	4.00	oz					
Northern, cooked, moist heat (Langoustine)	100.00	g	89	19.0	0.0	230.00	0.86
	85.05	g	76	16.2	0.0	195.61	0.73
	3.00	oz					
Spiny, mixed species, cooked, moist heat	100.00	g	143	26.4	3.1	208.00	1.94
	85.05	g	122	22.5	2.7	176.90	1.65
	3.00	oz					

CRAB

	SERVING QUANTITY	SERVING UNIT	CALORIES (kcal)	PROTEIN (g)	TOTAL CARBOHYDRATES (g)	POTASSIUM (mg)	TOTAL FAT (g)
blue, raw	100.00	g	87	18.1	0.0	329.00	1.08
	113.40	g	99	20.5	0.5	373.09	1.22
	4.00	oz					
blue, canned	100.00	g	83	17.9	0.0	259.00	0.74
	56.70	g	47	10.1	0.0	146.85	0.42
	2.00	oz					
dungeness, raw	100.00	g	86	17.4	0.7	354.00	0.97
	113.40	g	98	19.7	0.8	401.44	1.10
	4.00	oz					
dungeness, cooked, moist heat	100.00	g	110	22.3	1.0	408.00	1.24
	85.05	g	94	19.0	0.8	347.00	1.05
	3.00	oz					
alaska king, raw	100.00	g	84	18.3	0.0	204.00	0.60
	113.40	g	95	20.7	0.0	231.34	0.68
	4.00	oz					
alaska king, cooked, moist heat	100.00	g	97	19.4	0.0	262.00	1.54
	85.05	g	83	16.5	0.0	222.83	1.31
	3.00	oz					
imitation, crabmeat (Kani)	100.00	g	95	7.6	15.0	90.00	0.46
	85.05	g	81	6.5	12.8	76.54	0.39
	3.00	oz					
cakes	100.00	g	266	18.8	8.5	270.00	17.25
	60.00	g	160	11.3	5.1	162.00	10.35
	1.00	pc					

CATFISH

	SERVING QUANTITY	SERVING UNIT	CALORIES	PROTEIN	TOTAL CARBOHYDRATES	POTASSIUM	TOTAL FAT
channel, wild, raw	100.00	g	95	16.4	0.0	405.93	2.82
	113.40	g	108	18.6	0.0	357.97	3.20
	4.00	oz					
channel, farmed, raw	100.00	g	119	15.2	0.0	301.82	5.94
	85.05	g	101	13.0	0.0	256.70	5.05
	3.00	oz					
breaded, fried	100.00	g	229	18.1	8.0	340.00	13.33
	85.05	g	195	15.4	6.8	289.17	11.34
	3.00	oz					
wild, cooked, dry heat	100.00	g	105	18.5	0.0	419.00	2.85
	85.05	g	89	15.7	0.0	356.36	2.42
	3.00	oz					
farmed, cooked, dry heat	100.00	g	144	18.4	0.0	366.00	7.19
	85.05	g	122	15.7	0.0	311.28	6.12
	3.00	oz					

CRAYFISH/ CRAWFISH	SERVING QUANTITY	SERVING UNIT	CALORIES (kcal)	PROTEIN (g)	TOTAL CARBOHYDRATES (g)	POTASSIUM (mg)	TOTAL FAT (g)
Mixed species, farmed, raw	100.00	g	72	14.9	0.0	261.00	0.97
	113.40	g	82	16.8	0.0	295.97	1.10
	4.00	oz					
Mixed species, wild, raw	100.00	g	77	16.0	0.0	302.00	0.95
	113.40	g	87	18.1	0.0	342.47	1.08
	4.00	oz					
Mixed species, farmed, cooked, moist heat	100.00	g	87	17.5	0.0	238.00	0.22
	85.05	g	74	14.9	0.0	202.42	0.18
	3.00	oz					
mixed species, wild, cooked, moist heat	100.00	g	82	16.8	0.0	296.00	1.20
	85.05	g	70	14.3	0.0	251.75	1.02
	3.00	oz					

SQUID (CALAMARI)

	SERVING QUANTITY	SERVING UNIT	CALORIES (kcal)	PROTEIN (g)	TOTAL CARBOHYDRATES (g)	POTASSIUM (mg)	TOTAL FAT (g)
mixed species, fried	100.00	g	175	17.9	7.8	279.00	7.48
	85.05	g	149	15.3	6.6	237.29	6.36
	3.00	oz					
mixed species, raw	100.00	g	92	15.6	3.1	246.00	1.38
boneless	113.40	g	104	17.7	3.5	278.96	1.56
	4.00	oz					

CLAMS

	SERVING QUANTITY	SERVING UNIT	CALORIES (kcal)	PROTEIN (g)	TOTAL CARBOHYDRATES (g)	POTASSIUM (mg)	TOTAL FAT (g)
mixed species, raw	100.00	g	86	14.7	3.6	46.00	0.96
	85.05	g	73	12.5	3.0	39.12	0.82
	3.00	oz					
mixed species, breaded, fried	100.00	g	202	14.2	10.3	326.00	11.15
	85.05	g	172	12.1	8.8	277.26	9.48
	3.00	oz					
mixed species, canned, with liquid	100.00	g	2	0.4	0.1	149.00	0.02
	28.35	g	1	0.1	0.0	42.24	0.01
	1.00	oz					
mixed species, canned, drained	100.00	g	142	24.3	5.9	627.99	1.59
	56.70	g	81	13.8	3.4	356.07	0.90
	2.00	oz					

OYSTERS

	SERVING QUANTITY	SERVING UNIT	CALORIES	PROTEIN (g)	TOTAL CARBOHYDRATES (g)	POTASSIUM (mg)	TOTAL FAT (g)
ostrich, raw	100.00	g	125	21.6	0.0	297.00	3.67
	85.05	g	106	18.3	0.0	252.60	3.12
	3.00	oz					
ostrich, cooked	100.00	g	159	28.8	0.0	409.00	3.97
	85.05	g	135	24.5	0.0	347.85	3.38
	3.00	oz					
pacific, raw	100.00	g	81	9.5	5.0	168.00	2.30
	113.40	g	92	10.7	5.6	190.51	2.61
	4.00	oz					
pacific, cooked, moist heat	100.00	g	163	18.9	9.9	302.00	4.60
	85.05	g	139	16.1	8.4	256.85	3.91
	3.00	oz					
eastern, canned	100.00	g	68	7.1	3.9	229.00	2.47
	56.70	g	39	4.0	2.2	129.84	1.40
	2.00	oz					
eastern, farmed, raw	100.00	g	59	5.2	5.5	124.00	1.55
	85.05	g	50	4.4	4.7	105.46	1.32
	3.00	oz					
eastern, wild, raw	100.00	g	51	5.7	2.7	156.00	1.71
	113.40	g	58	6.5	3.1	176.90	1.94
	4.00	oz					
eastern, wild, breaded, fried	100.00	g	199	8.8	11.6	244.00	12.58
	85.05	g	169	7.5	9.9	207.52	10.70
	3.00	oz					
battered, breaded, fried, fast food	100.00	g	265	9.0	28.7	131.00	12.90
	85.05	g	225	7.7	24.4	111.41	10.97
	3.00	oz					

	SERVING QUANTITY	SERVING UNIT	CALORIES (kcal)	PROTEIN (g)	TOTAL CARBOHYDRATES (g)	POTASSIUM (mg)	TOTAL FAT (g)
MUSSELS							
blue, raw	100	g	86	11.9	3.7	320.00	2.24
	113.40	g	98	13.5	4.2	362.88	2.54
	4.00	oz					
blue, cooked, moist heat	100.00	g	172	23.8	7.4	268.00	4.48
	85.05	g	146	20.2	6.3	227.93	3.81
	3.00	oz					
atlantic or pacific, meat only	100.00	g	197	8.8	11.6	243.87	12.56
	85.05	g	167	7.5	9.9	207.41	10.69
	3.00	oz					
MACKEREL							
Atlantic or Boston, raw fillet	100.00	g	205	18.6	0.0	313.97	13.89
	113.40	g	232	21.1	0.0	356.04	15.75
	4.00	oz					
pacific and Jack, raw fillet	100.00	g	158	20.1	0.0	405.96	7.89
	113.40	g	179	22.8	0.0	460.36	8.95
	4.00	oz					
Atlantic Spanish, raw fillet	100.00	g	139	19.3	0.0	445.96	6.30
	113.40	g	158	21.9	0.0	505.71	7.14
	4.00	oz					
Jack, canned, solids, drained	100.00	g	156	23.2	0.0	194.00	6.30
	56.70	g	88	13.2	0.0	110.00	3.57
	2.00	oz					
Atlantic or Boston, cooked, dry heat	100.00	g	262	23.9	0.0	401.00	17.81
	85.05	g	223	20.3	0.0	341.05	15.15
	3.00	oz					
Atlantic, Spanish, cooked, dry heat	100.00	g	158	23.6	0.0	553.99	6.32
	85.05	g	134	20.1	0.0	471.17	5.38
	3.00	oz					
Pacific and Jack, mixed species, cooked	100.00	g	201	25.7	0.0	520.99	10.12
	85.05	g	171	21.9	0.0	443.11	8.61
	3.00	oz					

SCALLOPS	SERVING QUANTITY	SERVING UNIT	CALORIES (kcal)	PROTEIN (g)	TOTAL CARBOHYDRATES (g)	POTASSIUM (mg)	TOTAL FAT (g)
Mixed species, raw	100.00	g	69	12.1	3.2	205.00	0.49
	113.40	g	78	13.7	3.6	232.47	0.56
	4.00	oz					
Bay and Sea, steamed	100.00	g	111	20.5	5.4	314.00	0.84
	85.05	g	94	17.5	4.6	267.06	0.71
	3.00	oz					
mixed species, breaded and fried	100.00	g	216	18.1	10.1	333.00	10.94
	46.50	g	100	8.4	4.7	15.85	5.09
	3.00	pcs					
breaded, fried, fast food	100.00	g	268	10.9	26.7	204.00	13.47
	85.05	g	228	9.3	22.7	173.50	11.46
	3.00	oz					

HERRING

	SERVING QUANTITY	SERVING UNIT	CALORIES	PROTEIN (g)	TOTAL CARBOHYDRATES (g)	POTASSIUM (mg)	TOTAL FAT (g)
Pacific, raw	100.00	g	195	16.4	0.0	422.96	13.88
	113.40	g	221	18.6	0.0	479.64	15.74
	4.00	oz					
Atlantic, raw	100.00	g	158	18.0	0.0	326.97	9.04
	113.40	g	179	20.4	0.0	370.78	10.25
	4.00	oz					
Pacific, cooked, dry heat	100.00	g	250	21.0	0.0	541.99	17.79
	85.05	g	213	17.9	0.0	460.97	15.13
	3.00	oz					
Atlantic, cooked, dry heat	100.00	g	203	23.0	0.0	419.00	11.49
	85.05	g	173	19.6	0.0	356.36	9.86
	3.00	oz					
Roe or eggs, Pacific (Alaska Native)	100.00	g	74	9.6	4.5	na	1.93
	85.05	g	63	8.2	3.8	na	1.64
	3.00	oz					

Chapter 4: Dairy and Non-Dairy

Do you want to print the charts in letter-size (8.5x11")?

I have created downloadable printables of this chart. You can scan the QR code below or copy the link to your computer browser to be able to get your printable copies of the food charts

https://go.renaltracker.com/lowpotassiumprint

MILK

	SERVING QUANTITY	SERVING UNIT	CALORIES (kcal)	PROTEIN (g)	TOTAL CARBOHYDRATES (g)	POTASSIUM (mg)	TOTAL FAT (g)
(cow) whole	100	g	60	3.3	4.7	150.00	3.20
	244	g	146	8.0	11.4	366.00	7.81
	1	c					
2% reduced fat	100	g	50	3.4	4.9	159.00	1.90
	244	g	122	8.2	12.0	388.00	4.64
	1	c					
low fat (1%)	100	g	43	3.4	5.2	159.00	0.95
	244	g	105	8.3	12.7	388.00	2.32
	1	c					
skim, fat free	100	g	34	3.4	4.9	167.00	0.08
	244	g	83	8.4	11.9	407.00	0.20
	1	c					
lactose free, from whole milk	100	g	60	3.3	4.7	150.00	3.20
	244	g	146	8.0	11.4	366.00	7.81
	1	c					
Buttermilk, dried	100	g	387	34.3	49.0	1592.00	5.78
	6.5	g	25	2.2	3.2	103.00	0.38
	1	tbsp					
buttermilk, fluid, whole	100	g	62	3.2	4.9	135.00	3.31
	245	g	152	7.9	12.0	331.00	8.11
	1	c					
condensed, sweetened	100	g	321	7.9	54.4	371.00	8.70
	38	g	122	3.0	20.7	141.00	3.31
	1	fl oz					
evaporated, whole	100	g	134	6.8	10.0	303.00	7.56
	31.5	g	42	2.1	3.2	95.40	2.38
	1	fl oz					
malted	100	g	64	3.2	8.7	150.00	1.91
	256	g	164	8.2	22.2	384.00	4.89
	1	c					
chocolate	100	g	67	3.4	13.5	182.00	0.00
	248	g	166	8.4	33.4	451.00	0.00
	1	c					
strawberry (whole milk)	100	g	85	3.0	11.8	139.00	2.97
	248	g	211	7.5	29.3	345.00	7.37
	1	c					

MILK

	SERVING QUANTITY	SERVING UNIT	CALORIES (kcal)	PROTEIN (g)	TOTAL CARBOHYDRATES (g)	POTASSIUM (mg)	TOTAL FAT (g)
SOY	100	g	43	2.6	4.9	122.00	1.47
	244	g	105	6.3	12.0	298.00	3.59
	1	c					
soy, light	100	g	30	2.4	3.5	117.00	0.77
	244	g	73	5.8	8.6	285.00	1.88
	1	c					
soy, chocolate	100	g	63	2.3	10.0	143.00	1.53
	244	g	154	5.5	24.3	349.00	3.73
	1	c					
soy, non-fat	100	g	28	2.5	4.1	105.00	0.04
	244	g	68	6.0	10.1	256.00	0.10
	1	c					
RICE	100	g	47	0.3	9.2	27.00	0.97
	244	g	115	0.7	22.4	65.90	2.37
	1	c					
rice milk, unsweetened	100	g	47	0.3	9.2	27.00	0.97
	240	g	113	0.7	22.0	64.80	2.33
	8	fl oz					
ALMOND, unsweeteened	100	g	15	0.4	1.3	67.00	0.96
	244	g	37	1.0	3.2	163.00	2.34
	1	c					
almond, unsweetened, chocolate	100	g	16	0.5	1.5	71.00	1.00
	244	g	39	1.1	3.6	173.00	2.44
	1	c					
almond milk, sweeteend	100	g	30	0.4	5.2	64.00	0.93
	244	g	73	0.9	12.8	156.00	2.27
	1	c					
almond, sweetened, chocolate	100	g	41	0.4	8.3	67.00	0.95
	244	g	100	1.1	20.4	163.00	2.32
	1	c					
COCONUT	100	g	31	0.2	2.9	19.00	2.08
	244	g	76	0.5	7.1	46.40	5.08
	1	c					
GOAT, whole	100	g	69	3.6	4.5	204.00	4.14
	244	g	168	8.7	10.9	498.00	10.10
	1	c					

MILK SUBSTITUTE

	SERVING QUANTITY	SERVING UNIT	CALORIES (kcal)	PROTEIN (g)	TOTAL CARBOHYDRATES (g)	POTASSIUM (mg)	TOTAL FAT (g)
Non-dairy milk/creamer	100	g	29	1.0	3.8	80.00	1.17
	30.5	g	9	0.3	1.1	24.40	0.36
	1	fl oz					
imitation, non-soy	100	g	46	1.6	5.3	150.00	2.00
	244	g	112	3.9	12.9	366.00	4.88
	1	cup					
Kefir	100	g	52	3.6	7.5	159.00	0.96
	244	g	127	8.8	18.3	388.00	2.34
	1	c					
Sorbet	100	g	110	0.8	27.1	28.00	0.05
	80	g	88	0.6	21.7	22.40	0.04
	1	bar					

YOGURT

	SERVING QUANTITY	SERVING UNIT	CALORIES (kcal)	PROTEIN (g)	TOTAL CARBOHYDRATES (g)	POTASSIUM (mg)	TOTAL FAT (g)
coconut milk, yogurt	100	g	64	0.3	8.0	27.00	3.50
	170	g	109	0.5	13.5	45.90	5.95
	6	oz					
dressing	100	g	220	3.5	11.8	146.00	18.27
	15.4	g	34	0.5	1.8	22.50	2.81
	1	tbsp					
liquid	100	g	72	3.7	11.8	171.00	1.09
	245	g	176	9.1	28.9	419.00	2.67
	1	c					
plain, whole milk	100	g	61	3.5	4.7	155.00	3.25
	227	g	138	7.9	10.6	352.00	7.38
	8	oz					
Whole milk with fruit	100	g	87	3.1	12.4	146.00	2.87
	170	g	148	5.3	21.0	248.00	4.88
	6	oz					

YOGURT

YOGURT	SERVING QUANTITY	SERVING UNIT	CALORIES (kcal)	PROTEIN (g)	TOTAL CARBOHYDRATES (g)	POTASSIUM (mg)	TOTAL FAT (g)
whole milk, flavored (non-fruit)	100	g	77	3.3	9.4	147.00	3.10
	170	g	131	5.6	16.0	250.00	5.27
	6	oz					
non-fat milk, plain, vanilla	100	g	78	2.9	17.0	141.00	0.00
	227	g	177	6.7	38.7	320.00	0.00
	8	oz					
non-fat milk, fruit	100	g	83	5.1	15.0	234.00	0.17
	170	g	141	8.7	25.5	398.00	0.29
	6	oz					
Soy, yogurt, plain	100	g	94	3.5	16.0	47.00	1.80
	170	g	160	6.0	27.1	79.90	3.06
	6	oz					
Greek, plain, whole milk	100	g	97	9.0	4.0	141.00	5.00
	170	g	165	15.3	6.8	240.00	8.50
	6	oz					
Greek, fruit, whole milk	100	g	106	7.3	12.3	113.00	3.00
	170	g	180	12.5	20.9	192.00	5.10
	6	oz					
Greek, flavored, other than fruit	100	g	111	8.5	9.4	121.00	4.44
	170	g	189	14.4	15.9	206.00	7.55
	6	oz					
Greek, plain, low fat	100	g	73	10.0	3.9	141.00	1.92
	170	g	124	16.9	6.7	240.00	3.26
	6	oz					
Greek, LF, flavors other than fruit	100	g	95	8.6	9.5	123.00	2.50
	170	g	162	14.7	16.2	209.00	4.25
	6	oz					
Greek, non-fat (NF), plain	100	g	59	10.2	3.6	141.00	0.39
	170	g	100	17.3	6.1	240.00	0.66
	6	oz					
Greek, NF, flavors other than fruit	100	g	78	8.6	10.4	123.00	0.18
	170	g	133	14.7	17.6	209.00	0.31
	6	oz					
Frozen yogurt, chocolate	100	g	131	3.0	21.6	234.00	3.60
	160	g	210	4.8	34.6	374.00	5.76
1 scoop = small cup	1	scoop					

YOGURT	SERVING QUANTITY	SERVING UNIT	CALORIES (kcal)	PROTEIN (g)	TOTAL CARBOHYDRATES (g)	POTASSIUM (mg)	TOTAL FAT (g)
Frozen yogurt, vanilla	100	g	127	3.0	21.6	156.00	3.60
	160	g	203	4.8	34.6	250.00	5.76
1 scoop = small cup	1	scoop					
Frozen yogurt, soft serve, chocolate	100	g	160	4.3	24.9	237.00	5.76
	175	g	280	7.5	43.5	415.00	10.10
	1	c					
Frozn yogurt, soft serve, vanilla	100	g	159	4.0	24.2	211.00	5.60
	175	g	278	7.0	42.4	369.00	9.80
	1	c					
Frozn yogurt bar, vanilla	100	g	127	3.0	21.6	156.00	3.60
	65	g	83	2.0	14.0	101.00	2.34
	1	bar					
Frozn yogurt bar, chocolate	100	g	131	3.0	21.6	234.00	3.60
	65	g	85	2.0	14.0	152.00	2.34
	1	bar					
Frozn yogurt cone, vanilla	100	g	139	3.2	23.9	154.00	3.73
	125	g	174	4.0	29.9	192.00	4.66
	1	cone					
Frozn yogurt cone, chocolate	100	g	142	3.2	23.9	229.00	3.73
	125	g	178	4.0	29.9	286.00	4.66
	1	cone					
Frozn yogurt, waffle cone, vanilla	100	g	143	3.3	25.3	155.00	3.61
	255	g	365	8.4	64.5	395.00	9.20
	1	cone					
Frozn yogurt, waffle cone, choco	100	g	147	3.3	25.3	229.00	3.61
	255	g	375	8.4	64.5	584.00	9.20
	1	cone					

CHEESE

	SERVING QUANTITY	SERVING UNIT	CALORIES (kcal)	PROTEIN (g)	TOTAL CARBOHYDRATES (g)	POTASSIUM (mg)	TOTAL FAT (g)
mozzarella, from whole milk	100	g	299	22.2	2.4	76.00	22.14
shredded	112	g	335	24.8	2.7	85.10	24.80
	1	c					
mozzarella, part skim milk	100	g	254	24.3	2.8	84.00	15.92
	28.35	g	72	6.9	0.8	23.80	4.51
	1	oz					
Mozzarella, reduced sodium (shredded)	100	g	280	27.5	3.1	95.00	17.10
	113	g	316	31.1	3.5	107.00	19.30
	1	cup					
ricotta, from whole milk	100	g	158	7.8	6.9	230.00	11.00
	129	g	204	10.1	8.9	297.00	14.20
	0.5	c					
riccota, part skim milk	100	g	138	11.4	5.1	125.00	7.91
	124	g	171	14.1	6.4	155.00	9.81
	0.5	c					
cream cheese, regular	100	g	295	7.1	3.5	112.00	28.60
	28.35	g	84	2.0	1.0	31.80	8.11
	1	oz					
cream cheese, light	100	g	201	7.9	8.1	247.00	15.28
	28.35	g	57	2.2	2.3	70.00	4.33
	1	oz					
processed cheese food	100	g	307	16.1	8.9	295.00	23.06
	21	g	65	3.4	1.9	62.00	4.84
	1	slice					
Cottage cheese	100	g	84	11.0	4.3	120.00	2.30
	210	g	176	23.1	9.1	252.00	4.83
	1	cup					
cottage cheese, low fat	100	g	84	11.0	4.3	120.00	2.30
	226	g	190	24.9	9.7	271.00	5.20
	1	cup					
Monterey shredded	100	g	373	24.5	0.7	81.00	30.28
	113	g	421	27.7	0.8	91.50	34.20
	1	cup					
Cheddar	100	g	408	23.3	2.4	77.00	34.00
	21	g	86	4.9	0.5	16.20	7.14
	1	slice					

CHEESE

	SERVING QUANTITY	SERVING UNIT	CALORIES (kcal)	PROTEIN (g)	TOTAL CARBOHYDRATES (g)	POTASSIUM (mg)	TOTAL FAT (g)
Cheddar, reduced sodium	100	g	398	24.4	1.9	112.00	32.62
	21	g	84	5.1	0.4	23.50	6.85
	1	slice					
Cheddar, sharp sliced	100	g	410	24.3	2.1	76.00	33.82
	28	g	115	6.8	0.6	21.30	9.47
	1	oz					
Cheddar/ American cheese spread	100	g	290	16.4	8.7	242.00	21.23
	21	g	61	3.5	1.8	50.80	4.46
	1	wedge					
American	100	g	307	16.1	8.9	295.00	23.06
	21	g	65	3.4	1.9	62.00	4.84
	1	slice					
Brick	100	g	371	23.2	2.8	136.00	29.68
	17.2	g	64	4.0	0.5	23.40	5.10
	1	cubic inch					
Brie	100	g	334	20.8	0.5	152.00	27.68
	17	g	57	3.5	0.1	25.80	4.71
	1	cubic inch					
blue	100	g	353	21.4	2.3	256.00	28.74
	28.35	g	100	6.1	0.7	72.60	8.15
	1	oz					
Camembert 1 wedge = 1.33 oz	100	g	300	19.8	0.5	187.00	24.26
	38	g	114	7.5	0.2	71.10	9.22
	1	wedge					
Colby	100	g	394	23.8	2.6	127.00	32.11
	21	g	83	5.0	0.5	26.70	6.74
	1	slice					
Caraway	100	g	376	25.2	1.1	93.00	29.20
	28.35	g	107	7.1	0.9	26.40	8.28
	1	oz					
Edam	100	g	356	24.9	2.2	121.00	27.44
	21	g	75	5.2	0.5	25.40	5.76
	1	slice					
Feta	100	g	265	14.2	3.9	62.00	21.49
	17	g	45	2.4	0.7	10.50	3.62
	1	cubic inch					
Fontina	100	g	389	25.6	1.6	64.00	31.14
	21	g	82	5.4	0.3	13.40	6.54
	1	slice					
goat	100	g	364	21.6	0.1	158.00	29.84
	25	g	91	5.4	0.0	39.50	7.46
	1	cubic inch					

CHEESE

	Serving Quantity	Serving Unit	Calories (kcal)	Protein (g)	Total Carbohydrates (g)	Potassium (mg)	Total Fat (g)
Gouda	100	g	356	24.9	2.2	121.00	27.44
	28.35	g	101	7.0	0.6	34.30	7.78
	1	oz					
Gruyere	100	g	413	29.8	0.4	81.00	32.34
	21	g	87	6.3	0.1	17.00	6.70
	1	slice					
Blue or Roquefort	100	g	353	21.4	2.3	256.00	28.74
	17.3	g	61	3.7	0.4	44.30	4.97
	1	cubic inch					
Colby Jack	100	g	384	24.1	1.6	104.00	31.20
	21	g	81	5.1	0.3	21.80	6.55
	1	slice					
Parmesan, grated	100	g	420	29.6	12.4	184.00	28.00
	7.6	g	32	2.3	0.9	14.00	1.82
	1	tbsp					
Parmesan, hard	100	g	421	29.6	12.4	184.00	28.00
	10.3	g	43	3.1	1.3	19.00	2.88
	1	cubic inch					
Mexican blend shredded	100	g	358	23.5	1.8	85.00	28.51
	113	g	405	26.6	2.0	96.00	32.20
	1	cup					
Mexican blend, reduced fat shredded	100	g	282	24.7	3.4	93.00	19.40
	113	g	319	27.9	3.9	105.00	21.90
	1	cup					
Muenster	100	g	368	23.4	1.1	134.00	30.04
	21	g	77	5.0	0.2	28.10	6.31
	1	slice					
Neufchatel	100	g	253	9.2	3.6	152.00	22.78
	28.35	g	72	2.6	1.0	43.10	6.46
	1	oz					
Provolone	100	g	351	25.6	2.1	138.00	26.62
	21	g	74	5.4	0.4	29.00	5.59
	1	slice					
Romano	100	g	387	31.8	3.6	86.00	26.94
	28.35	g	110	9.0	1.0	24.40	7.64
	1	oz					
Swiss	100	g	393	27.0	1.4	71.00	31.00
	21	g	83	5.7	0.3	14.90	6.51
	1	slice					
Tilsiter/ Tilsit	100	g	340	24.4	1.9	65.00	25.98
	28.35	g	96	6.9	0.5	18.40	7.36
	1	oz					

CREAM

	SERVING QUANTITY	SERVING UNIT	CALORIES (kcal)	PROTEIN (g)	TOTAL CARBOHYDRATES (g)	POTASSIUM (mg)	TOTAL FAT (g)
sour cream, regular	100	g	198	2.4	4.6	125.00	19.35
	30	g	59	0.7	1.4	37.50	5.80
	1	container					
sour cream, light	100	g	136	3.5	7.1	212.00	10.60
	240	g	326	8.4	17.0	509.00	25.40
	1	cup					
sour cream, imitation	100	g	208	2.4	6.6	161.00	19.52
	240	g	499	5.8	15.9	386.00	46.80
	1	cup					
sour cream, fat free	100	g	74	3.1	15.6	129.00	0.00
	240	g	178	7.4	37.4	310.00	0.00
	1	cup					
heavy full cream	100	g	340	2.8	2.8	95.00	36.08
	30	g	102	0.9	1.0	28.50	10.80
	1	fl oz					
whipped	100	g	343	2.7	8.6	89.00	33.94
	40	g	137	1.1	3.4	35.60	13.60
	1	cup					
half and half	100	g	131	3.1	4.3	132.00	11.50
	30	g	39	0.9	1.3	39.60	3.45
	1	fl oz					
coffee, light cream	100	g	195	3.0	3.7	136.00	19.10
	11	g	21	0.3	0.4	15.00	2.10
	1	ind. container					

Chapter 5: Fats, Oils, and Nuts

Do you want to print the charts in letter-size (8.5x11")?

I have created downloadable printables of this chart. You can scan the QR code below or copy the link to your computer browser to be able to get your printable copies of the food charts

https://go.renaltracker.com/lowpotassiumprint

ALMOND	SERVING QUANTITY	UNIT SERVING	CALORIES (kcal)	PROTEIN (g)	TOTAL CARBOHYDRATES (g)	POTASSIUM (mg)	TOTAL FAT (g)
whole	100	g	579	21.2	21.6	733.00	49.9
	35.75	g	207	7.6	7.7	262.05	17.9
	0.25	c					
slivered	100	g	579	21.2	21.6	733.00	49.9
	27	g	156	5.7	5.8	197.91	13.5
	0.25	c					
ground	100	g	579	21.2	21.6	733.00	49.9
	23.75	g	138	5.0	5.1	174.09	11.9
	0.25	c					
paste (marzipan)	100	g	458	9.0	47.8	314.00	27.7
	28.38	g	130	2.6	13.6	89.10	7.9
	2	tbsp					
oil	100	g	884	0.0	0.0	0.00	100.0
	13.6	g	120	0.0	0.0	0.00	13.6
	1	tbsp					
butter, without salt added	100	g	614	21.0	18.8	748.00	55.5
	16	g	98	3.4	3.0	119.68	8.9
	1	tbsp					
dry roasted, without salt added	100	g	598	3.0	21.0	713.00	52.5
	34.5	g	206	7.2	7.3	245.99	18.1
	0.25	c					
oil roasted, without salt	100	g	607	21.2	17.7	699.00	55.2
	39.25	g	238	8.3	6.9	274.36	21.7
	0.25	c					
milk, unsweetened, shelf stable	100	g	15	0.4	1.3	67.00	1.0
	262	g	39	1.1	3.4	175.54	2.5
	1	c					
milk, sweetened, vanilla flavor ready-to-drink	100	g	38	0.4	6.6	50.00	1.0
	240	g	91	1.0	15.8	120.00	2.5
	1	c					
milk, chocolate flavor, unsweetened fortified Vit. D2 and E	100	g	21	0.8	1.3	96.00	1.5
	240	g	50	2.0	3.0	130.40	3.5
	1	c					

WALNUT

	SERVING QUANTITY	UNIT	CALORIES (kcal)	PROTEIN (g)	TOTAL CARBOHYDRATES (g)	POTASSIUM (mg)	TOTAL FAT (g)
english, halves	100	g	654	15.2	13.7	441.00	65.2
	25	g	164	3.8	3.4	110.25	16.3
	0.25	c					
english, ground	100	g	654	15.2	13.7	441.00	65.2
	20	g	131	3.1	2.7	88.20	13.0
	0.25	c					
english, chopped	100	g	654	15.2	13.7	441.00	65.2
	29.25	g	191	4.5	4.0	128.99	19.1
	0.25	c					
butternut or white walnut, dried	100	g	612	24.9	12.1	421.00	57.0
	120	g	734	29.9	14.5	505.20	68.4
	1	c					
black or american, dried, chopped	100	g	619	24.1	9.6	523.00	59.3
	31.25	g	193	7.5	3.0	163.44	18.5
	0.25	c					
black or american, dried, ground	100	g	604	23.5	9.3	509.92	57.9
	26.67	g	161	6.3	2.5	135.98	15.4
	0.33	c					
glazed	100	g	500	8.3	47.6	232.00	35.7
	28.35	g	142	2.4	13.5	65.77	10.1
	1	oz					
oil	100	g	884	0.0	0.0	0.00	100.0
	13.6	g	120	0.0	0.0	0.00	13.6
	1	tbsp					

PECANS	SERVING QUANTITY	SERVING UNIT	CALORIES (kcal)	PROTEIN (g)	TOTAL CARBOHYDRATES (g)	POTASSIUM (mg)	TOTAL FAT (g)
chopped	100	g	691	9.2	13.9	410.00	72.0
	109	g	753	10.0	15.1	446.90	78.5
	1	c					
halves	100	g	691	9.2	13.9	410.00	72.0
	24.75	g	171	2.3	3.4	101.48	17.8
	0.25	c					
halves, oil roasted	100	g	715	9.2	13.0	392.00	75.2
	110	g	787	10.1	14.3	431.20	82.8
	1	c					
dry roasted, without salt added	100	g	710	9.5	13.6	424.00	74.3
	28.35	g	201	2.7	3.8	120.20	21.1
	1	oz					

PISTACHIO

	SERVING QUANTITY	SERVING UNIT	CALORIES	PROTEIN (g)	TOTAL CARBOHYDRATES (g)	POTASSIUM (mg)	TOTAL FAT (g)
raw (1 oz = 49 kernels)	100	g	560	20.2	27.2	1,025	45.3
	123	g	689	24.8	33.4	1,260	55.7
	1	c					
dry roasted, no salt added	100	g	572	21.1	28.3	1,007	45.8
	123	g	704	25.9	34.8	1,238	56.4
	1	c					

MACADAMIA

	SERVING QUANTITY	SERVING UNIT	CALORIES	PROTEIN (g)	TOTAL CARBOHYDRATES (g)	POTASSIUM (mg)	TOTAL FAT (g)
whole or halves (1 oz = 10-12 kernels)	100	g	718	7.9	13.8	368.00	75.8
	134	g	962	10.6	18.5	493.12	101.5
	1	c					
dry roasted, without salt added	100	g	718	7.8	13.4	363.00	76.1
	33.5	g	241	2.6	4.5	121.61	25.5
	0.25	c					

CASHEW

	SERVING QUANTITY	UNIT	CALORIES (kcal)	PROTEIN (g)	TOTAL CARBOHYDRATES (g)	POTASSIUM (mg)	TOTAL FAT (g)
raw	100	g	553	18.2	30.2	660.00	43.9
	28.35	g	157	5.2	8.6	187.11	12.4
	1	oz					
oil roasted, no	100	g	580	16.8	29.9	632.00	47.8
salt added	129	g	748	21.7	38.5	815.28	61.6
	1	c					
dry roasted, no	100	g	574	15.3	32.7	565.00	46.4
salt aded	137	g	786	21.0	44.8	774.05	63.5
(halves and whole)	1	c					
butter, without	100	g	587	17.6	27.6	546.00	49.4
salt added	32	g	188	5.6	8.8	174.72	15.8
	2	tbsp					

HAZELNUT

	SERVING QUANTITY	UNIT	CALORIES (kcal)	PROTEIN (g)	TOTAL CARBOHYDRATES (g)	POTASSIUM (mg)	TOTAL FAT (g)
oil	100	g	884	0.0	0.0	0.00	100.0
	13.6	g	120	0.0	0.0	0.00	13.6
	1	tbsp					
whole (1 oz =	100	g	628	15.0	16.7	680.00	60.8
21 kernels)	33.75	g	212	5.1	5.6	229.50	20.5
	0.25	c					
blanched	100	g	629	13.7	17.0	658.00	61.2
	28.35	g	178	3.9	4.8	186.54	17.3
	1	oz					
chopped	100	g	628	15.0	16.7	680.00	60.8
	28.75	g	181	4.3	4.8	195.50	17.5
	0.25	c					
ground	100	g	628	15.0	16.7	680.00	60.8
	18.75	g	118	2.8	3.1	127.50	11.4
	0.25	c					
dry roasted,	100	g	646	15.0	17.6	755.00	62.4
without salt	28.35	g	183	4.3	5.0	214.04	17.7
added	1	oz					
spread, chocolate flavored	100	g	539	5.4	62.4	407.00	29.7

PEANUT	SERVING QUANTITY	UNIT SERVING	CALORIES (kcal)	PROTEIN (g)	TOTAL CARBOHYDRATES (g)	POTASSIUM (mg)	TOTAL FAT (g)
oil	100	g	884	0.0	0.0	0.00	100.0
	13.5	g	119	0.0	0.0	0.00	13.5
	1	tbsp					
all types	100	g	567	25.8	16.1	705.00	49.2
	36.5	g	207	9.4	5.9	257.33	18.0
	0.25	c					
all types, dry roasted, no salt added (1 oz = 28.35g)	100	g	587	24.4	21.4	634.00	49.7
	36.5	g	214	8.9	7.8	231.41	18.1
	0.25	c					
all types, oil roasted, no salt	100	g	599	28.0	15.3	726.00	52.5
	133	g	797	37.3	20.3	965.58	69.8
	1	c					
butter, smooth, reduced fat	100	g	520	25.9	36.7	669.00	34.0
	36	g	187	9.3	12.8	240.84	12.2
	2	tbsp					
butter, smooth, no salt added	100	g	598	22.2	22.3	558.00	51.4
	32	g	191	7.1	7.1	178.56	16.4
	2	tbsp					
butter, chunky, no salt added	100	g	589	24.1	21.6	745.00	49.9
	32	g	188	7.7	6.9	238.40	16.0
	2	tbsp					
butter, reduced sodium	100	g	590	24.0	21.8	747.00	49.9
	16	g	94	3.8	3.5	119.52	8.0
	1	tbsp					
sauce, made with PB, water & soy sauce	100	g	257	6.3	22.0	235.00	16.0
	18	g	46	1.1	4.0	42.30	2.9
	1	tbsp					
brittle	100	g	486	7.6	71.2	168.00	19.0
	42.53	g	207	3.2	30.3	71.44	8.1
	1.5	oz					
flour, defatted	100	g	327	52.2	34.7	1,290.00	0.6
	30	g	98	15.7	10.4	387.00	0.2
	0.5	c					

PINE	SERVING QUANTITY	UNIT	CALORIES (kcal)	PROTEIN (g)	TOTAL CARBOHYDRATES (g)	POTASSIUM (mg)	TOTAL FAT (g)
(Pinyon), dried	100	g	629	11.6	19.3	628.00	61.0
	28.35	g	178	3.3	5.5	178.04	17.3
	1	oz					
(Pignolia),	100	g	673	13.7	13.1	597.00	68.4
dried	8.6	g	58	1.2	1.1	51.34	5.9
	1	tbsp					
CHESTNUT							
Japanese	100	g	154	2.3	34.9	329.00	0.5
	28.35	g	44	0.6	9.9	93.27	0.2
	1	oz					
Chinese	100	g	224	4.2	49.1	447.00	1.1
	28.35	g	64	1.2	13.9	126.72	0.3
	1	oz					
European,	100	g	213	2.4	45.5	518.00	2.3
unpeeled	36.25	g	77	0.9	16.5	187.78	0.8
	0.25	c					
European,	100	g	196	1.6	44.2	484.00	1.3
peeled	28.35	g	56	0.5	12.5	137.21	0.4
	1	oz					
European,	100	g	245	3.2	53.0	592.00	2.2
roasted	28.35	g	69	0.9	15.0	167.83	0.6
	1	oz					
Japanese,	100	g	201	3.0	45.1	427.00	0.8
roasted	28.35	g	57	0.8	12.8	121.05	0.2
	1	oz					
Chinese,	100	g	239	4.5	52.4	477.00	1.2
roasted	28.35	g	68	1.3	14.8	135.23	0.3
	1	oz					
Chinese,	100	g	153	2.9	33.6	306.00	0.8
boiled and	28.35	g	43	0.8	9.5	86.75	0.2
steamed	1	oz					
European,	100	g	131	2.0	27.8	715.00	1.4
boiled and	28.35	g	37	0.6	7.9	202.70	0.4
steamed	1	oz					
Japanese,	100	g	56	0.8	12.6	119.00	0.2
boiled and	28.35	g	16	0.2	3.6	33.74	0.1
steamed	1	oz					

ACORN

	SERVING QUANTITY	UNIT	CALORIES (kcal)	PROTEIN (g)	TOTAL CARBOHYDRATES (g)	POTASSIUM (mg)	TOTAL FAT (g)
Nuts	100	g	387	6.2	40.8	539.00	23.9
	28.35	g	110	1.7	11.6	152.81	6.8
	1	oz					
flour	100	g	501	7.5	54.7	712.00	30.2
	28.35	g	142	2.1	15.5	201.85	8.6
	1	oz					
nuts, dried	100	g	509	8.1	53.7	709.00	31.4
	28.35	g	144	2.3	15.2	201.00	8.9
	1	oz					

CHIA

	SERVING QUANTITY	UNIT	CALORIES (kcal)	PROTEIN (g)	TOTAL CARBOHYDRATES (g)	POTASSIUM (mg)	TOTAL FAT (g)
seeds, dried	100	g	486	16.5	42.1	407.00	30.7
	28.35	g	138	4.7	11.9	115.38	8.7
	1	oz					

HEMP

	SERVING QUANTITY	UNIT	CALORIES (kcal)	PROTEIN (g)	TOTAL CARBOHYDRATES (g)	POTASSIUM (mg)	TOTAL FAT (g)
seeds, hulled	100	g	553	31.6	8.7	1,200.00	48.8
	30	g	166	9.5	2.6	360.00	14.6
	3	tbsp					

FLAXSEED

	SERVING QUANTITY	UNIT	CALORIES (kcal)	PROTEIN (g)	TOTAL CARBOHYDRATES (g)	POTASSIUM (mg)	TOTAL FAT (g)
seeds, whole	100	g	534	18.3	28.9	813.00	42.2
	10.3	g	55	1.9	3.0	83.70	4.3
	1	tbsp					
seeds, ground	7	g	37	1.3	2.0	56.90	3.0
	1	tbsp					
oil	100	g	884	0.1	0.0	0.00	100.0
	14	g	124	0.0	0.0	0.00	14.0
	1	tbsp					
oil with added sliced flaxseed	100	g	878	0.4	0.4	31.00	99.0
	13.7	g	120	0.1	0.1	4.25	13.6
	1	tbsp					
oil, cold pressed	100	g	884	0.1	0.0	0.00	100.0
	13.6	g	120	0.0	0.0	0.00	13.6
	1	tbsp					

SESAME	SERVING QUANTITY	UNIT	CALORIES (kcal)	PROTEIN (g)	TOTAL CARBOHYDRATES (g)	POTASSIUM (mg)	TOTAL FAT (g)
seeds, kernels,	100	g	567	17.0	26.0	406.00	48.0
toasted	128	g	726	21.7	33.3	519.68	61.4
	1	c					
butter or Tahini	100	g	592	17.4	21.5	459.00	53.0
	30	g	178	5.2	6.5	137.70	15.9
	2	tbsp					
seeds, whole,	100	g	573	17.7	23.5	468.00	49.7
dried	9	g	52	1.6	2.1	42.12	4.5
	1	tbsp					
butter or	100	g	595	17.0	21.2	414.00	53.8
Tahini, from	30	g	179	5.1	6.4	124.20	16.1
roasted/ toasted kernels	2	tbsp					

SUNFLOWER

	SERVING QUANTITY	UNIT	CALORIES (kcal)	PROTEIN (g)	TOTAL CARBOHYDRATES (g)	POTASSIUM (mg)	TOTAL FAT (g)
seeds, kernels,	100	g	619	17.2	20.6	491.00	56.8
toasted	33.5	g	207	5.8	6.9	164.49	19.0
	0.25	c					
seeds, kernels,	100	g	584	20.8	20.0	645.00	51.5
dried	36	g	210	7.5	7.2	232.20	18.5
	0.25	c					
seeds, kernels,	100	g	592	20.1	22.9	483.00	51.3
oil roasted	135	g	799	27.1	31.0	652.05	69.3
	1	c					
seeds, kernel,	100	g	582	19.3	24.1	850.00	49.8
dry roasted	32	g	186	6.2	7.7	272.00	15.9
	0.25	c					
butter, without	100	g	617	17.3	23.3	576.00	55.2
salt added	16	g	99	2.8	3.7	92.16	8.8
	1	tbsp					
oil, <60% /	100	g	884	0.0	0.0	0.00	100.0
>60%/ >70%	13.6	g	120	0.0	0.0	0.00	13.6
Linoleic	1	tbsp					
oil, industrial,	100	g	884	0.0	0.0	0.00	100.0
mid-oleic	13.6	g	120	0.0	0.0	0.00	13.6
for frying and salad dressings	1	tbsp					

OLIVE	SERVING QUANTITY	SERVING UNIT	CALORIES (kcal)	PROTEIN (g)	TOTAL CARBOHYDRATES (g)	POTASSIUM (mg)	TOTAL FAT (g)
oil, extra virgin,	100	g	884	0.0	0.0	1.00	100.0
virgin	14	g	124	0.0	0.0	0.14	14.0
	1	tbsp					
black,	100	g	116	0.8	6.0	8.00	10.9
kalamata	15	g	17	0.1	0.9	1.20	1.6
	3	pcs					
green	100	g	145	1.0	3.8	42.00	15.3
	15	g	22	0.2	0.6	6.30	2.3
	3	pcs					
spread	100	g	278	0.7	4.2	17.00	30.1
(tapenade)	16	g	45	0.1	0.7	2.72	4.8
	1	tbsp					
stuffed	100	g	128	1.0	4.0	58.00	13.2
	15	g	19	0.2	0.6	8.70	2.0
	3	pcs					
COCONUT							
fresh	100	g	354	3.3	15.2	356.00	33.5
	85	g	301	2.8	12.9	303.00	28.5
	1	c					
water,	100	g	18	0.2	4.2	165.00	0.0
unsweetened	240	g	43	0.5	10.2	396.00	0.0
	1	c					
milk	100	g	31	0.2	2.9	19.00	2.1
	244	g	76	0.5	7.1	46.40	5.1
	1	c					
milk/cream for	100	g	230	2.3	5.5	263.00	23.8
cooking	240	g	552	5.5	13.3	631.00	57.2
	1	c					
yogurt	100	g	64	0.3	8.0	27.00	3.5
	170	g	109	0.5	13.5	45.90	6.0
	6	oz					
cream,	100	g	357	1.2	53.2	101.00	16.3
canned,	37	g	132	0.4	19.7	37.40	6.0
sweetened	1/4	c					
oil	100	g	833	0.0	0.0	0.00	99.1
	14	g	117	0.0	0.0	0.00	13.9
	1	tbsp					
flaked,	100	g	456	3.1	51.9	361.00	28.0
shredded,	28	g	128	1.0	14.5	101.00	7.8
packed	2	tbsp					

SAFFLOWER	SERVING QUANTITY	UNIT	CALORIES (kcal)	PROTEIN (g)	TOTAL CARBOHYDRATES (g)	POTASSIUM (mg)	TOTAL FAT (g)
oil	100	g	884	0.0	0.0	0.00	100.0
	14	g	124	0.0	0.0	0.00	14.0
	1	tbsp					

CANOLA

oil	100	g	884	0.0	0.0	0.00	100.0
	14	g	124	0.0	0.0	0.00	14.0
	1	tbsp					

SOYBEAN

oil	100	g	884	0.0	0.0	0.00	100.0
	14	g	124	0.0	0.0	0.00	14.0
	1	tbsp					

BUTTER

stick	100	g	717	0.9	0.1	24.00	81.1
	14	g	100	0.1	0.0	3.36	11.4
	1	tbsp					
light, stick or tub	100	g	499	3.3	0.0	71.00	55.1
	14	g	70	0.5	0.0	9.94	7.7
	1	tbsp					
unsalted	100	g	717	0.9	0.1	24.00	81.1
	14	g	102	0.1	0.0	3.41	11.5
	1	tbsp					

GHEE

clarified butter	100	g	876	0.3	0.0	5.00	99.5
	14	g	123	0.0	0.0	0.70	13.9
	1	tbsp					

MARGARINE

stick	100	g	717	0.2	0.7	18.00	80.7
	14	g	100	0.0	0.1	2.52	11.3
	1	tbsp					

PUMPKIN	SERVING QUANTITY	SERVING UNIT	CALORIES (kcal)	PROTEIN (g)	TOTAL CARBOHYDRATES (g)	POTASSIUM (mg)	TOTAL FAT (g)
meat, 1" cubes	100	g	26	1.0	6.5	340.00	0.1
	116	g	30	1.2	7.5	394.40	0.1
	1	c					
flowers	100	g	15	1.0	3.3	173.00	0.1
	33	g	1	0.0	0.1	6.92	0.0
	1	c					
meat, boiled, drained, no salt added	100	g	20	0.7	4.9	230.00	0.1
	122.5	g	25	0.9	6.0	281.75	0.1
	0.5	c					
pumpkin pie spice powder	100	g	342	5.8	69.3	663.00	12.6
	1.7	g	6	0.1	1.2	11.27	0.2
	1	tsp					
seed sunfish, cooked dry heat	100	g	114	24.9	0.0	449.00	0.9
	85.05	g	97	21.2	0.0	381.87	0.8
	3	oz					
seeds, kernels, whole, roasted without salt added	100	g	446	18.6	53.8	919.00	19.4
	32	g	143	5.9	17.2	294.08	6.2
	0.5	c					
POPPYSEED							
oil	100	g	884	0.0	0.0	0.00	100.0
	13.6	g	120	0.0	0.0	0.00	13.6
	1	tbsp					
salad dressing, creamy	100	g	399	0.9	23.7	61.00	33.3
	33	g	132	0.3	7.8	20.13	11.0
	2	tbsp					

Chapter 6: Fruits

Do you want to print the charts in letter-size (8.5x11")?

I have created downloadable printables of this chart. You can scan the QR code below or copy the link to your computer browser to be able to get your printable copies of the food charts

https://go.renaltracker.com/lowpotassiumprint

BLUE BERRIES

	SERVING QUANTITY	SERVING UNIT	CALORIES (kcal)	PROTEIN (g)	TOTAL CARBOHYDRATES (g)	POTASSIUM (mg)	TOTAL FAT (g)
fresh	100.00	g	57	0.7	14.5	77.00	0.33
	145.00	g	83	1.1	21.0	111.65	0.48
	1.00	c					
sweetened, dried	100.00	g	317	2.5	80.0	214.00	2.50
	40.00	g	127	1.0	32.0	85.60	1.00
	0.25	c					
wild, frozen	100.00	g	57	0.0	13.9	68.00	0.16
	140.00	g	80	0.0	19.4	95.20	0.22
	1.00	c					
unsweetened, frozen	100.00	g	51	0.4	12.2	54.00	0.64
	155.00	g	79	0.7	18.9	83.70	0.99
	1.00	c					
canned, light syrup, drained	100.00	g	88	1.0	22.7	54.00	0.40
	244.00	g	215	2.5	55.3	131.76	0.98
	1.00	c					

STRAWBERRIES

	SERVING QUANTITY	SERVING UNIT	CALORIES (kcal)	PROTEIN (g)	TOTAL CARBOHYDRATES (g)	POTASSIUM (mg)	TOTAL FAT (g)
fresh, whole	100.00	g	32	0.7	7.7	153.00	0.30
	144.00	g	46	1.0	11.1	220.32	0.43
	1.00	c					
unsweetened, frozen (unthawed)	100.00	g	35	0.4	9.1	148.00	0.11
	149.00	g	52	0.6	13.6	220.52	0.16
	1.00	c					
sweetened, frozen, thawed	100.00	g	78	0.5	21.0	98.00	0.14
	127.50	g	99	0.7	26.8	124.95	0.18
	0.50	c					
fruit topping	100.00	g	254	0.2	66.3	51.00	0.10
	42.00	g	107	0.1	27.9	21.42	0.04
	2.00	tbsp					
pastry, 67pprox, enriched	100.00	g	371	5.4	47.8	83.00	18.50
	71.00	g	263	3.8	33.9	58.93	13.14
	1.00	pc					
Milkshake (fastfood)	100.00	g	113	3.4	18.9	182.00	2.80
	226.40	g	256	7.7	42.8	412.05	6.34
	8.00	fl oz					
yogurt 67pro, low fat	100.00	g	105	8.2	12.3	129.00	2.57
1 item = 1 container	150.00	g	158	12.3	18.4	193.50	3.86
	1.00	item					

RASPBERRIES

	SERVING QUANTITY	SERVING UNIT	CALORIES (kcal)	PROTEIN (g)	TOTAL CARBOHYDRATES (g)	POTASSIUM (mg)	TOTAL FAT (g)
raw	100.00	g	52	1.2	11.9	151.00	0.69
	123.00	g	64	1.5	14.7	185.73	0.80
	1.00	c					
frozen, unsweetend	100.00	g	56	1.2	12.6	184.00	0.81
	140.00	g	78	1.6	17.6	257.60	1.13
	1.00	c					
red, frozen, sweetened, unthawed	100.00	g	103	0.7	26.2	114.00	0.16
	125.00	g	129	0.9	32.7	142.50	0.20
	0.50	c					
puree, with seeds	100.00	g	55	na	11.5	195.00	0.97
juice concentrate	100.00	g	221	3.0	53.2	1,178.00	1.34

PEARS

	SERVING QUANTITY	SERVING UNIT	CALORIES	PROTEIN (g)	TOTAL CARBS (g)	POTASSIUM (mg)	TOTAL FAT (g)
whole, medium (2.5/lb)	100.00	g	57	0.4	15.2	116.00	0.14
	166.00	g	95	0.6	25.3	192.56	0.23
	1.00	pc					
halves, canned in water	100.00	g	29	0.2	7.8	53.00	0.03
	244.00	g	71	0.5	19.1	129.32	0.07
	1.00	c					
Asian	100.00	g	42	0.5	10.7	121.00	0.23
	122.00	g	51	0.6	13.0	147.62	0.28
	1.00	pc					

CRANBERRY

	SERVING QUANTITY	SERVING UNIT	CALORIES	PROTEIN (g)	TOTAL CARBS (g)	POTASSIUM (mg)	TOTAL FAT (g)
fresh, chopped	100.00	g	46	0.5	12.0	80.00	0.13
	55.00	g	25	0.3	6.6	44.00	0.07
	0.50	c					
dried, sweetened	100.00	g	308	0.2	82.8	49.00	1.09
	40.00	g	123	0.1	33.1	19.60	0.44
	0.33	c					
juice, unsweetened	100.00	g	46	0.4	12.2	77.00	0.13
	253.00	g	116	1.0	30.9	194.81	0.33
	1.00	c					
juice, cran cocktail	100.00	g	54	0.0	13.5	14.00	0.10
	253.00	g	137	0.0	34.2	35.42	0.25
	8.00	fl oz					
sauce, canned, sweetened	100.00	g	159	0.9	40.4	28.00	0.15
	69.25	g	110	0.6	28.0	19.39	0.10
	0.25	c					

CHERRIES

	SERVING QUANTITY	SERVING UNIT	CALORIES (kcal)	PROTEIN (g)	TOTAL CARBOHYDRATES (g)	POTASSIUM (mg)	TOTAL FAT (g)
sweet, without pits	100.00	g	63	1.1	16.0	222.00	0.20
	154.00	g	97	1.6	24.7	341.88	0.31
	1.00	c					
sour red, without pits	100.00	g	50	1.0	12.2	173.00	0.30
	155.00	g	78	1.6	18.9	268.15	0.47
	1.00	c					
juice, tart	100.00	g	59	0.3	13.7	161.00	0.54
	269.00	g	159	0.8	36.9	433.09	1.45
	1.00	c					
Pitanga or Surinam	100.00	g	33	0.8	7.5	103.00	0.40
	173.00	g	57	1.4	13.0	178.19	0.69
	1.00	c					
tart, dried, sweetened	100.00	g	333	1.3	80.5	376.00	0.73
	40.00	g	133	0.5	32.2	150.40	0.29
	0.25	c					
maraschino, canned, drained	100.00	g	165	0.2	42.0	21.00	0.21
	5.00	g	8	0.0	2.1	1.05	0.01
	1.00	pc/ item					
sweet, canned in juice, pitted	100.00	g	54	0.9	13.8	131.00	0.02
	250.00	g	135	2.3	34.5	327.50	0.05
	1.00	c					
sweet, canned in water	100.00	g	46	0.8	11.8	131.00	0.13
	248.00	g	114	1.9	29.2	324.88	0.32
	1.00	c					
sweet, frozen, sweetened thawed	100.00	g	89	1.2	22.4	199.00	0.13
	259.00	g	231	3.0	57.9	515.41	0.34
	1.00	c					
pie filling, canned	100.00	g	115	0.4	28.0	105.00	0.07
	74.00	g	85	0.3	20.7	77.70	0.05
1/8 of 21 oz can = 1 svg	1.00	svg					
pie fillings, low calorie	100.00	g	53	0.8	12.0	118.00	0.16
	264.00	g	140	2.2	31.6	311.52	0.42
	1.00	c					
sour red, canned in water, drained	100.00	g	42	0.7	10.5	115.00	0.21
	168.00	g	71	1.2	17.6	193.20	0.35
	1.00	c					
sour red, frozen unthawed	100.00	g	46	0.9	11.0	124.00	0.44
	155.00	g	71	1.4	17.1	192.20	0.68
	1.00	c					
sour red, canned in light syrup	100.00	g	75	0.7	19.3	95.00	0.10
	126.00	g	95	0.9	24.3	119.70	0.13
	0.50	c					

APPLE

	SERVING QUANTITY	SERVING UNIT	CALORIES (kcal)	PROTEIN (g)	TOTAL CARBOHYDRATES (g)	POTASSIUM (mg)	TOTAL FAT (g)
Gala, raw, with skin	100.00	g	57	0.3	13.7	108.00	0.12
	172.00	g	98	0.4	23.5	185.76	0.21
	1.00	pc, med					
fuji, raw, with skin	100.00	g	63	0.2	15.2	109.00	0.18
	192.00	g	121	0.4	29.2	209.28	0.35
	1.00	pc, med					
golden delicious, with skin	100.00	g	57	0.3	13.6	100.00	0.15
	169.00	g	96	0.5	23.0	169.00	0.25
	1.00	pc, med					
granny smith, w/ skin, raw	100.00	g	58	0.4	13.6	120.00	0.19
	167.00	g	97	0.7	22.7	200.40	0.32
	1.00	pc, med					
juice, frozen concentrate	100.00	g	47	0.1	11.5	126.00	0.10
	239.00	g	112	0.3	27.6	301.14	0.24
	8.00	fl oz					
applesauce, sweetened, canned	100.00	g	68	0.2	17.5	75.00	0.17
	123.00	g	84	0.2	21.5	92.25	0.21
	0.50	c					
applesauce, unsweetened, canned	100.00	g	42	0.2	11.3	74.00	0.10
	122.00	g	51	0.2	13.8	90.28	0.12
	0.50	c					

BLACKBERRIES

	SERVING QUANTITY	SERVING UNIT	CALORIES (kcal)	PROTEIN (g)	TOTAL CARBOHYDRATES (g)	POTASSIUM (mg)	TOTAL FAT (g)
raw	100.00	g	43	1.4	9.6	162.00	0.49
	144.00	g	62	2.0	13.8	233.28	0.71
	1.00	c					
frozen, unsweetened	100.00	g	64	1.2	15.7	140.00	0.43
	151.00	g	97	1.8	23.7	211.40	0.65
	1.00	c					
canned, heavy syrup	100.00	g	92	1.3	23.1	99.00	0.14
	256.00	g	236	3.4	59.1	253.44	0.36
	1.00	c					

PINE APPLE

	SERVING QUANTITY	SERVING UNIT	CALORIES (kcal)	PROTEIN (g)	TOTAL CARBOHYDRATES (g)	POTASSIUM (mg)	TOTAL FAT (g)
traditional varieties, diced	100.00	g	45	0.6	18.3	125.00	0.13
	155.00	g	70	0.9	11.8	193.75	0.20
	1.00	c					
sweetened, frozen, chunks	100.00	g	86	0.4	22.2	100.00	0.10
	245.00	g	211	1.0	54.4	245.00	0.25
	1.00	c					
canned in water	100.00	g	32	0.4	8.3	127.00	0.09
crushed, sliced, or chunks	246.00	g	79	1.1	20.4	312.42	0.22
	1.00	c					
canned in juice	100.00	g	60	0.4	15.7	122.00	0.08
crushed, sliced, or chunks	249.00	g	149	1.1	39.1	303.78	0.20
	1.00	c					
extra sweet variety, diced	100.00	g	51	0.5	13.5	108.00	0.11
	155.00	g	79	0.8	20.9	167.40	0.17
	1.00	c					
juice, unsweetened, canned	100.00	g	53	0.4	12.9	130.00	0.12
	250.00	g	133	0.9	32.2	325.00	0.30
	8.00	fl oz					
canned in light syrup	100.00	g	52	0.4	13.5	105.00	0.12
crushed, sliced, or chunks	126.00	g	66	0.5	17.0	132.30	0.15
	0.50	c					
juice, unsweetened, frozen concentrate	100.00	g	179	1.3	44.3	472.00	0.10
	288.00	g	387	2.8	95.7	1,019.52	0.22
	1.00	c					
juice, 71pprox.71ned with Vit A, C & E	100.00	g	50	0.4	12.2	132.00	0.14
	250.00	g	125	0.9	30.5	330.00	0.35
	1.00	c					

GRAPE-FRUIT	SERVING QUANTITY	SERVING UNIT	CALORIES (kcal)	PROTEIN (g)	TOTAL CARBOHYDRATES (g)	POTASSIUM (mg)	TOTAL FAT (g)
fresh	100.00	g	32	0.6	8.1	139.00	0.10
	153.33	g	49	1.0	12.4	213.13	0.15
	0.67	c					
white, fresh, small (3.5 diameter)	100.00	g	33	0.7	8.4	148.00	0.10
	118.00	g	39	0.8	9.9	174.64	0.12
	0.50	pc					
pink or red	100.00	g	42	0.8	10.7	135.00	0.14
	153.33	g	64	1.2	16.4	207.00	0.21
	0.67	c					
juice, white	100.00	g	39	0.5	9.2	162.00	0.10
	247.00	g	96	1.2	22.7	400.14	0.25
	8.00	fl oz					
juice, pink	100.00	g	39	0.5	9.2	162.00	0.10
	247.00	g	96	1.2	22.7	400.14	0.25
	1.00	c					
juice, unsweetened, pink, canned	100.00	g	37	0.6	7.5	141.00	0.66
	247.20	g	91	1.4	18.6	348.55	1.63
	8.00	fl oz					
ELDERBERRIES							
fresh	100.00	g	73	7.0	6.00	39.00	
	145.00	g	106	1.0	8.70	56.55	
	1.00	c					
GOOSEBERRIES							
fresh	100.00	g	44	0.9	1.00	27.00	
	150.00	g	66	1.3	1.50	40.50	
	1.00	c					
canned in light syrup	100.00	g	73	0.7	2.00	7.00	
	252.00	g	184	1.6	5.04	17.64	
	1.00	c					
KIWI (Chinese gooseberries)							
fresh, medium, without skin	100.00	g	61	1.1	3.00	34.00	
	76.00	g	46	0.9	2.28	25.84	
	1.00	pc					
LOGANBERRIES							
frozen	100.00	g	55	1.5	1.00	26.00	
	147.00	g	81	2.2	1.47	38.22	
	1.00	c					

GRAPE

	SERVING QUANTITY	SERVING UNIT	CALORIES (kcal)	PROTEIN (g)	TOTAL CARBOHYDRATES (g)	POTASSIUM (mg)	TOTAL FAT (g)
red or green, seedless	100.00	g	69	0.7	18.1	191.00	0.16
	151.00	g	104	1.1	27.3	288.41	0.24
	1.00	c					
juice, unsweetened, plus Vit.C	100.00	g	60	0.4	14.8	104.00	0.13
	252.80	g	152	0.9	37.3	262.90	0.33
	8.00	fl oz					
fruit mixed/ fruit cocktail, light, drained	100.00	g	55	0.4	14.3	85.00	0.08
juice, sweetened, frozen concentrate 6 fl oz can	100.00	g	179	0.7	44.4	74.00	0.31
	216.00	g	387	1.4	95.8	159.84	0.67
	1.00	can/item					
seedless, Thompson, canned in water	100.00	g	40	0.5	10.3	107.00	0.11
	245.00	g	98	1.2	25.2	262.15	0.27
	1.00	c					
jelly	100.00	g	266	0.2	70.0	54.00	0.02
1 packet= 14g (0.5oz)	21.00	g	56	0.0	14.7	11.34	0.00
	1	tbsp					

ORANGE

	SERVING QUANTITY	SERVING UNIT	CALORIES (kcal)	PROTEIN (g)	TOTAL CARBOHYDRATES (g)	POTASSIUM (mg)	TOTAL FAT (g)
whole, 2-5/8" diameter	100.00	g	47	0.9	11.8	181.00	0.12
	131.00	g	62	1.2	15.4	237.11	0.16
	1.00	pc/ item					
Valencia (California)	100.00	g	49	1.0	11.9	179.00	0.30
	135.00	g	66	1.4	16.1	241.65	0.41
	0.75	c					
Navel (California)	100.00	g	49	0.9	12.5	166.00	0.15
	123.75	g	61	1.1	15.5	205.43	0.19
	0.75	c					
Clementines	100.00	g	47	0.9	12.0	177.00	0.15
	74.00	g	35	0.6	8.9	130.98	0.11
	1.00	pc/ item					
orange sections	100.00	g	47	0.9	11.8	181.00	0.12
	135.00	g	63	1.3	15.9	244.35	0.16
	0.75	c					
juice	100.00	g	45	0.7	10.4	200.00	0.20
	248.00	g	112	1.7	25.8	496.00	0.50
	8.00	fl oz					
Florida, sections 1 fruit = 141g	100.00	g	46	0.7	11.5	169.00	0.21
	138.75	g	64	1.0	16.0	234.49	0.29
	0.75	c					
soda	100.00	g	48	0.0	12.3	2.00	0.00
	248.00	g	119	0.0	30.5	4.96	0.00
	8.00	fl oz					
marmalade	100.00	g	246	0.3	66.3	37.00	0.00
	20.00	g	49	0.1	13.3	7.40	0.00
	1.00	tbsp					
juice, frozen	100.00	g	95	0.5	23.2	100.00	0.00
	238.40	g	70	0.4	17.2	74.00	0.00
	1.00	c					
orange peel zest	100.00	g	97	1.5	25.0	212.00	0.20
	2.00	g	2	0.0	0.5	4.24	0.00
	1.00	tsp					
juice, unsweetened, canned	100.00	g	47	0.7	11.0	184.00	0.15
	249.00	g	117	1.7	27.4	458.16	0.37
	8.00	fl oz					
Mandarin, canned in juice	100.00	g	37	0.6	5.00	10.00	
	249.00	g	92	1.5	12.45	24.90	
	1.00	c					
juice, light, no pulp	100.00	g	21	0.2	4.00	4.00	
	240.00	g	50	0.5	9.60	9.60	
	8.00	fl oz					
Mandarin, canned in light syrup	100.00	g	61	0.5	6.00	10.00	
	252.00	g	154	1.1	15.12	25.20	
	1.00	c					

LEMON

	SERVING QUANTITY	SERVING UNIT	CALORIES (kcal)	PROTEIN (g)	TOTAL CARBOHYDRATES (g)	POTASSIUM (mg)	TOTAL FAT (g)
whole, without seeds	100.00	g	20	1.2	10.7	145.00	0.30
	108.00	g	22	1.3	11.6	156.60	0.32
	1.00	pc/ item					
peeled, 2-1/8" in diameter)	100.00	g	29	1.1	9.3	138.00	0.30
	58.00	g	17	0.6	5.4	80.04	0.17
	1.00	pc/ item					
juice, fresh	100.00	g	22	0.4	6.9	103.00	0.24
	30.50	g	7	0.1	2.1	31.42	0.07
	1.00	fl oz					
peel or zest	100.00	g	47	1.5	16.0	160.00	0.30
	2.00	g	1	0.0	0.3	3.20	0.01
	1.00	tsp					
pudding mix 1 svg = ½ c	100.00	g	363	0.1	91.8	5.00	0.50
1 package = 85g	21.20	g	77	0.0	19.5	1.06	0.11
	1.00	svg					
juice, canned	100.00	g	17	0.5	5.6	109.00	0.07
	30.50	g	5	0.1	1.7	33.25	0.02
	1.00	fl oz					
soda, lemon lime	100.00	g	40	0.1	24.9	1.00	0.02
	245.60	g	98	0.1	10.1	2.46	0.05
	8.00	fl oz					
juice, unsweetened, frozen	100.00	g	22	0.5	6.5	89.00	0.32
	5.08	g	1	0.0	0.3	4.52	0.02
	1.00	tsp					
pudding, ready to eat	100.00	g	125	0.1	25.0	1.00	3.00
1 can = 5 oz	142.00	g	178	0.1	35.5	1.42	4.26
	1.00	can/ item					
tea, black, sweetened, ready to drink	100.00	g	45	0.0	10.8	14.00	0.22
	271.00	g	122	0.0	29.3	37.94	0.60
	1.00	c					

LIME

	SERVING QUANTITY	SERVING UNIT	CALORIES (kcal)	PROTEIN (g)	TOTAL CARBOHYDRATES (g)	POTASSIUM (mg)	TOTAL FAT (g)
whole, 2" in diameter	100.00	g	30	0.7	10.5	102.00	0.20
	67.00	g	20	0.5	7.1	68.34	0.13
	1.00	pc/ item					
juice, fresh	100.00	g	25	0.4	8.4	117.00	0.07
	5.13	g	1	0.0	0.4	6.01	0.00
	1.00	tsp					
juice, unsweetened, canned	100.00	g	21	0.3	6.7	75.00	0.23
	246.00	g	52	0.6	16.5	184.50	0.57
	1.00	c					
frozen ice dessert	100.00	g	128	0.4	32.6	3.00	0.00
	99.00	g	127	0.4	32.3	2.97	0.00
	0.50	c					

LYCHEE

whole, fresh	100.00	g	66	0.8	16.5	171.00	0.44
	142.50	g	94	1.2	23.6	243.68	0.63
	0.75	c					
dried	100.00	g	277	3.8	70.7	1,110.00	1.20
	40.00	g	111	1.5	28.3	444.00	0.48
	16.00	pcs/ items					

MANGO

whole, fresh	100.00	g	60	0.8	15.0	168.00	0.38
	207.00	g	124	1.7	31.0	347.76	0.79
	1.00	pc/ item					
dired, sweetened	100.00	g	319	2.5	78.6	279.00	1.18
nectar, canned	100.00	g	51	0.1	13.1	24.00	0.06
	251.00	g	128	0.3	32.9	60.24	0.15
	1.00	c					

PEACHES

	SERVING QUANTITY	SERVING UNIT	CALORIES (kcal)	PROTEIN (g)	TOTAL CARBOHYDRATES (g)	POTASSIUM (mg)	TOTAL FAT (g)
raw, medium (77pprox. 4/lb)	100.00	g	39	0.9	9.5	190.00	0.25
	150.00	g	59	1.4	14.3	285.00	0.38
	1.00	pc/ item					
dried	100.00	g	325	4.9	83.2	1,351.00	1.03
	38.67	g	126	1.9	32.2	522.39	0.40
	0.33	c					
slices	100.00	g	39	0.9	9.5	190.00	0.25
	154.00	g	60	1.4	14.7	292.60	0.39
	1.00	c					
nectar, canned	100.00	g	49	0.1	11.6	30.00	0.57
	249.00	g	122	0.3	28.9	74.70	1.42
	8.00	fl oz					
pie, prepared 1/6 of 8-in. pie	100.00	g	224	1.9	33.0	125.00	10.00
	117.00	g	262	2.2	38.5	146.25	11.70
	1.00	slice					
slices, sweetened, frozen	100.00	g	94	0.6	24.0	130.00	0.13
	125.00	g	118	0.8	30.0	162.50	0.16
	0.50	c					
halves/ slices, canned in water	100.00	g	24	0.4	6.1	99.00	0.06
	122.00	g	29	0.5	7.5	120.78	0.07
	0.50	c					
halves/ slices, canned in juice	100.00	g	44	0.6	11.6	128.00	0.03
	124.00	g	55	0.8	14.4	158.72	0.04
	0.50	c					
canned in extra light syrup	100.00	g	42	0.4	11.1	74.00	0.10
	123.50	g	52	0.5	13.7	91.39	0.12
	0.50	c					
canned in heavy syrup	100.00	g	75	0.4	20.1	85.00	0.10
	242.00	g	182	1.0	48.6	205.70	0.24
	1.00	c					
canned in light syrup, drained	100.00	g	61	0.6	15.7	87.00	0.15
fruit cocktail, canned light syrup with solids and liquid	100.00	g	55	0.4	14.3	85.00	0.08

APRICOT

	SERVING QUANTITY	SERVING UNIT	CALORIES (kcal)	PROTEIN (g)	TOTAL CARBOHYDRATES (g)	POTASSIUM (mg)	TOTAL FAT (g)
whole, fresh	100.00	g	48	1.4	11.1	259.00	0.39
	140.00	g	67	2.0	15.6	362.60	0.55
	4.00	pcs/ items					
jam or preserves	100.00	g	242	0.7	64.4	77.00	0.20
	20.00	g	48	0.1	12.9	15.40	0.04
1 packet = 0.5 oz = 14g	1.00	tbsp					
nectar, canned	100.00	g	56	0.2	13.6	67.00	0.45
	251.00	g	141	0.4	34.2	168.17	1.13
	8.00	fl oz					
sweetened, frozen	100.00	g	98	0.7	25.1	229.00	0.10
	242.00	g	237	1.7	60.7	554.18	0.24
	1.00	c					
dehydrated, sulfured	100.00	g	320	4.9	82.9	1,850.00	0.62
	30.00	g	96	1.5	24.9	555.00	0.19
	0.25	c					
dried, halves, sulfured	100.00	g	241	3.4	62.6	1,162.00	0.51
	43.33	g	104	1.5	27.1	503.53	0.22
	0.33	c					
halves w/ skin, canned in juice	100.00	g	48	0.6	12.3	165.00	0.04
	244.00	g	117	1.5	30.1	402.60	0.10
	1.00	c					
halves with skin, canned in light syrup	100.00	g	63	0.5	16.5	138.00	0.05
	253.00	g	159	1.3	41.7	349.14	0.13
	1.00	c					

PLUM

	SERVING QUANTITY	SERVING UNIT	CALORIES (kcal)	PROTEIN (g)	TOTAL CARBOHYDRATES (g)	POTASSIUM (mg)	TOTAL FAT (g)
whole, fresh, sliced	100.00	g	46	0.7	11.4	157.00	0.28
	165.00	g	76	1.2	18.8	259.05	0.46
	1.00	c					
sauce	100.00	g	184	0.9	42.8	259.00	1.04
	19.00	g	35	0.2	8.1	49.21	0.20
	1.00	tbsp					
purple, pitted, canned in water	100.00	g	41	0.4	11.0	126.00	0.01
	249.00	g	102	1.0	27.5	313.74	0.02
	1.00	c					
purple, canned in juice	100.00	g	58	0.5	15.2	154.00	0.02
	252.00	g	146	1.3	38.2	388.08	0.05
	1.00	c					

CANTALOUPE MELON	SERVING QUANTITY	SERVING UNIT	CALORIES (kcal)	PROTEIN (g)	TOTAL CARBOHYDRATES (g)	POTASSIUM (mg)	TOTAL FAT (g)
composite, raw	100.00	g	31	0.7	7.5	202.35	0.20
	165.50	g	51	1.1	12.5	334.89	0.33
	1.00	c					
honeydew, balls 1 slice = 125g	100.00	g	36	0.5	9.1	228.00	0.14
	132.75	g	48	0.7	12.1	302.67	0.19
	0.75	c					
Navajo	100.00	g	21	0.8	4.1	140.00	0.20
	85.05	g	18	0.7	3.5	119.07	0.17
	3.00	oz					
melon balls, frozen, unthawed	100.00	g	33	0.8	7.9	280.00	0.25
	173.00	g	57	1.5	13.7	484.40	0.43
	1.00	c					
BANANA							
medium, 77.8 in long	100.00	g	89	1.1	22.8	358.00	0.33
	118.00	g	105	1.3	27.0	422.44	0.39
	1.00	pc/ item					
dehydrated, powder	100.00	g	346	3.9	88.3	1,491.00	1.81
	6.20	g	21	0.2	5.5	92.44	0.11
	1.00	tbsp					
chips, dried	100.00	g	519	2.3	58.4	536.00	14.29
	42.53	g	221	1.0	24.8	227.93	33.60
	1.50	oz					
pudding, mix	100.00	g	366	0.0	93.0	17.00	0.40
mix to make ½ c	22.00	g	81	0.0	20.5	3.74	0.09
1 package= 88g = 3 ½ oz	1.00	svg					
pudding, ready to eat	100.00	g	127	2.4	21.2	110.00	3.60
1 can = 5 oz	142.00	g	180	3.4	30.1	156.20	5.11
	5.00	oz					

WATER MELON	SERVING QUANTITY	SERVING UNIT	CALORIES (kcal)	PROTEIN (g)	TOTAL CARBOHYDRATES (g)	POTASSIUM (mg)	TOTAL FAT (g)
raw, balls	100.00	g	30	0.6	7.6	112.00	0.15
	154.00	g	46	0.9	11.6	172.00	0.23
	1.00	c					
juice, 100%,	100.00	g	30	0.6	7.6	112.00	0.15
no ice	30.00	g	9	0.2	2.3	33.60	0.05
	1.00	fl oz					
seeds, kernels,	100.00	g	557	28.3	15.3	648.00	47.37
dried	28.35	g	158	8.0	4.3	184.00	13.40
	1.00	oz					

FIG

raw	100.00	g	74	0.8	19.2	232.00	0.30
	50.00	g	37	0.4	9.6	116.00	0.15
	1.00	pc/ item					
dried	100.00	g	249	3.3	63.9	680.00	0.92
	8.00	g	20	0.3	5.1	54.40	0.07
	1.00	pc					
canned	100.00	g	75	0.6	19.4	157.00	0.24
	250.00	g	188	1.4	48.4	392.00	0.60
	1.00	c					
dried, stewed	100.00	g	107	1.4	27.6	294.00	0.40
	259.00	g	277	3.7	71.4	761.00	1.04
	1.00	c					
canned, water pack, solids/liquids	100.00	g	53	0.4	14.0	103.00	0.10
	248.00	g	131	1.0	34.7	255.00	0.25
	1.00	c					
canned, light syrup pack, solids/liquids	100.00	g	69	0.4	18.0	102.00	0.10
	252.00	g	174	1.0	45.2	257.00	0.25
	1.00	c					

GUAVA

raw	100.00	g	68	2.6	14.3	417.00	0.95
	55.00	g	37	1.4	7.9	229.00	0.52
	1.00	pc/ item					
nectar	100.00	g	48	0.3	13.3	33.00	0.07
no ice	31.00	g	15	0.1	4.1	10.20	0.02
	1.00	fl oz					
paste	100.00	g	280	0.1	77.6	69.00	0.27
	20.00	g	56	0.0	14.5	13.80	0.05
	1.00	tbsp					

PAPAYA

	SERVING QUANTITY	SERVING UNIT	CALORIES (Kcal)	PROTEIN (g)	TOTAL CARBOHYDRATES (g)	POTASSIUM (mg)	TOTAL FAT (g)
whole, fresh, cubes	100.00	g	43	0.5	10.8	182.00	0.26
	140.00	g	60	0.7	15.2	254.80	0.36
	1.00	c					
nectar, canned	100.00	g	57	0.2	14.5	31.00	0.15
	250.00	g	143	0.4	36.3	77.50	0.38
	8.00	fl oz					
canned with heavy syrup, drained	100.00	g	206	0.1	55.8	67.00	0.55
	39.00	g	80	0.1	21.8	26.13	0.21
	1.00	pc/ chunk					

NECTARINE

	SERVING QUANTITY	SERVING UNIT	CALORIES (Kcal)	PROTEIN (g)	TOTAL CARBOHYDRATES (g)	POTASSIUM (mg)	TOTAL FAT (g)
whole, fresh, slices	100.00	g	44	1.1	10.6	201.00	0.32
	138.00	g	61	1.5	14.7	277.38	0.44
	1.00	c					

PERSIMMON

	SERVING QUANTITY	SERVING UNIT	CALORIES (Kcal)	PROTEIN (g)	TOTAL CARBOHYDRATES (g)	POTASSIUM (mg)	TOTAL FAT (g)
whole, fresh	100.00	g	127	0.8	33.5	310.00	0.40
	25.00	g	32	0.2	8.4	77.50	0.10
	1.00	pc/ item					
Japanese, fresh, 2-1/2" in diameter	100.00	g	70	0.6	18.6	161.00	0.19
	168.00	g	118	1.0	31.2	270.48	0.32
	1.00	pc/item					
Japanese, dried	100.00	g	274	1.4	73.4	802.00	0.59
	34.00	g	93	0.5	25.0	272.68	0.20
	1.00	pc/ item					

PURPLE PASSION FRUIT/ GRANADILLA

	SERVING QUANTITY	SERVING UNIT	CALORIES (Kcal)	PROTEIN (g)	TOTAL CARBOHYDRATES (g)	POTASSIUM (mg)	TOTAL FAT (g)
whole, fresh - no refuse	100.00	g	97	2.2	23.4	348.00	0.70
	18.00	g	18	0.4	4.2	62.60	0.13
	1.00	pc/ fruit					
nectar, no ice	100.00	g	67	1.2	17.4	112.00	0.06
	31.00	g	21	0.1	5.4	34.70	0.02
	1.00	fl oz					
juice, purple passion fruit	100.00	g	51	0.4	13.6	278.00	0.05
	30.90	g	16	0.1	4.2	85.90	0.02
	1.00	fl oz					
juice, yellow passion fruit	100.00	g	60	0.7	14.5	278.00	0.18
	30.90	g	19	0.2	4.5	85.90	0.06
	1.00	fl oz					

PRUNE	SERVING QUANTITY	SERVING UNIT	CALORIES (kcal)	PROTEIN (g)	TOTAL CARBOHYDRATES (g)	POTASSIUM (mg)	TOTAL FAT (g)
puree	100.00	g	257	2.1	65.1	852.00	0.20
	28.35	g	73	0.6	18.5	241.54	0.06
	1.00	oz					
dried	100.00	g	240	2.2	63.9	732.00	0.38
	42.50	g	102	0.9	27.2	311.10	0.16
	0.25	c					
juice, canned	100.00	g	71	0.6	17.5	276.00	0.03
	256.00	g	182	1.6	44.7	706.56	0.08
	8.00	fl oz					
dehydrated, stewed	100.00	g	113	1.2	29.7	353.00	0.24
	36.40	g	41	0.5	10.8	128.49	0.09
	0.13	c					
dehydrated, low moisture	100.00	g	339	3.7	89.1	1,058.00	0.73
	33.00	g	112	1.2	29.4	349.14	0.24
	0.25	c					

RHUBARB

	SERVING QUANTITY	SERVING UNIT	CALORIES	PROTEIN (g)	TOTAL CARBOHYDRATES (g)	POTASSIUM (mg)	TOTAL FAT (g)
whole, fresh, diced	100.00	g	21	0.9	4.5	288.00	0.20
	81.33	g	17	0.7	3.7	234.24	0.16
	0.67	c					
diced, frozen	100.00	g	21	0.6	5.1	108.00	0.11
	137.00	g	29	0.8	7.0	147.96	0.15
	1.00	c					
frozen, cooked with sugar	100.00	g	116	0.4	31.2	96.00	0.05
	120.00	g	139	0.5	37.4	115.20	0.06
	0.50	c					

POMEGRANATE

	SERVING QUANTITY	SERVING UNIT	CALORIES	PROTEIN (g)	TOTAL CARBOHYDRATES (g)	POTASSIUM (mg)	TOTAL FAT (g)
whole, fresh, 4" in diameter	100.00	g	83	1.7	18.7	236.00	1.17
	282.00	g	234	4.7	52.7	665.52	3.30
	1.00	pc/item					
juice, bottled	100.00	g	54	0.2	13.1	214.00	0.29
	251.20	g	136	0.4	33.0	537.57	0.73
	8.00	fl oz					

	SERVING QUANTITY	SERVING UNIT	CALORIES (kcal)	PROTEIN (g)	TOTAL CARBOHYDRATES (g)	POTASSIUM (mg)	TOTAL FAT (g)
DATES							
whole, dried	100.00	g	282	2.5	75.0	656.00	0.39
	8.00	g	23	0.2	6.0	52.50	0.03
	1.00	pc/item					
Medjool, pitted	100.00	g	277	1.8	75.0	696.00	0.15
	24.00	g	67	0.4	18.0	167.00	0.04
	1.00	pc/item					
candy	100.00	g	379	4.2	58.1	540.00	18.04
	28.35	g	107	1.2	16.5	153.00	5.11
	1.00	oz					
POMELO							
whole, fresh	100.00	g	38	0.8	9.6	216.00	0.04
section	190.00	g	72	1.4	18.3	410.00	0.08
	1.00	c					
MANGOSTEEN							
canned, syrup pack	100.00	g	73	0.4	17.9	48.00	0.58
drained	196.00	g	143	0.8	35.1	94.10	1.14
	1.00	c					
JACKFRUIT							
raw, fresh	100.00	g	95	1.7	23.3	448.00	0.64
slices	165.00	g	157	2.8	38.4	739.00	1.06
	1.00	c					
canned, syrup pack drained	100.00	g	92	0.4	23.9	96.00	0.14
	178.00	g	164	0.6	42.6	171.00	0.25
	1.00	c					
DURIAN							
raw or frozen	100.00	g	147	1.5	27.1	436.00	5.33
chopped or diced	243.00	g	357	3.6	65.8	1,060.00	13.00
	1.00	c					
SOURSOP							
raw, pulp	100.00	g	66	1.0	16.8	278.00	0.30
	225.00	g	148	2.3	37.9	626.00	0.68
	1.00	c					
nectar	100.00	g	59	0.1	14.9	25.00	0.17
no ice, pure	31.00	g	18	0.0	4.6	7.75	0.05
	1.00	fl oz					

PLANTAIN	SERVING QUANTITY	SERVING UNIT	CALORIES (kcal)	PROTEIN (g)	TOTAL CARBOHYDRATES (g)	POTASSIUM (mg)	TOTAL FAT (g)
ripe, raw, fresh	100.00	g	122	1.3	31.9	487.00	0.35
	180.00	g	220	2.3	57.4	877.00	0.63
	1.00	pc/ item					
green, raw, fresh	100.00	g	152	1.3	36.7	431.00	0.07
	267.00	g	406	3.3	97.9	1,150	0.19
	1.00	pc/item					
green, boiled	100.00	g	121	1.1	29.2	289.00	0.08
	137.00	g	166	1.5	39.9	396.00	0.11
	1.00	c					
green, fried	100.00	g	309	1.5	49.2	482.00	11.81
	118.00	g	365	1.8	58.0	569.00	13.90
	1.00	c					
yellow, raw, fresh	100.00	g	122	1.3	31.9	487.00	0.35
	270.00	g	329	3.5	86.1	1,310	0.95
	1.00	pc/ item					
yellow, baked	100.00	g	155	1.5	41.4	477.00	0.16
	139.00	g	215	2.1	57.5	663.00	0.22
	1.00	c					
chips	100.00	g	531	2.3	63.8	786.00	29.59
	28.35	g	151	0.6	18.1	223.00	8.39
	1.00	oz					
AVOCADO							
fresh, raw	100.00	g	160	2.0	8.5	485.00	14.66
mashed/	230.00	g	368	4.6	19.6	1,120	33.70
pureed	1.00	c					
oil	100.00	g	884	0.0	0.0	0.00	100.00
	14.00	g	124	0.0	0.0	0.00	14.00
	1.00	tbsp					
dressing	100.00	g	427	1.9	7.4	58.00	43.33
	15.30	g	65	0.3	1.1	8.87	6.63
	1.00	tbsp					
California, raw/fresh no seed and skin	100.00	g	167	2.0	8.6	507.00	15.41
	136.00	g	227	2.7	11.8	690.00	21.00
	1.00	pc/ item					
Florida, fresh/ raw no seed and skin	100.00	g	120	2.2	7.8	351.00	10.06
	304.00	g	365	6.8	23.8	1,070	30.60
	1.00	pc/ item					
Guacamole	100.00	g	155	2.0	8.5	472.00	14.18
	15.00	G	23	0.3	1.3	70.80	2.13
	1.00	tbsp					

TAMARIND	SERVING QUANTITY	SERVING UNIT	CALORIES (kcal)	PROTEIN (g)	TOTAL CARBOHYDRATES (g)	POTASSIUM (mg)	TOTAL FAT (g)
fresh, raw	100.00	g	239	2.8	62.5	628.00	0.60
	2.00	g	5	0.1	1.3	12.60	0.01
	1.00	pc/item					
candy	100.00	g	331	0.0	92.0	309.00	0.00
	22.00	g	73	0.0	20.2	68.00	0.00
	1.00	tbsp					
dried	100.00	g	254	2.5	66.2	565.00	0.57
	160.00	g	406	4.0	106.0	904.00	0.91
	1.00	c					

SAPODILLA							
fresh/raw	100.00	g	83	0.4	20.0	193.00	1.10
	170.00	g	141	0.8	33.9	328.00	1.87
	1.00	pc/item					

SUGAR APPLE
(Sweetsop)

fresh, raw	100.00	g	94	2.1	23.6	247.00	0.29
(2-7/8" in diameter)	155.00	g	146	3.2	36.6	383.00	0.45
	1.00	pc/item					

STARFRUIT

fresh/raw	100.00	g	31	1.0	6.7	133.00	0.33
	90.00	g	28	0.9	6.1	120.00	0.30
	1.00	pc/item					

Chapter 7: Vegetables

Do you want to print the charts in letter-size (8.5x11")?

I have created downloadable printables of this chart. You can scan the QR code below or copy the link to your computer browser to be able to get your printable copies of the food charts

https://go.renaltracker.com/lowpotassiumprint

PEPPER

	SERVING QUANTITY	SERVING UNIT	CALORIES (kcal)	PROTEIN (g)	TOTAL CARBOHYDRATES (g)	POTASSIUM (mg)	TOTAL FAT (g)
bell, sweet yellow, 3 in diameter	100.00	g	27	1.0	6.3	212.00	
	186.00	g	50	1.9	11.8	394.32	
	1.00	pc					
bell, sweet green, chopped	100.00	g	20	0.9	4.6	175.00	
	74.50	g	15	0.6	3.5	130.38	
	0.50	c					
bell, sweet green, sauteed	100.00	g	116	0.8	4.2	134.00	
bell, sweet red, chopped	100.00	g	26	1.0	6.0	211.00	
	74.50	g	19	0.7	4.5	157.20	
	0.50	c					
bell, sweet red, sauteed	100.00	g	133	1.0	6.6	193.00	
bell, sweet red, chopped, frozen, drained, boiled, no salt added	100.00	g	16	1.0	3.3	72.00	
	85.05	g	14	0.8	2.8	61.24	
	3.00	oz					
jalapeno, sliced	100.00	g	29	0.9	6.5	248.00	
	22.50	g	7	0.2	1.5	55.80	
	0.13	c					
serrano, chopped	100.00	g	32	1.7	6.7	305.00	
	26.25	g	8	0.5	1.8	80.06	
	0.25	c					
black, ground	100.00	g	251	10.4	64.0	1,329	
	2.10	g	5	0.2	1.3	27.91	
	1.00	tsp					
white, ground	100.00	g	296	10.4	68.6	73.00	
	2.40	g	7	0.3	1.7	1.75	
	1.00	tsp					
hot chilli, red	100.00	g	40	1.9	8.8	322.00	
	45.00	g	18	0.8	4.0	144.90	
	1.00	pc					

ASPARAGUS	SERVING QUANTITY	SERVING UNIT	CALORIES (kcal)	PROTEIN (g)	TOTAL CARBOHYDRATES (g)	POTASSIUM (mg)	TOTAL FAT (g)
boiled,	100.00	g	22	2.4	4.1	224.00	0.22
drained	90.00	g	20	2.2	3.7	201.60	0.20
	0.50	c					
frozen	100.00	g	24	3.2	4.1	253.00	0.23
	87.00	g	21	2.8	3.6	220.11	0.20
	6.00	pcs					
frozen, boiled,	100.00	g	18	3.0	1.9	172.00	0.42
drained	90.00	g	16	2.7	1.7	154.80	0.38
	0.50	c					
canned,	100.00	g	19	2.1	2.5	172.00	0.65
drained	121.00	g	23	2.6	3.0	208.12	0.79
	0.50	c					

BEANS

	SERVING QUANTITY	SERVING UNIT	CALORIES	PROTEIN	TOTAL CARBS	POTASSIUM	TOTAL FAT
green wax, raw	100.00	g	31	1.8	7.0	211.00	
	82.50	g	26	1.5	5.8	174.08	
	0.75	c					
green wax,	100.00	g	33	1.8	7.5	186.00	
frozen	82.67	g	27	1.5	6.2	153.76	
	0.67	c					
green wax,	100.00	g	35	1.9	7.9	146.00	
boiled,	125.00	g	44	2.4	9.9	182.50	
drained	1.00	c					
green wax,	100.00	g	21	1.1	4.2	96.00	
canned,	135.00	g	28	1.4	5.7	129.60	
drained	1.00	c					

CARROTS

	SERVING QUANTITY	SERVING UNIT	CALORIES	PROTEIN	TOTAL CARBS	POTASSIUM	TOTAL FAT
strips, slices	100.00	g	41	0.9	9.6	320.00	
	122.00	g	50	1.1	11.7	390.40	
	1.00	c					
grated	100.00	g	41	0.9	9.6	320.00	
	82.50	g	34	0.8	7.9	264.00	
	0.75	c					
sliced, boiled,	100.00	g	35	0.8	8.2	235.00	
drained, no salt	78.00	g	27	0.6	6.4	183.30	
	0.50	c					
frozen	100.00	g	36	0.8	7.9	235.00	
	85.33	g	31	0.7	6.7	200.53	
	0.67	c					
baby	100.00	g	35	0.6	8.2	237.00	
	80.00	g	28	0.5	6.6	189.60	
	8.00	pcs					
juice, canned	100.00	g	40	1.0	9.3	292.00	
	236.00	g	94	2.2	21.9	689.12	
	8.00	fl oz					

MUSHROOM	SERVING QUANTITY	SERVING UNIT	CALORIES (kcal)	PROTEIN (g)	TOTAL CARBOHYDRATES (g)	POTASSIUM (mg)	TOTAL FAT (g)
Shitake, raw	100.00	g	34	2.2	6.8	304.00	
	19.00	g	6	0.4	1.3	57.76	
	1.00	pc					
Shitake, dried	100.00	g	296	9.6	75.4	1,534.00	
	32.40	g	96	3.1	24.4	497.02	
	9.00	pcs					
Shitake, cooked	100.00	g	56	1.6	14.4	117.00	
	72.50	g	41	1.1	10.4	84.83	
	0.50	c					
Shitake, stir fried	100.00	g	39	3.5	7.7	326.00	
	108.00	g	42	3.7	8.3	352.08	
	1.00	c					
Portabella/Portabello	100.00	g	22	2.1	3.9	364.00	
Portabello, grilled	100.00	g	29	3.3	4.4	437.00	
White, raw	100.00	g	22	3.0	3.3	318.00	
	96.00	g	21	3.0	3.1	305.28	
	1.00	c					
white, sliced, stir-fried	100.00	g	26	3.6	4.0	396.00	
	108.00	g	28	3.9	4.4	427.68	
	1.00	c					

LETTUCE

	SERVING QUANTITY	SERVING UNIT	CALORIES (kcal)	PROTEIN (g)	TOTAL CARBOHYDRATES (g)	POTASSIUM (mg)	TOTAL FAT (g)
romaine, shredded	100.00	g	17	1.2	3.3	8.00	30.00
	70.50	g	12	0.9	2.3	5.64	21.15
	1.50	c					
butterhead, medium leaves	100.00	g	13	1.4	2.2	5.00	33.00
	82.50	g	11	1.1	1.8	4.13	27.23
	11.00	pcs					
Red Leaf, shredded	100.00	g	13	1.3	2.3	25.00	28.00
	28.00	g	4	0.4	0.6	7.00	7.84
	1.00	c					
Iceberg, shredded or chopped	100.00	g	14	0.9	3.0	10.00	20.00
	108.00	g	15	1.0	3.2	10.80	21.60
	1.50	c					
Iceberg, loose leaves, medium	100.00	g	14	0.9	3.0	10.00	20.00
	80.00	g	11	0.7	2.4	8.00	16.00
	10.00	pcs					

BROCCOLI	SERVING QUANTITY	SERVING UNIT	CALORIES (kcal)	PROTEIN (g)	TOTAL CARBOHYDRATES (g)	POTASSIUM (mg)	TOTAL FAT (g)
florets, raw	100.00	g	28	3.0	5.1	325.00	0.35
	71.00	g	20	2.1	3.6	230.75	0.25
	1.00	c					
Cooked, no salt	100.00	g	35	2.4	7.2	293.00	0.41
	78.00	g	27	1.9	5.6	228.54	0.32
	0.50	c					
frozen, spears	100.00	g	29	3.1	5.4	250.00	0.34
	85.05	g	25	2.6	4.6	212.62	0.29
	3.00	oz					
CAULIFLOWER							
green, raw	100.00	g	31	3.0	6.1	300.00	0.30
	64.00	g	20	1.9	3.9	192.00	0.19
	1.00	c					
cooked, no salt	100.00	g	32	3.0	6.3	278.00	0.31
	62.00	g	20	1.9	3.9	172.36	0.19
	0.50	c					
CUCUMBER							
sliced, raw	100.00	g	15	0.7	3.6	147.00	0.11
	52.00	g	8	0.3	1.9	76.44	0.06
	0.50	c					
sliced	100.00	g	15	0.7	3.6	147.00	0.11
	78.00	g	12	0.5	2.8	114.66	0.09
	0.75	c					
BEETS							
raw	100.00	g	43	1.6	9.6	325.00	0.17
	90.67	g	39	1.5	8.7	294.67	0.15
	0.67	c					
whole or sliced, boiled, drained, no salt	100.00	g	44	1.7	10.0	305.00	0.18
whole, canned	100.00	g	30	0.7	7.1	159.00	0.09
	246.00	g	74	1.8	17.6	391.14	0.22
	1.00	c					
sliced, canned, drained	100.00	g	31	0.9	7.2	148.00	0.14
	85.00	g	26	0.8	6.1	125.80	0.12
	0.50	c					

POTATOES	SERVING QUANTITY	SERVING UNIT	CALORIES (kcal)	PROTEIN (g)	TOTAL CARBOHYDRATES (g)	POTASSIUM (mg)	TOTAL FAT (g)
russet, flesh and skin	100.00	g	79	2.1	18.1	417.00	0.08
russet, flesh and skin, baked	100.00	g	95	2.6	21.4	550.00	0.13
	173.00	g	164	4.6	37.1	951.50	0.22
	1.00	pc					
white, flesh and skin	100.00	g	69	1.7	15.7	407.00	0.10
white, flesh and skin, baked	100.00	g	92	2.1	21.1	544.00	0.15
	173.00	g	159	3.6	36.5	941.12	0.26
	1.00	pcs					
french fries, frozen	100.00	g	147	2.2	24.8	408.00	4.66
	71.50	g	105	1.6	17.7	291.72	3.33
	11.00	pcs					
sweet, cubed	100.00	g	86	1.6	20.1	337.00	0.05
	99.75	g	86	1.6	20.1	336.16	0.05
	0.75	c					
sweet, boiled, mashed	100.00	g	76	1.4	17.7	230.00	0.14
	328.00	g	249	4.5	58.1	754.40	0.46
	1.00	c					
sweet, frozen, baked	100.00	g	100	1.7	23.4	377.00	0.12
	117.33	g	117	2.0	27.5	442.35	0.14
	0.67	c					
sweet, baked, peeled	100.00	g	90	2.0	20.7	475.00	0.15
	0.50	c					
chips, unsalted	100.00	g	536	7.0	52.9	1,275.00	34.60
	28.35	g	152	2.0	15.0	361.46	9.81
	1.00	oz					
hash browns, frozen	100.00	g	82	2.1	17.7	285.00	0.62
	70.00	g	57	1.4	12.4	199.50	0.43
	0.33	c					
wedges, frozen	100.00	g	129	2.7	25.5	394.00	2.20

COLLARDS	SERVING QUANTITY	SERVING UNIT	CALORIES (kcal)	PROTEIN (g)	TOTAL CARBOHYDRATES (g)	POTASSIUM (mg)	TOTAL FAT (g)
chopped, raw	100.00	g	32	3.0	5.4	213.00	0.61
	90.00	g	29	2.7	4.9	191.70	0.55
	2.50	c					
boiled, drained	100.00	g	33	2.7	5.7	117.00	0.72
	95.00	g	31	2.6	5.4	111.15	0.68
	0.50	c					
frozen, chopped, raw	100.00	g	33	2.7	6.5	253.00	0.37
	85.05	g	28	2.3	5.5	215.17	0.31
	3.00	oz					
frozen, chopped, boiled/ drained	100.00	g	36	3.0	7.1	251.00	0.41
	85.00	g	31	2.5	6.0	213.35	0.35
	0.50	c					
EGGPLANT/AUBERGINE							
boiled, drained, no salt	100.00	g	35	0.8	8.7	123.00	0.23
cut in 1" cubes	99.00	g	35	0.8	8.6	121.77	0.23
	1.00	c					
pickled	100.00	g	49	0.9	9.8	12.00	0.70
	`136	g	67	1.2	13.3	16.32	0.95
	1.00	c					
JICAMA (YAMBEAN)							
raw	100.00	g	38	0.7	8.8	150.00	0.09
	86.67	g	33	0.6	7.6	130.00	0.08
	0.67	c					
boiled, drained, no salt	100.00	g	38	0.7	8.8	135.00	0.09
1 svg= 3oz	85.05	g	32	0.6	7.5	114.82	0.08
	3.00	oz					

	SERVING QUANTITY	SERVING UNIT	CALORIES (kcal)	PROTEIN (g)	TOTAL CARBOHYDRATES (g)	POTASSIUM (mg)	TOTAL FAT (g)
ARUGULA							
raw, leaves	100.00	g	25	2.6	3.7	369.00	0.66
	80.00	g	20	2.1	2.9	295.20	0.53
	4.00	c					
salad mixed	100.00	g	18	1.5	3.3	298.76	0.27
baby greens	41.25	g	7	0.6	1.4	123.24	0.11
Arugula,butterhead, endives, Radicchio	1.00	c					
ENDIVE OR ESCAROLE							
raw, chopped	100.00	g	17	1.3	3.4	314.00	0.20
	87.50	g	15	1.1	2.9	274.75	0.18
	1.75	c					
Chicory, Witlof	100.00	g	17	0.9	4.0	211.00	0.10
or Belgium	90.00	g	15	0.8	3.6	189.90	0.09
	1.00	c					
OKRA							
raw	100.00	g	33	1.9	7.5	299.00	0.19
	75.00	g	25	1.5	5.6	224.25	0.14
	0.75	c					
sliced, boiled,	100.00	g	22	1.9	4.5	135.00	0.21
drained, n.s.	80.00	g	18	1.5	3.6	108.00	0.17
	0.50	c					
frozen	100.00	g	30	1.7	6.6	211.00	0.25
	85.05	g	26	1.4	5.6	179.45	0.21
	3.00	oz					
frozen, boiled,	100.00	g	29	1.6	6.4	184.00	0.24
drained, no salt sliced	92.00	g	27	1.5	5.9	169.28	0.22
	0.50	c					
PUMPKIN							
fruit/meat, raw,	100.00	g	26	1.0	6.5	340.00	0.10
cut 1" cube	116.00	g	30	1.2	7.5	394.40	0.12
	1.00	c					
boiled, drained,	100.00	g	20	0.7	4.9	230.00	0.07
mashed, n.s.	122.50	g	25	0.9	6.0	281.75	0.09
	0.50	c					
flowers	100.00	g	15	0.0	3.3	173.00	0.07
	33.00	g	1	0.0	0.1	6.92	0.00
	1.00	c					
flowers, boiled,	100.00	g	15	1.1	3.3	106.00	0.08
drained	89.33	g	13	1.0	3.0	5.36	0.07
	0.67	c					
seeds (squash	100.00	g	559	30.2	10.7	809.00	49.05
kernels), dried	34.50	g	193	10.4	3.7	279.11	16.92
	0.25	c					
seeds	100.00	g	446	18.6	53.8	919.00	19.40
(pumkin/squash), whole,	32.00	g	143	5.9	17.2	294.08	6.21
roasted no salt added	0.50	c					

SWISS CHARD	SERVING QUANTITY	SERVING UNIT	CALORIES (kcal)	PROTEIN (g)	TOTAL CARBOHYDRATES (g)	POTASSIUM (mg)	TOTAL FAT (g)
raw	100.00	g	19	1.8	3.7	379.00	0.20
	36.00	g	7	0.7	1.4	136.44	0.07
	1.00	c					
boiled, drained, no salt	100.00	g	20	1.9	4.1	549.00	0.08
	175.00	g	35	3.3	7.2	960.75	0.14
	1.00	c					
SPINACH							
raw, chopped	100.00	g	23	2.9	3.6	558.00	0.39
	90.00	g	21	2.6	3.3	502.20	0.35
	3.00	c					
frozen	100.00	g	29	3.6	4.2	346.00	0.57
	78.00	g	23	2.8	3.3	269.88	0.44
	0.50	c					
chopped, boiled, drained, no salt	100.00	g	23	3.0	3.8	466.00	0.26
	90.00	g	21	2.7	3.4	419.40	0.23
	0.50	c					
mustard (Tendergreens)	100.00	g	22	2.2	3.9	449.00	0.30
	150.00	g	33	3.3	5.9	673.50	0.45
	1.00	c					
mustard, boiled, drained, no salt	100.00	g	16	1.7	2.8	285.00	0.20
	180.00	g	29	3.1	5.0	513.00	0.36
	1.00	c					
TOMATILLOS							
chopped	100.00	g	32	1.0	5.8	268.00	1.02
	132.00	g	42	1.3	7.7	353.76	1.35
	1.00	c					
TURNIPS							
raw	100.00	g	28	0.9	6.4	191.00	0.10
	130.00	g	34	1.1	7.8	233.02	0.12
	1.00	c					
frozen	100.00	g	16	1.0	2.9	137.00	0.16
	85.05	g	14	0.9	2.5	116.52	0.14
	3.00	oz					
cubed, boiled, drained, no salt	100.00	g	22	0.7	5.1	177.00	0.08
	156.00	g	34	1.1	7.9	276.12	0.12
	1.00	c					
frozen, boiled, drained, no salt	100.00	g	23	1.5	4.4	182.00	0.24
	78.00	g	18	1.2	3.4	141.96	0.19

WATER CHESTNUTS	SERVING QUANTITY	SERVING UNIT	CALORIES (kcal)	PROTEIN (g)	TOTAL CARBOHYDRATES (g)	POTASSIUM (mg)	TOTAL FAT (g)
fresh, raw, Chinese (Matai) slices	100.00	g	97	1.4	23.9	584.00	0.10
	62.00	g	60	0.9	14.8	362.08	0.06
	0.50	c					
canned with liquid Chinese (Matai)	100.00	g	50	0.9	12.3	118.00	0.06
	70.00	g	35	0.6	8.6	82.60	0.04
	0.50	c					

WATERCRESS

raw, chopped	100.00	g	11	2.3	1.3	330.00	0.10
	34.00	g	4	0.8	0.4	112.20	0.03
	1.00	c					

YAM

raw, in cubes	100.00	g	118	1.5	28.0	816.00	0.17
	112.50	g	133	1.7	31.4	918.00	0.19
	0.75	c					
baked or broiled, drained, no salt cubed	100.00	g	116	1.5	27.5	670.00	0.14
	68.00	g	79	1.0	18.7	455.60	0.10
	0.50	c					
Hawaiin Mountain, raw cubed	100.00	g	67	1.3	16.3	418.00	0.10
	68.00	g	46	0.9	11.1	284.24	0.07
	0.50	c					
Hawaiian Mountain, steamed cubed	100.00	g	82	1.7	20.0	495.00	0.08
	145.00	g	119	2.5	29.0	717.75	0.12
	1.00	c					

MIXED VEGETABLES

frozen	100.00	g	72	3.3	13.5	212.00	0.52
	72.00	g	52	2.4	9.7	152.64	0.37
	0.50	c					
frozen, boiled, drained, no salt added	100.00	g	65	2.9	13.1	169.00	0.15
	91.00	g	59	2.6	11.9	153.79	0.14
	0.50	c					
canned, drained	100.00	g	49	2.6	9.3	291.00	0.25
	163.00	g	80	4.2	15.1	474.33	0.41
	1.00	c					

BRUSSEL SPROUTS

raw	100.00	g	43	3.4	9.0	389.00	0.30
	88.00	g	38	3.0	7.9	342.00	0.26
	1.00	c					

TOMATO

	SERVING QUANTITY	SERVING UNIT	CALORIES (kcal)	PROTEIN (g)	TOTAL CARBOHYDRATES (g)	POTASSIUM (mg)	TOTAL FAT (g)
red, whole medium 2.6 in diameter	100.00	g	18	0.9	3.9	237.00	
	123.00	g	22	1.1	4.8	291.51	
	1.00	pc					
diced or chopped	100.00	g	18	0.9	3.9	237.00	
	90.00	g	16	0.8	3.5	213.30	
	0.50	c					
yellow, chopped	100.00	g	15	1.0	3.0	258.00	
	92.67	g	14	0.9	2.8	239.08	
	0.67	c					
orange, chopped	100.00	g	16	1.2	3.2	212.00	
	79.00	g	13	0.9	2.5	167.48	
	0.50	c					
green	100.00	g	23	1.2	5.1	204.00	
	90.00	g	21	1.1	4.6	183.60	
	0.50	c					
whole, canned	100.00	g	16	0.8	3.5	191.00	
	240.00	g	38	1.9	8.3	458.40	
	1.00	c					
sauce, canned, no salt	100.00	g	24	1.2	5.3	297.00	
	244.00	g	59	2.9	13.0	724.68	
	1.00	c					
crushed, canned	100.00	g	32	1.6	7.3	293.00	
	56.70	g	18	0.9	4.1	166.13	
	2.00	oz					
paste, canned	100.00	g	82	4.3	18.9	1,014.00	
	32.80	g	27	1.4	6.2	332.59	
	2.00	tbsp					
puree, canned, no salt	100.00	g	38	1.7	9.0	439.00	
	250.00	g	95	4.1	22.5	1,097.50	
	1.00	c					
sun dried, in oil, drained	100.00	g	213	5.1	23.3	1,565.00	
	27.50	g	59	1.4	6.4	430.38	
	0.25	c					
Ketchup, low sodium	100.00	g	101	1.0	27.4	281.00	
	15.00	g	15	0.2	4.1	42.15	
	1.00	tbsp					
juice, canned	100.00	g	17	0.9	3.5	217.00	
	243.00	g	41	2.1	8.6	527.31	
	8.00	fl oz					
cherry, sweet, raw	100.00	g	63	1.1	16.0	222.00	
	138.00	g	87	1.5	22.1	306.00	
	1.00	c					

CABBAGE	SERVING QUANTITY	SERVING UNIT	CALORIES (kcal)	PROTEIN (g)	TOTAL CARBOHYDRATES (g)	POTASSIUM (mg)	TOTAL FAT (g)
green, chopped	100.00	g	25	1.3	5.8	170.00	
	89.00	g	22	1.1	5.2	151.30	
	1.00	c					
green shredded, sliced	100.00	g	25	1.3	5.8	170.00	
	87.50	g	22	1.1	5.1	148.75	
	1.25	c					
green, shredded, boiled, drained, no salt added	100.00	g	23	1.3	5.5	196.00	
	75.00	g	17	1.0	4.1	147.00	
	0.50	c					
chinese, shredded, raw	100.00	g					
	76.00	g	12	0.9		181.00	
	1.00	c					
chinese, cooked, no salt	100.00	g					
	75.00	g	17	1.0		147.00	
	0.50	c					
red, shredded	100.00	g	31	1.4	7.4	243.00	
	87.50	g	27	1.3	6.5	212.63	
	1.25	c					
red, shredded, boiled, drained, no salt added	100.00	g	29	1.5	6.9	262.00	
	75.00	g	27	1.1	5.2	196.50	
	0.50	c					
Bok Choy or White Mustard, shredded	100.00	g	13	1.5	2.2	252.00	
	87.50	g	11	1.3	1.9	220.50	
	1.25	c					
Bok Choy/ Pak Choi, shredded, boiled, drained	100.00	g	12	1.6	1.8	371.00	
	85.00	g	10	1.3	1.5	315.35	
	0.50	c					
Kimchi	100.00	g	15	1.1	2.4	151.00	
	150.00	g	23	1.7	3.6	226.50	
	1.00	c					

CORN

	SERVING QUANTITY	SERVING UNIT	CALORIES (kcal)	PROTEIN (g)	TOTAL CARBOHYDRATES (g)	POTASSIUM (mg)	TOTAL FAT (g)
white, sweet	100.00	g	390	7.8	86.6	88.00	
	25.00	g	98	2.0	21.7	22.00	
	1.00	c					
white, steamed	100.00	g	386	9.7	75.2	532.00	
(Navajo)	85.05	g	328	8.3	64.0	452.47	
	3.00	oz					
white, stew, steamed (Navajo)	100.00	g	112	8.8	10.8	177.00	
	85.05	g	95	7.5	9.2	150.54	
	3.00	oz					
sweet, boiled, drained	100.00	g	94	3.1	22.3	251.00	0.74
	82.00	g	77	2.6	18.3	205.82	0.61
	0.50	c					
flour, white, whole grain	100.00	g	361	6.9	76.9	315.00	3.86
	29.25	g	106	2.0	22.5	92.14	1.13
	0.25	c					
yellow, sweet, boiled, drained	100.00	g	96	3.4	21.0	218.00	1.50
	82.00	g	79	2.8	17.2	178.76	1.23
	0.50	c					
yellow, sweet, on the cob	100.00	g	86	3.3	18.7	270.00	1.35
	154.00	g	77	2.9	16.8	243.00	1.22
	1.00	c					
yellow, sweet, creamed, canned	100.00	g	72	1.7	18.1	134.00	0.42
	128.00	g	92	2.2	23.2	171.52	0.54
	0.50	c					
yellow, sweet, kernels, frozen	100.00	g	88	3.0	20.7	213.00	0.78
	82.00	g	72	2.5	17.0	174.66	0.64
	0.50	c					
yellow, sweet, canned with liquid	100.00	g	61	2.0	13.9	136.00	0.77
	128.00	g	78	2.5	17.7	174.08	0.99
	0.50	c					
tortilla, no salt added	100.00	g	222	5.7	46.6	154.00	2.50
	26.00	g	58	1.5	12.1	40.04	0.65
	1.00	pc					

PEAS

	SERVING QUANTITY	SERVING UNIT	CALORIES (kcal)	PROTEIN (g)	TOTAL CARBOHYDRATES (g)	POTASSIUM (mg)	TOTAL FAT (g)
green	100.00	g	81	5.4	14.5	244.00	0.40
	72.50	g	59	3.9	10.5	176.90	0.29
	0.50	c					
green, frozen	100.00	g	77	5.2	13.6	153.00	0.40
	72.00	g	55	3.8	9.8	110.16	0.29
	0.50	c					
green, boiled, drained	100.00	g	84	5.4	15.6	271.00	0.22
	80.00	g	67	4.3	12.5	216.80	0.18
	0.50	c					
green, canned, drained	100.00	g	68	4.5	11.4	106.00	0.80
	87.50	g	60	3.9	9.9	92.75	0.70
	0.50	c					
green, frozen, boiled, drained	100.00	g	78	5.2	14.3	110.00	0.27
	80.00	g	62	4.1	11.4	88.00	0.22
	0.50	c					
split, boiled, no salt added	100.00	g	118	8.3	21.1	362.00	0.39
	98.00	g	116	8.2	21.0	354.76	0.38
	0.50	c					
sugar or snow peas, whole fresh	100.00	g	42	2.8	7.6	200.00	0.20
	78.75	g	33	2.2	6.0	157.50	0.16
	1.25	c					
snow/sugar, frozen	100.00	g	42	2.8	7.6	200.00	0.20
	78.75	g	33	2.2	6.0	157.50	0.16
	1.25	c					
snow/sugar, boiled, drained	100.00	g	42	3.3	7.1	240.00	0.23
	80.00	g	34	2.6	5.6	192.00	0.18
	0.50	c					
snow/sugar, frozen, boiled, drained	100.00	g	52	3.5	9.0	217.00	0.38
	80.00	g	42	2.8	7.2	173.60	0.30
	0.50	c					

ARTI-CHOKES

	Serving Quantity	Serving Unit	Calories	Protein (g)	Total Carbohydrates (g)	Potassium (mg)	Total Fat (g)
whole, boiled, drained	100.00	g	53	2.9	12.0	286.00	0.34
med size	120.00	g	64	3.5	14.3	343.20	0.41
	1.00	pc					
hearts, boiled, drained	100.00	g	53	2.9	11.9	286.00	0.34
	84.00	g	45	2.4	10.0	240.24	0.29
	0.50	c					
Globe or French, frozen	100.00	g	45	3.1	9.2	264.00	0.50
boiled, drained	80.00	g	36	2.5	7.3	211.20	0.40
1 svg = 1/3 of 9oz package	1.00	svg					

ALFALFA

	Serving Quantity	Serving Unit	Calories	Protein (g)	Total Carbohydrates (g)	Potassium (mg)	Total Fat (g)
sprouts	100.00	g	23	4.0	2.1	79.00	0.69
	33.00	g	8	1.3	0.7	26.07	0.23
	1.00	c					

CELERY

	Serving Quantity	Serving Unit	Calories	Protein (g)	Total Carbohydrates (g)	Potassium (mg)	Total Fat (g)
stalk	100.00	g	14	0.7	3.0	260.00	0.17
medium 7.5 - 8 in long	80.00	g	11	0.6	2.4	208.00	0.14
	2.00	stalks					
diced, chopped	100.00	g	14	0.7	3.0	260.00	0.17
	101.00	g	14	0.7	3.0	262.60	0.17
	1.00	c					
celeriac or celery root	100.00	g	42	1.5	9.2	300.00	0.30
	78.00	g	33	1.2	7.2	234.00	0.23
	0.50	c					
seeds	100.00	g	392	18.1	41.4	1,400	25.27
	2.00	g	8	0.4	0.8	28.00	0.51
	1.00	tsp					
flakes, dried	100.00	g	319	11.3	68.7	4,388	2.10
	28.35	g	90	3.2	18.1	1,244	0.60
	1.00	oz					

KALE

	SERVING QUANTITY	SERVING UNIT	CALORIES (kcal)	PROTEIN (g)	TOTAL CARBOHYDRATES (g)	POTASSIUM (mg)	TOTAL FAT (g)
raw, chopped	100.00	g	35	2.9	4.4	348.00	1.49
	83.75	g	29	2.5	3.7	291.45	1.25
	1.25	c					
chopped, boiled, drained, no salt	100.00	g	36	2.9	5.3	144.00	1.21
	65.00	g	23	1.9	3.5	93.60	0.79
	0.50	c					
scotch, raw, chopped	100.00	g	42	2.8	8.3	450.00	0.60
	83.75	g	35	2.4	7.0	376.88	0.50
	1.25	c					
scotch, boiled, drained, chopped, no salt	100.00	g	28	1.9	5.6	274.00	0.41
	86.67	g	24	1.7	4.9	237.47	0.36
	0.67	c					
frozen, raw 1 pack=10 oz/ 284g	100.00	g	28	2.7	4.9	333.00	0.46
	85.05	g	24	2.3	4.2	283.21	0.39
	3.00	oz					
frozen, chopped, boiled, drained, no salt	100.00	g	36	2.9	5.3	144.00	1.21
	65.00	g	23	1.9	3.5	93.60	0.79
	0.50	c					

MUSTARD GREENS

	SERVING QUANTITY	SERVING UNIT	CALORIES (kcal)	PROTEIN (g)	TOTAL CARBOHYDRATES (g)	POTASSIUM (mg)	TOTAL FAT (g)
raw, chopped	100.00	g	27	2.9	4.7	384.00	0.42
	84.00	g	23	2.4	3.9	322.56	0.35
	1.50	c					
boiled, drained, chopped, no salt	100.00	g	26	2.6	4.5	162.00	0.47
	70.00	g	18	1.8	3.2	113.40	0.33
	0.50	c					
frozen 1 pack=10oz/284g	100.00	g	20	2.5	3.4	170.00	0.27
	73.00	g	15	1.8	2.5	124.10	0.20
	0.50	c					
frozen, boiled, drained, no salt 1 pack = 10oz/ 212g	100.00	g	19	2.3	3.1	139.00	0.25
	75.00	g	14	1.7	2.3	104.25	0.19
	0.50	c					

SQUASH	SERVING QUANTITY	SERVING UNIT	CALORIES (kcal)	PROTEIN (g)	TOTAL CARBOHYDRATES (g)	POTASSIUM (mg)	TOTAL FAT (g)
winter,	100.00	g	34	1.0	8.6	350.00	0.13
all varieties cubes	116.00	g	39	1.1	10.0	406.00	0.15
	1.00	c					
butternut	100.00	g	45	1.0	11.7	352.00	0.10
cubes	140.00	g	63	1.4	16.4	492.80	0.14
	1.00	c					
winter,	100.00	g	57	1.8	14.4	212.00	0.10
butternut,	85.05	g	48	1.5	12.3	180.30	0.09
frozen	3.00	oz					
summer,	100.00	g	16	1.2	3.4	262.00	0.18
all varieties sliced	84.75	g	14	1.0	2.8	222.05	0.15
	0.75	c					
KOHLRABI							
raw	100.00	g	27	1.7	6.2	350.00	0.10
	135.00	g	36	2.3	8.4	472.50	0.14
	1.00	c					
boiled,	100.00	g	29	1.8	6.7	340.00	0.11
drained, sliced	165.00	g	48	3.0	11.0	561.00	0.18
	1.00	c					
LEEKS							
raw	100.00	g	61	1.5	14.2	180.00	0.30
	89.00	g	54	1.3	12.6	160.20	0.27
	1.00	c					
boiled, drained,	100.00	g	31	0.8	7.6	87.00	0.20
chopped or diced	26.00	g	8	0.2	2.0	22.62	0.05
	0.25	c					
CASSAVA/YUCCA/MANIOC							
raw	100.00	g	160	1.4	38.1	271.00	0.28
	103.00	g	165	1.4	39.2	279.13	0.29
	0.50	c					
RADISH							
oriental (Daikon),	100.00	g	18	0.6	4.1	227.00	0.10
7" long	338.00	g	61	2.0	13.9	767.26	0.34
	1.00	pc					
oriental, boiled,	100.00	g	17	0.7	3.4	285.00	0.24
drained, no salt	73.50	g	13	0.5	2.5	209.48	0.18
sliced	0.50	c					
sprouts	100.00	g	43	3.8	3.6	86.00	2.53
	38.00	g	16	1.5	1.4	32.68	0.96
	1.00	c					

TURNIP GREENS	SERVING QUANTITY	SERVING UNIT	CALORIES (kcal)	PROTEIN (g)	TOTAL CARBOHYDRATES (g)	POTASSIUM (mg)	TOTAL FAT (g)
raw, turnip greens, chopped	100.00	g	32	1.5	7.1	296.00	0.30
	82.50	g	26	1.2	5.9	244.20	0.25
	1.50	c					
frozen	100.00	g	22	2.5	3.7	184.00	0.31
	82.00	g	18	2.0	3.0	150.88	0.25
	0.50	c					
canned	100.00	g	14	1.4	2.4	141.00	0.30
	78.00	g	11	1.1	1.9	109.98	0.23
	0.33	c					
chopped, boiled, drained, no salt	100.00	g	20	1.1	4.4	203.00	0.23
	144.00	g	29	1.6	6.3	292.32	0.33
	1.00	c					
canned, with no salt	100.00	g	19	1.4	2.8	141.00	0.30
	144.00	g	27	2.0	4.1	203.04	0.43
	1.00	c					
frozen, chopped, boiled, drained, no salt added	100.00	g	29	3.4	5.0	224.00	0.42
	164.00	g	48	5.5	8.2	367.36	0.69
	1.00	c					
RUTABAGA							
raw, cubes	100.00	g	37	1.1	8.6	305.00	0.16
	93.33	g	35	1.0	8.1	284.67	0.15
	0.67	c					
boiled, drained, no salt cubed	100.00	g	30	0.9	6.8	216.00	0.18
	170.00	g	51	1.6	11.6	367.20	0.31
	1.00	c					
boiled, drained, mashed	100.00	g	30	0.9	6.8	216.00	0.18
	160.80	g	48	1.5	11.0	347.33	0.29
	0.67	c					
PARSNIPS							
raw, sliced	100.00	g	75	1.2	18.0	375.00	0.30
	88.67	g	67	1.1	16.0	332.50	0.27
	0.67	c					
boiled, drained, sliced, no salt	100.00	g	71	1.3	17.0	367.00	0.30
	78.00	g	55	1.0	13.3	286.26	0.23
	0.50	c					

Chapter 8: Herbs and Spices

Do you want to print the charts in letter-size (8.5x11")?

I have created downloadable printables of this chart. You can scan the QR code below or copy the link to your computer browser to be able to get your printable copies of the food charts

https://go.renaltracker.com/lowpotassiumprint

		SERVING QUANTITY	SERVING UNIT	CALORIES (kcal)	PROTEIN (g)	TOTAL CARBOHYDRATES (g)	POTASSIUM (mg)	TOTAL FAT (g)
SAGE								
	ground	100	g	315	10.6	60.7	1070	12.8
	Ground (1 tbsp)	2	g	6.3	0.212	1.21	21.4	0.256
CINNAMON								
	ground	100	g	247	3.99	80.6	431	1.24
	ground (1 tbsp)	7.8	g	19.3	0.311	6.29	33.6	0.097
CUMIN								
	seed	100	g	375	17.8	44.2	1790	22.3
	Seed	6	g	22.5	1.07	2.65	107	1.34
		1	tbsp					
NUTMEG								
	ground	100	g	525	5.84	49.3	350	36.3
	ground	7	g	36.8	0.409	3.45	24.5	2.54
		1	tbsp					
CLOVES								
	ground	100	g	274	5.97	65.5	1020	13
	ground	6.5	g	17.8	0.388	4.26	66.3	0.845
		1	tbsp					
PARSLEY								
	fresh	100	g	36	2.97	6.33	554	0.79
	dried	100	g	292	26.6	50.6	2680	5.48
CORIANDER								
	seed	100	g	298	12.4	55	1270	17.8
	leaves, raw	100	g	23	2.13	3.67	521	0.52
THYME								
	fresh	100	g	101	5.56	24.4	609	1.68
	dried	100	g	276	9.11	63.9	814	7.43
LEMON GRASS								
	raw	100	g	99	1.82	25.3	723	0.49

ONION	SERVING QUANTITY	SERVING UNIT	CALORIES (kcal)	PROTEIN (g)	TOTAL CARBOHYDRATES (g)	POTASSIUM (mg)	TOTAL FAT (g)
red, raw	100	g	44	0.94	9.93	197	0.1
1 onion	197	g	86.7	1.85	19.6	388	0.197
white, raw	100	g	36	0.89	7.68	141	0.13
yellow, raw	100	g	38	0.83	8.61	182	0.05
1 onion	143	g	54.3	1.19	12.3	260	0.071

GARLIC

raw	100	g	149	6.36	33.1	401	0.5
3 cloves	9	g	13.4	0.572	2.98	36.1	0.045

GINGER

raw	100	g	80	1.82	17.8	415	0.75

SPRING ONIONS

raw	100	g	32	1.83	7.34	276	0.19
1 large	25	g	8	0.458	1.84	69	0.048

CHIVES

raw	100	g	30	3.27	4.35	296	0.73

BASIL

fresh	100	g	23	3.15	2.65	295	0.64
dried	100	g	233	23	47.8	2630	4.07

OREGANO

dried	100	g	265	9	68.9	1260	4.28

ROSEMARY

fresh	100	g	131	3.31	20.7	668	5.86
dried	100	g	331	4.88	64.1	995	15.2

MARJORAM

dried	100	g	271	12.7	60.6	1520	7.04

FENNEL

	SERVING QUANTITY	SERVING UNIT	CALORIES (kcal)	PROTEIN (g)	TOTAL CARBOHYDRATES (g)	POTASSIUM (mg)	TOTAL FAT (g)
bulb, raw	100	g	31	1.24	7.3	414	0.2
seed	100	g	345	15.8	52.3	1690	14.9
seed	(1 tbsp, whole) 5.8	g	20	0.916	3.03	98	0.864

DILL

fresh	100	g	43	3.46	7.02	738	1.12
dried	100	g	253	20	55.8	3310	4.36
dried	(1 tbsp) 3.1	g	7.84	0.62	1.73	103	0.135

ANISE

seed	100	g	337	17.6	50	1440	15.9
seed	(1 tbsp, whole) 6.7	g	22.6	1.18	3.35	96.5	1.06

CARDAMOM

ground	100	g	311	10.8	68.5	1120	6.7
ground	(1 tbsp) 5.8	g	18	0.626	3.97	65	0.389

CAYENNE

ground	100	g	318	12	56.6	2010	17.3
ground	(1 tbsp) 5.3	g	16.9	0.636	3	107	0.917

CURRY POWDER

	100	g	325	14.3	55.8	1170	14
	(1 tbsp) 6.3	g	20.5	0.901	3.52	73.7	0.882

PAPRIKA

ground	100	g	282	14.1	54	2280	12.9
ground	(1 tbsp) 6.8	g	19.2	0.959	3.67	155	0.877

CELERY

celery, raw	100	g	14	0.69	2.97	260	0.17

SAFFRON

	SERVING QUANTITY	SERVING UNIT	CALORIES (kcal)	PROTEIN (g)	TOTAL CARBOHYDRATE (g)	POTASSIUM (mg)	TOTAL FAT (g)
	100	g	310	11.4	65.4	1720	5.85
	(1 tbsp) 2.1	g	6.51	0.239	1.37	36.1	0.123

PEPPER, BLACK

	SERVING QUANTITY	SERVING UNIT	CALORIES	PROTEIN	TOTAL CARBOHYDRATE	POTASSIUM	TOTAL FAT
ground	100	g	251	10.4	64	1330	3.26
ground	(1 tbsp, ground) 6.9	g	17.3	0.718	4.42	91.8	0.225

PEPPER, WHITE

	SERVING QUANTITY	SERVING UNIT	CALORIES	PROTEIN	TOTAL CARBOHYDRATE	POTASSIUM	TOTAL FAT
ground	100	g	296	10.4	68.6	73	2.12
ground	(1 tbsp, ground) 7.1	g	21	0.738	4.87	5.18	0.151

TARRAGON

	SERVING QUANTITY	SERVING UNIT	CALORIES	PROTEIN	TOTAL CARBOHYDRATE	POTASSIUM	TOTAL FAT
dried	100	g	295	22.8	50.2	3020	7.24
dried, leaves	(1 tbsp, leaves) 1.8	g	5.31	0.41	0.904	54.4	0.13
dried, ground	(1 tbsp, ground) 4.8	g	14.2	1.09	2.41	145	0.348

HORSERADISH

	SERVING QUANTITY	SERVING UNIT	CALORIES	PROTEIN	TOTAL CARBOHYDRATE	POTASSIUM	TOTAL FAT
	100	g	48	1.18	11.3	246	0.69
	(1 tbsp) 15	g	7.2	0.177	1.7	36.9	0.103

Part 2. Meal Planning and Recipes

Chapter 9: Low Potassium Meal Plan

Creating a Low Potassium Meal Plan

Equipped with a full list of food items that you can refer to when planning your meal, here are some general guidelines I would recommend so that you will be more well-prepared on your next visit to your dietitian. You may use this as a checklist in making those informed choices about your low-potassium meal plan for CKD:

- ✓ Understand Potassium Levels in Foods:

Potassium is found in many foods, especially fruits and vegetables. It's important to know which foods are high in potassium and limit them in your diet. Foods high in potassium include bananas, oranges, potatoes, spinach, and tomatoes.

- ✓ Portion Control:

Even low-potassium foods can become high in potassium if you eat a large amount of them. Keep your portions moderate to small.

- ✓ Leaching Vegetables:

I've discussed about this in the beginning of the book on *page 353* but I find it a very important thing to emphasize. You can pick out foods to include in your meal plans that you can apply leaching with. Remember, this does not necessarily remove all the potassium content in your food, but it could very well help in keeping you within your limits by minimizing it

✓ Choose Low-Potassium Foods:

Include more low-potassium foods in your meal plan such as apples, berries, grapes, pears, plums, pineapples, cabbage, cucumber, eggplant, onions and bell peppers.

✓ Limit Dairy Intake:

Dairy products are high in potassium. Limit your intake or opt for non-dairy alternatives like almond milk or rice milk.

✓ Limit Protein Intake:

While protein is essential for health, too much can make the kidneys work harder and can contribute to kidney damage over time. Aim for moderate protein intake.

✓ Avoid Salt Substitutes:

Many salt substitutes are high in potassium. Instead of using these products, try flavoring your food with herbs and spices.

✓ Regular Check-ups:

Regular check-ups are crucial to monitor your potassium levels and adjust your diet accordingly.

5-Day Low Potassium Sample Meal Plan

DAY 1

- Breakfast: 1 cup of cooked oatmeal, 1 slice of whole grain toast, and 1 small apple
- Lunch: Grilled chicken salad (with lettuce, cucumber, carrots, and vinegar dressing)
- Dinner: Baked fish with lemon, steamed green beans, and a small portion of white rice
- Snack: A handful of blueberries

DAY 2

- Breakfast: Scrambled eggs (made with egg whites), 1 slice of whole grain toast, and a small pear
- Lunch: Turkey sandwich (with lettuce and mayonnaise on whole grain bread) and cucumber slices
- Dinner: Grilled chicken breast, steamed cauliflower, and a small portion of couscous
- Snack: A handful of grapes

DAY 3

- Breakfast: Whole grain cereal with almond milk and a small peach
- Lunch: Tuna salad (made with mayonnaise) on whole grain bread and raw carrot sticks
- Dinner: Baked cod, steamed broccoli, and a small portion of quinoa
- Snack: A handful of strawberries

DAY 4

- Breakfast: Egg white omelette with bell peppers and onions, and a slice of whole grain toast
- Lunch: Grilled chicken wrap (with lettuce and mayonnaise in a whole grain tortilla) and raw bell pepper slices
- Dinner: Baked salmon, steamed zucchini, and a small portion of brown rice
- Snack: A handful of raspberries

DAY 5

- Breakfast: Cooked oatmeal with a handful of blueberries, and 1 slice of whole grain toast
- Lunch: Turkey and cheese sandwich (with lettuce and mayonnaise on whole grain bread) and cucumber slices
- Dinner: Grilled chicken breast, steamed asparagus, and a small portion of white rice
- Snack: A small apple

Remember to drink plenty of water throughout the day, unless your doctor has advised otherwise. Also, avoid adding extra salt to your meals - use herbs and spices for flavor instead. For protein portions, aim for about 3 ounces per meal (about the size of a deck of cards).

Low Potassium Dietary Recommendations

Sure, here are the low-potassium dietary recommendations and sample meal plans for each stage of Chronic Kidney Disease (CKD). Keep in mind that these are general guidelines and may not suit everyone. Always consult with your healthcare provider or dietitian before making any changes to your diet.

1. Early Stage Kidney Disease:

In the early stages of CKD (stages 1-2), the kidneys are still able to regulate potassium levels in the body, so a low-potassium diet may not be necessary unless recommended by your healthcare provider.

Recommendations:
- Maintain a balanced diet rich in fruits, vegetables, lean proteins, and whole grains.
- Limit high-sodium foods.
- Stay hydrated.

2. Mid-stage Kidney Disease:

In the mid-stages of CKD (stages 3-4), the kidneys start losing their ability to regulate potassium levels in the body. A low-potassium diet becomes important.

Recommendations:
- Limit high-potassium foods like bananas, oranges, potatoes, spinach, and tomatoes.
- Include more low-potassium foods like apples, berries, grapes, pears, plums, pineapples, cabbage, cucumber, eggplant, onions and bell peppers.
- Continue limiting high-sodium foods.
- Monitor protein intake

3. Late Stage Kidney Disease:

In the late stages of CKD (stages 4-5), the kidneys have a significantly reduced ability to regulate potassium levels in the body. A low-potassium diet is crucial.

Recommendations:
- Strictly limit high-potassium foods.
- Leach vegetables to remove some of the potassium.
- Limit protein intake and choose high-quality sources.
- Avoid salt substitutes as they often contain potassium.
- Monitor fluid intake as recommended by your healthcare provider.

Remember that these are general guidelines and individual needs may vary. Always consult with your healthcare provider or dietitian for personalized advice.

Chapter 10: Low Potassium Recipes

Spicy Deviled Egg

MAKES: 1 SERVING

Aesthetically irresistible, this egg appetizer dish is made so meticulously to perfection.

INGREDIENTS

- 1 hard-boiled egg
- 1 teaspoon pimentos
- 1/4 teaspoon dry mustard
- 1 tablespoon mayonnaise
- 1/4 teaspoon black pepper
- paprika (to garnish)

DIRECTIONS

1. Cut egg lengthwise and remove yolk.
2. Mix yolk, pimentos, dry mustard, mayonnaise, and black pepper.
3. Place mixture inside egg whites in equal parts.
4. Sprinkle eggs with paprika.

NUTRIENT ANALYSIS | PER SERVING

Calories (kCal):	116.0
Proteins (g):	7.0
Carbohydrates (g):	4.0
Fats (g):	8.0
Potassium (mg):	83.0
Phosphorus (mg):	95.0
Sodium (mg):	78.0

Baked Egg Cups

MAKES: 1 SERVING

Very enticing dish, perfect for breakfast and can be taken also as appetizer.

INGREDIENTS

- 6 slices low-sodium bacon
- 1/3 cup onion
- 1/3 cup mushrooms
- 1/3 cup bell pepper
- 12 large eggs
- 1/4 teaspoon black pepper

DIRECTIONS

1. Preheat oven to 3500 F. Line muffin tin with paper muffin wrappers. Dice vegetables.
2. Cook bacon until crisp. Crumble cooked bacon and combine with diced vegetables in a large bowl.
3. Spoon mixture into cups, filling them 2/3 of the way, leaving room to add the egg mixture.
4. In another bowl, beat together eggs and black pepper.
5. Pour egg mixture into each muffin cup. Leave 1/4 inch at the top.
6. Bake 25 minutes, or until muffins have risen and are firm.
7. Remove muffins from pan and serve.

NUTRIENT ANALYSIS

	PER SERVING
Calories (kCal):	80.0
Proteins (g):	7.0
Carbohydrates (g):	1.0
Fats (g):	5.0
Potassium (mg):	92.0
Phosphorus (mg):	101.0
Sodium (mg):	78.0

Apple Muffins

MAKES: 12 SERVINGS

Bake a batch of delicious breakfast apple muffins that are low in fat and calories.

INGREDIENTS

- 12 muffin papers
- 1-1/2 cups raw apple
- 2 eggs
- 1 cup sugar
- 1/2 cup canola oil
- 1/4 cup water
- 1 tablespoon vanilla
- 1-1/2 cups all purpose white flour
- 1 teaspoon baking soda
- 1-1/2 teaspoons cinnamon

DIRECTIONS

1. Preheat oven to 400° F and place muffin papers in muffin pan. Peel and cut apple into small pieces.
2. Beat eggs in a large bowl. Add sugar, oil and water; mix well. Add vanilla.
3. In a separate bowl, combine flour, baking soda and 1 teaspoon cinnamon.
4. Stir flour mixture into egg mixture. Batter will be lumpy. Fold in apple pieces.
5. Fill muffin cups 3/4 full. Mix remaining 1/2 teaspoon cinnamon with 1 teaspoon sugar. Sprinkle on top of muffins.
6. Bake for 20 minutes or until lightly browned.

NUTRIENT ANALYSIS

	PER SERVING
Calories (kCal):	162.0
Proteins (g):	3.0
Carbohydrates (g):	15.0
Fats (g):	10.0
Potassium (mg):	46.0
Phosphorus (mg):	34.0
Sodium (mg):	117.0

Crab Cakes

MAKES: 6 SERVINGS

A rather peculiar seafood recipe that you can have as an appetizer, or as part of your lunch and dinner main course

INGREDIENTS

- 1 egg (egg substitute or egg white optional)
- 1/3 cup green or red pepper, finely chopped
- 1/3 cup low sodium crackers
- 1/4 cup reduced fat mayonnaise
- 1 tablespoon dry mustard
- 1 teaspoon crushed red pepper or black pepper
- 2 tablespoons lemon juice
- 1 teaspoon garlic powder
- 2 tablespoon vegetable oil

DIRECTIONS

1. Combine all ingredients.
2. Divide into 6 balls and form patties.
3. Heat vegetable oil in pan at medium heat or oven at 350°F.
4. Fry patties 4-5 minutes or bake 15 minutes in oven.
5. Serve warm.

NUTRIENT ANALYSIS — PER SERVING

Calories (kCal):	101.0
Proteins (g):	2.0
Carbohydrates (g):	5.0
Fats (g):	9.0
Potassium (mg):	72.0
Phosphorus (mg):	43.0
Sodium (mg):	67.0

Baked Flounder Teriyaki

MAKES: 4 SERVINGS

Teriyaki is a Japanese dish of meat or fish that is grilled or broiled after being soaked in a seasoned soy sauce marinade.

INGREDIENTS

- 6 small flounder or other lean fish fillets
- 1/3 cup dry sherry or apple juice
- 2 tablespoon chopped green onions
- 3 tablespoon lemon juice
- 2 teaspoons finely chopped gingerroot
- 2 teaspoon honey
- 1 teaspoon vegetable oil
- 1/4 teaspoon pepper
- 2 cloves garlic, finely chopped.

DIRECTIONS

1. Spray rectangular pan, 13 x 9 x 2 inches, with non-stickcooking spray.
2. Place fish in pan. Mix remaining ingredients; spoon over fish.
3. Cover with aluminum foil and refrigerate 1 hour.
4. Heat oven to 350 degrees. Bake covered 15-20 minutes or until fish flakes easily with fork.

NUTRIENT ANALYSIS	PER SERVING
Calories (kCal):	105.0
Proteins (g):	20.0
Carbohydrates (g):	2.0
Fats (g):	2.0
Potassium (mg):	90.0
Phosphorus (mg):	80.0
Sodium (mg):	85.0

Basic Rice Pilaf

MAKES: 6 SERVINGS

This is a dish that is made of seasoned rice and vegetables. You may also add bits of meat, chicken and seafood for variety.

INGREDIENTS

- 2 ounces vermicelli noodles, uncooked
- 2 tablespoons unsalted butter
- 1 cup parboiled rice, uncooked
- 2 cups water
- 1 cube chicken-flavor bouillon
- 1 tablespoon Onion and Herb seasoning blend

DIRECTIONS

1. In a skillet over medium heat, melt butter.
2. Break vermicelli noodles into 2" pieces and cook, stirring often until noodles begin to brown.
3. Add rice and stir to coat rice evenly with remaining melted butter.
4. Crush chicken bouillon and add to skillet along with water and herb seasoning. Stir to blend ingredients.
5. Cover and bring to a boil. Reduce to low heat and cook 20 minutes. Do not remove the cover.
6. Turn off heat and allow to sit covered for an additional 5 minutes.
7. Fluff with a fork and serve.

NUTRIENT ANALYSIS

	PER SERVING
Calories (kCal):	180.0
Proteins (g):	4.0
Carbohydrates (g):	30.0
Fats (g):	5.0
Potassium (mg):	87.0
Phosphorus (mg):	68.0
Sodium (mg):	154.0

Egg Salad

MAKES: 8 SERVINGS

This simple egg recipe is best to start your meal or as a side dish to your vegetable

INGREDIENTS

- 2 tablespoons mayonnaise
- 1 teaspoon dry mustard
- ½ teaspoon black pepper
- 3 boiled eggs, chopped
- 1 tablespoon regular pickle relish
- paprika

DIRECTIONS

1. Mix together mayonnaise, mustard, pepper, eggs, and pickle relish. Mix well.
2. Sprinkle with paprika.

NUTRIENT ANALYSIS	PER SERVING
Calories (kCal):	58.0
Proteins (g):	3.0
Carbohydrates (g):	5.0
Fats (g):	1.0
Potassium (mg):	28.0
Phosphorus (mg):	36.0
Sodium (mg):	58.0

Apple Bars

MAKES: 18 SERVINGS

Can be made in large quantity, this healthy go-to apple dessert doesn't spoil very easily when stored well.

INGREDIENTS

- 3/4 cup unsalted butter
- 1 cup granulated sugar
- 1 cup sour cream
- 1 teaspoon vanilla extract
- 1 teaspoon baking soda
- 1/2 teaspoon salt
- 2 cups all-purpose white flour
- 2 medium apples
- 1/2 cup brown sugar
- 1 teaspoon cinnamon
- 2 tablespoons milk
- 1 cup powdered sugar

DIRECTIONS

1. Preheat oven to 350° F.
2. Peel and chop apples.
3. Cream together 1/2 cup butter and white sugar or Splenda.
4. Add sour cream, vanilla, baking soda, salt and flour. Stir to mix; add chopped apples.
5. Pour batter into a greased 9" x 13" baking pan.
6. In a small bowl, crumble 2 tablespoons softened butter, brown sugar and cinnamon together. Sprinkle over top of batter.
7. Bake for 35 to 40 minutes. Let cool completely.
8. To make icing, combine 2 tablespoons melted butter, milk (or milk substitute) and powdered sugar. Drizzle over top; and cut dessert into 18 bars.

NUTRIENT ANALYSIS	PER SERVING
Calories (kCal):	246.0
Proteins (g):	2.0
Carbohydrates (g):	35.0
Fats (g):	11.0
Potassium (mg):	72.0
Phosphorus (mg):	27.0
Sodium (mg):	140.0

Minted Lemonade

MAKES: 5 SERVINGS

Add flavor to your usual lemonade by dropping in some mint leaves.

INGREDIENTS

- 6 tablespoons fresh lemon juice
- 1/2 cup sugar
- 6 mint leaves
- 3-1/2 cups cold water

DIRECTIONS

1. In a 1-quart pitcher, mix lemon juice, sugar and mint leaves. Add 3-1/2 cups of cold water to fill the pitcher.
2. Chill until cold.
3. Serve in a 6-ounce glass with a sprig of mint to garnish.

NUTRIENT ANALYSIS	PER SERVING
Calories (kCal):	80.0
Proteins (g):	0.0
Carbohydrates (g):	21.0
Fats (g):	0.0
Potassium (mg):	34.0
Phosphorus (mg):	2.0
Sodium (mg):	0.0

Apple-Ginger Sparkler

MAKES: 12 SERVINGS

Add a zing to an apple beverage by adding ginger to the mixture.

INGREDIENTS

- 2 cups sugar
- 1 six-inch piece fresh ginger, finely diced
- 2 cups water
- ice cubes
- 4 cups sparkling apple cider
- 6 cinnamon sticks, cut in half
- 12 pieces crystallized ginger

DIRECTIONS

1. To prepare ginger syrup, place sugar*, grate ginger and water in a medium saucepan; bring to boil. Reduce heat to low and simmer for 1 hour until ginger flavor is strong.
2. Strain mixture and refrigerate to chill.
3. To prepare Ginger-Apple Sparkler, place one tablespoon ginger syrup in each glass (use short tumblers).
4. Fill with ice cubes, pour in 1/2-cup cider and stir to combine.
5. Garnish with cinnamon stick and crystallized ginger.

NUTRIENT ANALYSIS	PER SERVING
Calories (kCal):	185.0
Proteins (g):	0.0
Carbohydrates (g):	47.0
Fats (g):	0.0
Potassium (mg):	110.0
Phosphorus (mg):	7.0
Sodium (mg):	25.0

Pickled Okra

MAKES: 16 SERVINGS

Fermented okras can last for more than a month when stored properly.

INGREDIENTS

- 20 ounces frozen okra
- 2 teaspoons dill seed
- 2 dried red peppers
- 2 whole chili peppers, canned
- 4 garlic cloves
- 1-1/4 cups white vinegar
- 1/2 cup water

DIRECTIONS

1. Thaw and drain okra.
2. Sterilize two one-pint jars and lids.
3. Place 1-teaspoon dill seed into each jar. Pack okra into jars.
4. To each jar add 1 red pepper, 1 chili pepper and 2 cloves of garlic.
5. Combine vinegar and water and bring to a boil, simmer for 5 minutes.
6. Pour hot mixture over okra in each jar. Cap jar and cool.
7. Refrigerate and okra pickles will be ready to serve in 2 weeks.

NUTRIENT ANALYSIS	PER SERVING
Calories (kCal):	14.0
Proteins (g):	1.0
Carbohydrates (g):	2.0
Fats (g):	0.0
Potassium (mg):	98.0
Phosphorus (mg):	19.0
Sodium (mg):	19.0

Chapter 11:
Embracing the Journey

Coping with Chronic Kidney Disease, Dietary Adjustments, and Lifestyle Modifications

Living with Chronic Kidney Disease (CKD) is undeniably challenging. It demands a significant shift in your dietary habits, lifestyle, and overall perspective on life. However, it's essential to remember that this journey is not one you must traverse alone. This chapter aims to provide you with effective coping strategies, support networks, resources, and professional encouragement to help you navigate this new terrain.

Coping Strategies and Overcoming Struggles

Adapting to a low-potassium CKD diet may initially seem overwhelming. The key is to take small steps and make gradual changes. Start by reducing your intake of high-potassium foods while increasing low-potassium alternatives. For instance, swap bananas (high in potassium) for apples (lower in potassium).

It's also crucial to maintain a balanced diet despite the restrictions. Consult with a dietitian who can help create a personalized meal plan that caters to your nutritional needs without compromising on taste.

Lifestyle modifications are another aspect of managing CKD. Regular exercise, while taking into account your physical limitations, can significantly improve your health and mood. Incorporate mild activities such as walking or yoga into your daily routine.

Remember that it's okay to have bad days. Allow yourself to feel frustrated or upset but don't dwell on these feelings. Instead, focus on what you can control and let go of what you can't.

Finding the Right Support Networks

Support networks play an integral role in managing CKD. They provide emotional assistance, practical advice, and a sense of community. Consider joining local support groups where you can connect with others navigating similar experiences. The American Association of Kidney Patients (AAKP), for example, offers numerous local chapters across the country.

Online forums like the National Kidney Foundation's community on HealthUnlocked provide a platform to share experiences and advice. These virtual communities can be particularly beneficial for those who may not have access to local support groups.

Utilizing Resources

There are numerous resources available to assist you on your CKD journey. The National Kidney Foundation (NKF) and the American Kidney Fund (AKF) offer comprehensive guides on diet, exercise, and overall CKD management.

Apps like My Food Coach, developed by the NKF, help you track your diet, providing food suggestions based on your specific dietary needs. Similarly, the AKF's Kidney Kitchen offers a range of kidney-friendly recipes and cooking tips.

Conclusion

As a Nephrology Nurse and Dietitian with a decade of experience, I want to reassure you that living with CKD is manageable with the right approach and mindset. It's essential to maintain regular appointments with your healthcare team who can monitor your progress and make necessary adjustments to your treatment plan.

Remember, you are more than your diagnosis. With determination, support, and the right resources, you can live a fulfilling life while managing CKD.

In conclusion, coping with CKD involves dietary and lifestyle changes, finding supportive networks, utilizing available resources, and maintaining a positive outlook. This journey may seem daunting at first, but remember that each small step brings you closer to better health and improved quality of life. Embrace this journey with courage, resilience, and hope. You are not alone; we are here to walk this path with you.

References

BIDMC Food Prioritization Project by https://www.renaltracker.com
Food List Reference: USDA FoodData Central – https://www.fdc.nal.usda.gov

Potassium in Your CKD Diet

>National Kidney Foundation: https://www.kidney.org/atoz/content/potassium-ckd-diet

High potassium (hyperkalemia): Causes, prevention and treatment

>American Kidney Fund: https://www.kidneyfund.org/living-kidney-disease/health-problems-caused-kidney-disease/high-potassium-hyperkalemia-causes-prevention-and-treatment

CKD food and Nutrition

>Mayo Clinic: https://www.mayoclinic.org/diseases-conditions/chronic-kidney-disease/expert-answers/food-and-nutrition/faq-20058408

Recipes

>1. Fool-Proof Kidney Dieting for First Timers by Rachelle Gordon, BSN RN
>2. CKD Diet Recipes (50 Renal Dietitian Created Recipes for Kidney Disease Patients)

Low Potassium Food List Index

	Page		*Page*
CARBOHYDRATES	**357**	**FATS (NUTS AND OILS)**	
Amaranth	359	Olive	412
Barley	361	Peanut	408
Breads	363	Pecans	406
Cereals	362	Pine	409
Couscous	361	Pistachios	406
Crackers	366	Poppyseed	414
Grits	361	Pumpkin	414
Oats	359	Safflower	413
Pancake	367	Sesame	411
Pasta	368	Soybean	413
Polenta (cornmeal)	361	Sunflower	411
Quinoa	361	Walnut	405
Rice	358	**FRUITS**	**415**
Waffle	367	Apple	*419*
Wheat	360	Apricot	*427*
FATS (NUTS AND OILS)	**403**	Avocado	*433*
Acorn	410	Banana	
Almond	404	Blackberries	*419*
Butter	413	Blueberries	*416*
Canola	413	Canteloupe/ Melon	*428*
Cashew	407	Cherries	*418*
Chestnut	409	Coconut	*412*
Chia	410	Cranberry	*417*
Coconut	412	Dates	*432*

Flaxseed	410	Durian	*432*
Ghee	413	Elderberries	*421*
Hazelnut	407	Fig	*429*
Hemp	410	Gooseberries	*421*
Macadamia	406	Grapefruit	*421*
Margarine	413	Grapes	*422*

Low Potassium Food List Index

FRUITS	Page	HERBS AND SPICES	Page
	415		
Guava	429	Anise	456
Jackfruit	432	Basil	455
Kiwi	421	Cardamom	456
Lemon	424	Cayenne	456
Lime	425	Celery	456
Loganberries	421	Chives	455
Lychee	425	Cinnamon	454
Mango	425	Cloves	454
Mangosteen	432	Coriander	454
Nectarine	430	Cumin	454
Orange	423	Curry Powder	456
Papaya	430	Dill	456
Peaches	426	Fennel	456
Pears	417	Fennel Seeds	456
Persimmon	430	Garlic	455
Pineapple	419	Ginger	455
Plantain	433	Horseradish	457
Plum	427	Lemon grass	454
Pomegranate	431	Marjoram	455
Pomelo	432	Nutmeg	454
Prune	431	Onion	455
PurplePassionFruit/Granadilla	430	Oregano	455
Raspberries	417	Paprika	456
Rhubarb	431	Parsley	454

Sapodilla	*434*	Pepper, black	457
Soursop	*432*	Pepper, white	457
Starfruit (Carambola)	*434*	Rosemary	455
Strawberries	*416*	Saffron	457
Sugar apple (sweetsop)	*434*	Sage	454
Tamarind	*434*	Spring Onions	455
Watermelon	*429*	Tarragon	457
		Thyme	454

Low Potassium Food List Index

	Page		Page
ANIMAL PROTEIN		**MILKS AND CHEESE**	**393**
Anchovies	384	Cheeses	399
Beef	380	Cream	402
Carp	386	Milk	394
Catfish	388	Milk Sub	395
Chicken	374	Yogurt	396
Clams	390	**VEGETABLES**	
Cod	384	Alfalfa	449
Crab	388	Artichokes	449
Crayfish/Crawfish	389	Arugula	442
Eggs	373	Asparagus	437
Flatfish	387	Beans	437
Halibut	387	Beets	439
Herring	392	Broccoli	439
Lamb	381	Brussel Sprouts	444
Lobster	387	Cabbage	446
Mackerel	391	carrots	437
Mahi-Mahi	386	Cassava/ Yucca/Manioc	451
Mussels	391	Cauliflower	439
Oysters	390	Celery	449
Pangasius (Cream Dory) (Swai)	385	Collards	441
Pollock	385	Corn	447
Pork	377	Cucumber	439
Salmon	383	Eggplant (aubergine)	441
Sardines	385	Endive or Escarole	442
Scallops	392	Jicama (Yambean)	441

Shrimp	384	Kale	450
Squid (Calamari)	389	Kohlrabi	451
Tilapia	385	Leeks	451
Trout	386	Lettuce	438
Tuna	383	Mixed Vegetables	444
Turkey	376	Mushroom	438
Veal	381	Mustard Greens	450

Low Potassium Food List Index

	Page
VEGETABLES	**435**
Okra	442
Parsnips	452
Peas	448
Pepper	436
Potatoes	440
Pumpkin	442
Radish	451
Rutabaga	452
Spinach	443
Squash	451
Swiss Chard	443
Tomatillos	443
Tomato	445
Turnip Greens	452
Turnips	443
Waterchestnuts	444
Watercress	444
Yam	444
VEGETABLES PROTEIN	**370**
Beans	371
Chickpeas	372
Edamame	370
Spirulina	370
Tempeh	370
Tofu	370

From the Author

As we reach the conclusion of this book, I sincerely hope it has served as a valuable guide, one you'll frequently refer to when navigating the complexities of Low Potassium CKD dieting.

To all those bravely fighting kidney disease, my deepest wish is that you emerge victorious in this battle through self-empowerment and control.

Your decision to choose this book may seem simple, but it carries profound significance for me. Although our paths may not have crossed personally, your support is genuinely appreciated.

If this book has contributed positively to your journey, please consider sharing your experience by writing a review on Amazon. You can do so by scanning the provided code or manually entering the link into your web browser.

https://go.renaltracker.com/book3review

Cheering for your best kidney health!

Janeth Kingston, BSN RN

THE KIDNEY-FRIENDLY LOW-SODIUM DIET GUIDE
Essential Food List

Manage Kidney Disease with Delicious, Low-Sodium Meals and Recipes

Janeth Kingston, BSN RN

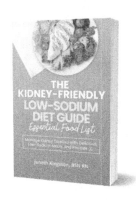

The Kidney-Friendly Low-Sodium Diet Guide Essential Food List

Manage Kidney Disease with Delicious, Low-Sodium Meals and Recipes

Janeth Kingston, BSN RN

Introduction

Welcome to The **Kidney-Friendly Low-Sodium Diet Guide: Essential Food List!** If you're reading this, you are likely seeking to improve your health and manage chronic kidney disease (CKD) through dietary changes. This guide is designed to provide you with comprehensive information about the importance of a low-sodium diet, practical food lists, and delicious recipes tailored to your unique needs.

With nearly 37 million adults in the United States living with CKD, many are searching for effective ways to manage their condition through nutrition. The right dietary choices can significantly influence kidney health, helping to reduce symptoms, slow disease progression, and enhance overall well-being.

Author's Journey: Janeth Kingston's Story

I'm Janeth Kingston, a dedicated nephrology nurse with over a decade of experience in the field. My mission is to improve the lives of those living with CKD, and I have devoted my career to this pursuit, both in the U.S. and Europe. Recognized for my expertise, my research has been awarded by the American Society of Nephrology through their prestigious KidneyX program.

Throughout my nursing career, I have witnessed the challenges faced by individuals managing kidney disease, particularly in adhering to dietary restrictions. This realization motivated me to create a resource that simplifies the complexities of dietary management, making it accessible and practical for everyone.

This book is structured to provide you with a wealth of information and practical tools. Here's how to make the most of it:

Comprehensive Food List: In Chapter 4, you will find a detailed low-sodium food list categorized by food groups. Each entry will include serving sizes and important macronutrient (macros) and micronutrient (micros) information to help you make informed choices.

Chapter 1: Understanding Kidney Health

Overview of Chronic Kidney Disease (CKD)

Chronic Kidney Disease (CKD) is a progressive condition characterized by the gradual loss of kidney function over time. According to the Centers for Disease Control and Prevention (CDC), approximately 37 million adults in the United States are affected by CKD, with many unaware of their condition until it reaches advanced stages.

CKD can result from various factors, including diabetes, hypertension, and glomerulonephritis. As kidney function declines, the body's ability to filter waste and excess fluids diminishes, leading to a buildup of toxins in the bloodstream. This can cause a range of complications, including cardiovascular disease, anemia, and bone disease.

The Importance of Diet in Managing Kidney Health

Diet plays a crucial role in the management of CKD. A well-balanced diet can help control symptoms, slow disease progression, and reduce the risk of complications. For individuals with CKD, dietary management often involves:

Limiting Sodium Intake: Reducing sodium can help manage blood pressure and decrease fluid retention, which is vital for kidney health.

Controlling Protein Consumption: While protein is essential for overall health, excess protein can lead to an increased burden on the kidneys. It's important to choose high-quality protein sources and monitor intake.

Balancing Potassium and Phosphorus: Many individuals with CKD need to limit potassium and phosphorus to prevent complications, such as heart problems and bone disease.

By making informed dietary choices, individuals with CKD can significantly improve their quality of life and health outcomes.

Understanding Sodium's Role in Kidney Disease

Sodium plays a critical role in fluid balance and blood pressure regulation. However, for individuals with CKD, excessive sodium intake can be particularly harmful. The kidneys are responsible for filtering excess sodium from the body, but as kidney function declines, they become less effective at this task. This can lead to fluid retention, increased blood pressure, and ultimately strain on the heart and kidneys.

Research indicates that a high sodium diet can exacerbate hypertension and worsen kidney function. Therefore, managing sodium intake is essential for those with CKD. The American Heart Association recommends that individuals limit sodium intake to 1,500 mg per day for optimal heart health. For those with kidney disease, adhering to these guidelines can help control blood pressure and reduce the risk of complications.

Understanding the intricacies of kidney health is vital for effectively managing chronic kidney disease. By recognizing the importance of dietary choices, particularly in relation to sodium, individuals can take proactive steps to improve their health outcomes.

As you continue your journey toward better health, remember that informed dietary choices can make a significant difference in managing kidney disease.

The Importance of Diet in Managing Kidney Disease

Diet plays a crucial role in the management of Chronic Kidney Disease (CKD), as it directly impacts kidney function, overall health, and the progression of the disease. According to the Kidney Disease: Improving Global Outcomes (KDIGO) guidelines, dietary management is an essential aspect of care for patients with CKD. Here are key dietary considerations according to KDIGO recommendations:

Protein Intake

Moderation is Key: KDIGO recommends that patients with CKD should manage their protein intake carefully. While protein is essential for maintaining muscle mass and overall health, excessive protein can increase the workload on the kidneys.

High-Quality Protein Sources: Patients are encouraged to consume high-quality protein sources, such as lean meats, fish, and eggs, while moderating the intake of red and processed meats. These sources provide essential amino acids without excessive amounts of waste products that the kidneys must filter.

Sodium Reduction

Limit Sodium Intake: The KDIGO guidelines emphasize the importance of reducing sodium intake to help manage blood pressure and prevent fluid retention. High sodium levels can lead to hypertension, which is detrimental to kidney health.

Recommended Sodium Levels: A sodium intake of less than 2,300 mg per day is recommended for individuals with CKD. Those with hypertension or fluid retention may benefit from a more stringent limit of 1,500 mg per day.

Potassium and Phosphorus Management

Monitor Potassium: Patients with CKD may experience difficulties excreting potassium, leading to hyperkalemia (high potassium levels), which can cause serious heart problems. KDIGO advises monitoring potassium intake, particularly for patients with advanced CKD or those receiving certain medications.

Phosphorus Control: Elevated phosphorus levels can lead to bone disease and cardiovascular issues in CKD patients. KDIGO recommends limiting phosphorus intake through diet, particularly from high-phosphorus foods such as dairy products, nuts, seeds, and certain whole grains. Patients are encouraged to choose low-phosphorus alternatives and consider phosphate binders if necessary, as they can help manage phosphorus levels effectively.

Fluid Intake

Individualized Fluid Management: For individuals with CKD, fluid intake may need to be monitored and adjusted based on kidney function and the presence of fluid retention or edema. KDIGO guidelines suggest that patients work with healthcare providers to determine their specific fluid needs, particularly in later stages of CKD.

Avoiding Excessive Fluids: Managing fluid intake is crucial to prevent complications such as hypertension and heart failure. Patients should be educated on the importance of balancing fluid intake with their overall dietary plan.

Balanced Nutrient Intake

Focus on Nutrient-Dense Foods: The KDIGO guidelines emphasize the importance of a balanced diet rich in fruits and vegetables that are low in potassium, healthy fats, and whole grains (within limits). These foods can provide essential vitamins and minerals while supporting overall health.

Micronutrient Supplementation: In some cases, patients may require supplementation of specific vitamins and minerals, especially if their dietary intake is restricted. KDIGO suggests monitoring micronutrient levels and providing supplementation if deficiencies are identified.

Overall Dietary Patterns

Mediterranean-Inspired Diet: Although not specifically stated in KDIGO guidelines, a Mediterranean-style diet can be beneficial for kidney health. This dietary pattern emphasizes whole, minimally processed foods, including fruits, vegetables, whole grains, healthy fats (like olive oil), and lean proteins. This approach aligns well with the goals of managing kidney health, as it promotes anti-inflammatory properties and supports cardiovascular health, which is particularly important for CKD patients.

Behavioral and Lifestyle Considerations

Education and Support: Patient education is crucial in dietary management. Understanding the impact of diet on kidney health empowers patients to make informed choices. Support groups and community resources can provide additional encouragement and accountability.

Mindful Eating: Encouraging mindful eating practices can help individuals better connect with their food choices and recognize hunger and fullness cues. This can lead to healthier eating habits and improved dietary adherence.

In summary, diet plays an essential role in the management of chronic kidney disease, and the KDIGO guidelines provide a framework for making informed dietary choices. By focusing on protein moderation, sodium reduction, potassium and phosphorus management, fluid balance, and nutrient-dense foods, individuals can significantly improve their health outcomes and quality of life.

Chapter 2: The Basics of a Low-Sodium Diet

What is a Low-Sodium Diet?

A low-sodium diet is a dietary approach that restricts the intake of sodium, typically to less than 2,300 mg per day, with further reductions to 1,500 mg per day recommended for individuals with chronic kidney disease (CKD), hypertension, or those at risk for cardiovascular diseases. Sodium is an essential mineral that plays a critical role in fluid balance, nerve function, and muscle contraction. However, excessive sodium intake can lead to increased blood pressure, fluid retention, and a higher risk of heart disease and stroke.

For individuals with CKD, managing sodium intake is crucial because the kidneys' ability to excrete excess sodium diminishes as kidney function declines. This can lead to complications such as hypertension and worsening kidney function.

How to Read Food Labels for Sodium Content

Understanding how to read food labels is essential for successfully managing a low-sodium diet. Here's how to navigate food labels to monitor sodium intake effectively:

Check the Serving Size: Always look at the serving size at the top of the nutrition label. Sodium content is often listed per serving, so be aware of how much you are actually consuming based on your portion size.

Look at the Sodium Amount: Find the sodium content in milligrams (mg) listed on the label. Foods are generally categorized as follows:

Low Sodium: 140 mg or less per serving

Very Low Sodium: 35 mg or less per serving

Sodium-Free: Less than 5 mg per serving

Consider Daily Values: The % Daily Value (%DV) indicates how much a nutrient in a serving contributes to a daily diet based on a 2,000-calorie diet. For sodium, 5% DV or less is considered low, while 20% DV or more is considered high. This can help you gauge whether a food product fits into your low-sodium diet.

Ingredient List: Examine the ingredient list for hidden sources of sodium. Ingredients such as sodium bicarbonate, sodium nitrite, and monosodium glutamate (MSG) are common additives that can increase sodium levels. Opt for products with fewer processed ingredients to minimize sodium intake.

Choose Whole Foods: Whenever possible, focus on whole, unprocessed foods, which naturally contain lower levels of sodium. Fresh fruits, vegetables, whole grains, and lean proteins are excellent choices that can fit into a low-sodium lifestyle.

Common Sources of Sodium in the Diet

Understanding where sodium commonly appears in the diet can help you make informed choices. Here are some typical sources of sodium to watch out for:

Processed Foods: Many processed foods contain added sodium for flavor and preservation. This includes:

Canned soups and broths: Often high in sodium to enhance flavor.

Frozen meals: These can contain significant sodium levels to prolong shelf life.

Snack foods: Chips, pretzels, and crackers often have added salt.

Condiments and Sauces: Many condiments are surprisingly high in sodium, including:

Soy sauce: Contains a high amount of sodium; opt for low-sodium versions if needed.

Ketchup and barbecue sauce: Often loaded with added sugars and sodium.

Pickles and olives: Curing processes typically involve salt, increasing their sodium content.

Deli Meats and Processed Meats: Items such as bacon, ham, salami, and other deli meats are often cured with salt and can be very high in sodium. Even "low-sodium" options can still contain significant amounts, so it's important to read labels carefully.

Cheese: Many types of cheese, especially processed varieties, can contain high levels of sodium. Cheese is often used in dishes for flavor, but it can contribute significantly to daily sodium intake.

Bread and Bakery Products: Bread, rolls, and baked goods can contain added sodium. Even if they don't taste salty, the sodium content can add up, especially if you consume multiple servings throughout the day.

Restaurant and Fast Food: Meals prepared outside the home are often higher in sodium than homemade meals. Many restaurants use salt liberally to enhance flavor, and portion sizes can also contribute to higher sodium intake.

Salt Substitutes: While some salt substitutes may be marketed as healthier options, they can contain potassium chloride, which some individuals need to limit based on kidney function. Always consult with a healthcare provider before using salt substitutes.

Understanding the nuances of a low-sodium diet is essential for managing kidney health and preventing complications associated with excess sodium intake. By learning to read food labels effectively and being aware of common sources of sodium, you can make informed dietary choices.

Chapter 3: Essential Foods for a Kidney-Friendly Diet

Comprehensive Low-Sodium Food List by Category

This section provides a detailed list of kidney-friendly foods that can help you maintain a balanced diet while managing sodium intake. These foods are not only low in sodium but also rich in nutrients essential for kidney health.

Fruits and Vegetables

Fruits	Vegetables
Apples	Spinach (cooked)
Berries (blueberries, strawberries, raspberries)	Kale (cooked)
Cantaloupe	Zucchini
Peaches	Broccoli (cooked)
Pears	Cauliflower (cooked)
Melons (honeydew, watermelon)	Carrots
Plums	Bell peppers (various colors)
Grapes	Asparagus

Oranges	Green beans
Kiwi	Sweet potatoes (in moderation)

Whole Grains

Quinoa
Brown rice
Oats (rolled or steel-cut)
Barley
Millet

Proteins (Meat, Dairy, Plant-Based)

Meat	Dairy	Plant-Based
Skinless chicken breast	Plain Greek yogurt	Tofu (firm or soft)
Lean cuts of beef (e.g., sirloin)	Low-fat cottage cheese	Lentils (in moderation)
Turkey	Hard cheeses (e.g., cheddar, mozzarella)	Chickpeas (in moderation)
Fish (e.g., salmon, cod, tilapia)	Almond milk (unsweetened)	Edamame (in moderation)
Shellfish (e.g., shrimp, crab)	Low-fat cream cheese	Quinoa (as a protein source)

Healthy Fats

Olive oil
Avocado oil
Coconut oil
Nuts (in moderation) (e.g., almonds, walnuts)
Seeds (in moderation) (e.g., chia seeds, flaxseeds)

Herbs and Spices for Flavoring

Herbs and Spices	
Basil	Parsley
Oregano	Garlic
Thyme	Ginger
Rosemary	Turmeric
Dill	Black pepper

Foods to Avoid and Alternatives

Understanding which foods to avoid is just as important as knowing what to include in your diet. Here's a list of high-sodium and potentially harmful foods to limit or eliminate, along with suitable alternatives.

Foods to Avoid

CATEGORY	FOODS TO AVOID	ALTERNATIVES
Processed Foods	Canned soups (high in sodium)	Homemade soups with low-sodium broth

	Frozen meals (high in sodium)	Freshly prepared meals or homemade frozen meals
Deli Meats	Salami, bologna, and other processed meats	Grilled chicken or turkey breast
	Bacon	Turkey bacon or lean ham
Condiments	Soy sauce (regular)	Low-sodium soy sauce or coconut aminos
	Ketchup and barbecue sauce	Homemade sauces with fresh ingredients
Snack Foods	Chips, pretzels, and salted nuts	Air-popped popcorn or raw vegetables with hummus
High-Sodium Cheese	Processed cheese products	Fresh cheese (like mozzarella or feta) in moderation
Fast Food	Burgers, fries, and other high-sodium options	Homemade versions using low-sodium ingredients
High-Sodium Sauces	Packaged salad dressings	Homemade vinaigrettes with olive oil and vinegar

By focusing on the right foods and avoiding high-sodium options, you can create a balanced and kidney-friendly diet that supports your health.

Chapter 4: The Low-Sodium Food List Chart

Now, we have come to the heart of this book. I take so much pride in this chapter with the help of my team of nurses and dietitians who helped with making this food list chart come together. Unlike most and many sources online in this day and age, where even charts like these can be generated through-AI, my team really put in some elbow grease and dedication to make sure that what you get is curated information. Well, a bit of a disclaimer here, I find AI really helpful in areas that will benefit from quick information, but there will be always things that meticulous research and real human "touch" are ultimately necessary.

Now, How to use the charts?

Refer to the charts to check for the macronutrient and micronutrient values according to the general standard recommendations I have mentioned or as set by your dietitian.

1. The foods are categorized: Vegetables, vegetable proteins, Fruits, Carbohydrates, Milks and Cheeses, Fats and Oils, Animal Proteins, and Herbs & Spices.

2. Each food item is given at least 1 corresponding serving size. We have standardized the serving size to 100 grams, but you will also find other alternative serving sizes to most food items in the charts.
    a. For reference:

G/g = grams	c = cup
mg = milligrams	tsp = teaspoon
svg = serving	tbsp = tablespoon
fl oz = fluid ounce	pc = piece

3. How to read/apply the chart?

   For example, you are only allowed to have around 140mg of Potassium for your snack, and you have 1 peach on hand. Looking at the chart, 1 piece medium-sized raw peach is 150grams, with 285 mg of Potassium. If you have a scale handy, you may want to weigh 75grams only of the peach you have. Or you can just simply slice the peach into half and just eat half of it.

PEACHES	SERVING QUANTITY	SERVING UNIT	CALORIES (kcal)	PROTEIN (g)	TOTAL CARBOHYDRATES (g)	SODIUM (mg)	POTASSIUM (mg)	PHOSPHORUS (mg)	TOTAL FAT (g)
raw, medium	100.00	g	39	0.9	9.5	0.00	190.0	20.00	0.25
approx.	150.00	g	59	1.4	14.3	0.00	285.0	30.00	0.38
	1.00	pc/ item							

A. Vegetables

Hey there!

Do you need to print out this Food List?

You can download a printable version of this chart by scanning the QR code below or copying the link on your computer browser.

https://go.renaltracker.com/printfoodlist

ASPARAGUS	SERVING QUANTITY	SERVING UNIT	CALORIES (kcal)	PROTEIN (g)	TOTAL CARBOHYDRATES (g)	SODIUM (mg)	POTASSIUM (mg)	PHOSPHORUS (mg)	TOTAL FAT (g)
boiled, drained	100.00	g	22	2.4	4.1	14.00	224.0	54.00	0.22
	90.00	g	20	2.2	3.7	12.60	201.6	48.60	0.20
	0.50	c							
frozen	100.00	g	24	3.2	4.1	8.00	253.0	64.00	0.23
	87.00	g	21	2.8	3.6	6.96	220.1	55.68	0.20
	6.00	pcs							
frozen, boiled, drained	100.00	g	18	3.0	1.9	3.00	172.0	49.00	0.42
	90.00	g	16	2.7	1.7	2.70	154.8	44.10	0.38
	0.50	c							
canned, drained	100.00	g	19	2.1	2.5	287.0	172.0	43.00	0.65
	121.00	g	23	2.6	3.0	347.2	208.1	52.03	0.79
	0.50	c							
BEANS									
green wax, raw	100.00	g	31	1.8	7.0	6.00	211.0	38.00	
	82.50	g	26	1.5	5.8	4.95	174.1	31.35	
	0.75	c							
green wax, frozen	100.00	g	33	1.8	7.5	3.00	186.0	32.00	
	82.67	g	27	1.5	6.2	2.48	153.7	26.45	
	0.67	c							
green wax, boiled, drained	100.00	g	35	1.9	7.9	1.00	146.0	29.00	
	125.00	g	44	2.4	9.9	1.25	182.5	36.25	
	1.00	c							
green wax, canned, drained	100.00	g	21	1.1	4.2	268.0	96.00	22.00	
	135.00	g	28	1.4	5.7	361.8	129.6	29.70	
	1.00	c							
CARROTS									
strips, slices	100.00	g	41	0.9	9.6	69.00	320.0	35.00	
	122.00	g	50	1.1	11.7	84.18	390.4	42.70	
	1.00	c							
grated	100.00	g	41	0.9	9.6	69.00	320.0	35.00	
	82.50	g	34	0.8	7.9	56.93	264.0	28.88	
	0.75	c							
sliced, boiled drained, no salt	100.00	g	35	0.8	8.2	58.00	235.0	30.00	
	78.00	g	27	0.6	6.4	45.24	183.3	23.40	
	0.50	c							
frozen	100.00	g	36	0.8	7.9	68.00	235.0	33.00	
	85.33	g	31	0.7	6.7	58.03	200.5	28.16	
	0.67	c							
baby	100.00	g	35	0.6	8.2	78.00	237.0	28.00	
	80.00	g	28	0.5	6.6	62.40	189.6	22.40	
	8.00	pcs							

TOMATO	SERVING QUANTITY	SERVING UNIT	CALORIES (kcal)	PROTEIN (g)	TOTAL CARBOHYDRATES (g)	SODIUM (mg)	POTASSIUM (mg)	PHOSPHORUS (mg)
red, whole	100.00	g	18	0.9	3.9	5.00	237	24.00
medium 2.6 in	123.00	g	22	1.1	4.8	6.15	292	29.52
diameter	1.00	pc						
diced or	100.00	g	18	0.9	3.9	5.00	237	24.00
chopped	90.00	g	16	0.8	3.5	4.50	213	21.60
	0.50	c						
yellow,	100.00	g	15	1.0	3.0	23.00	258	36.00
chopped	92.67	g	14	0.9	2.8	21.31	239	33.36
	0.67	c						
orange,	100.00	g	16	1.2	3.2	42.00	212	29.00
chopped	79.00	g	13	0.9	2.5	33.18	167	22.91
	0.50	c						
green	100.00	g	23	1.2	5.1	13.00	204	28.00
	90.00	g	21	1.1	4.6	11.70	183	25.20
	0.50	c						
whole, canned	100.00	g	16	0.8	3.5	115	191	17.00
	240.00	g	38	1.9	8.3	276	458	40.80
	1.00	c						
sauce, canned,	100.00	g	24	1.2	5.3	11.00	297	27.00
no salt	244.00	g	59	2.9	13.0	26.84	725	65.88
	1.00	c						
crushed,	100.00	g	32	1.6	7.3	186	293	32.00
canned	56.70	g	18	0.9	4.1	106	166	18.14
	2.00	oz						
paste, canned	100.00	g	82	4.3	18.9	790	1,014	83.00
	32.80	g	27	1.4	6.2	259	333	27.22
	2.00	tbsp						
puree, canned,	100.00	g	38	1.7	9.0	28.00	439	40.00
no salt	250.00	g	95	4.1	22.5	70.00	1,098	100.00
	1.00	c						
sun dried, in	100.00	g	213	5.1	23.3	266	1,565	139.00
oil, drained	27.50	g	59	1.4	6.4	73.15	430	38.23
	0.25	c						
Ketchup, low	100.00	g	101	1.0	27.4	20.00	281	26.00
sodium	15.00	g	15	0.2	4.1	3.00	42.15	3.90
	1.00	tbsp						
juice, canned	100.00	g	17	0.9	3.5	253	217	19.00
	243.00	g	41	2.1	8.6	614	527	46.17
	8.00	fl oz						
cherry, sweet,	100.00	g	63	1.1	16.0	0.00	222	21.00
raw	138.00	g	87	1.5	22.1	0.00	306	29.00
	1.00	c						

PEPPER

	SERVING QUANTITY	SERVING UNIT	CALORIES (kcal)	PROTEIN (g)	TOTAL CARBOHYDRATES (g)	SODIUM (mg)	POTASSIUM (mg)	PHOSPHORUS (mg)	TOTAL FAT (g)
bell, sweet yellow, 3 in diameter	100.00	g	27	1.0	6.3	2.00	212.0	24.00	
	186.00	g	50	1.9	11.8	3.72	394.3	44.64	
	1.00	pc							
bell, sweet green, chopped	100.00	g	20	0.9	4.6	3.00	175.0	20.00	
	74.50	g	15	0.6	3.5	2.24	130.3	14.90	
	0.50	c							
bell, sweet green, sauteed	100.00	g	116	0.8	4.2	17.00	134.0	15.00	
bell, sweet red, chopped	100.00	g	26	1.0	6.0	4.00	211.0	26.00	
	74.50	g	19	0.7	4.5	2.98	157.2	19.37	
	0.50	c							
bell, sweet red, sauteed	100.00	g	133	1.0	6.6	21.00	193.0	23.00	
bell, sweet red, chopped, frozen, drained, boiled, no salt added	100.00	g	16	1.0	3.3	4.00	72.00	13.00	
	85.05	g	14	0.8	2.8	3.40	61.24	11.06	
	3.00	oz							
jalapeno, sliced	100.00	g	29	0.9	6.5	3.00	248.0	26.00	
	22.50	g	7	0.2	1.5	0.68	55.80	5.85	
	0.13	c							
serrano, chopped	100.00	g	32	1.7	6.7	10.00	305.0	40.00	
	26.25	g	8	0.5	1.8	2.63	80.06	10.50	
	0.25	c							
black, ground	100.00	g	251	10.4	64.0	20.00	1,329	158.0	
	2.10	g	5	0.2	1.3	0.42	27.91	3.32	
	1.00	tsp							
white, ground	100.00	g	296	10.4	68.6	5.00	73.00	176.0	
	2.40	g	7	0.3	1.7	0.12	1.75	4.22	
	1.00	tsp							
Hot chilli, red	100.00	g	40	1.9	8.8	9.00	322.0	43.00	
	45.00	g	18	0.8	4.0	4.05	144.9	19.35	
	1.00	pc							

CABBAGE

	SERVING QUANTITY	SERVING UNIT	CALORIES (kcal)	PROTEIN (g)	TOTAL CARBOHYDRATES (g)	SODIUM (mg)	POTASSIUM (mg)	PHOSPHORUS (mg)	TOTAL FAT (g)
green, chopped	100.00	g	25	1.3	5.8	18.00	170.0	26.00	
	89.00	g	22	1.1	5.2	16.02	151.3	23.14	
	1.00	c							
green shredded, sliced	100.00	g	25	1.3	5.8	18.00	170.0	26.00	
	87.50	g	22	1.1	5.1	15.75	148.7	22.75	
	1.25	c							
green, shredded, boiled, drained, no salt added	100.00	g	23	1.3	5.5	8.00	196.0	33.00	
	75.00	g	17	1.0	4.1	6.00	147.0	24.75	
	0.50	c							
chinese, shredded, raw	100.00	g							
	76.00	g	12	0.9		6.84	181.0	22.04	
	1.00	c							
chinese, cooked, no salt	100.00	g							
	75.00	g	17	1.0		6.00	147.0	24.75	
	0.50	c							
red, shredded	100.00	g	31	1.4	7.4	27.00	243.0	30.00	
	87.50	g	27	1.3	6.5	23.63	212.6	26.25	
	1.25	c							
red, shredded, boiled, drained, no salt added	100.00	g	29	1.5	6.9	28.00	262.0	33.00	
	75.00	g	27	1.1	5.2	21.00	196.5	24.75	
	0.50	c							
Bok Choy or White Mustard, shredded	100.00	g	13	1.5	2.2	65.00	252.0	37.00	
	87.50	g	11	1.3	1.9	56.88	220.5	32.38	
	1.25	c							
Bok Choy/ Pak Choi, shredded, boiled, drained	100.00	g	12	1.6	1.8	34.00	371.0	29.00	
	85.00	g	10	1.3	1.5	28.90	315.3	24.65	
	0.50	c							
Kimchi	100.00	g	15	1.1	2.4	498.0	151.0	24.00	
	150.00	g	23	1.7	3.6	747.0	226.5	36.00	
	1.00	c							

	SERVING QUANTITY	SERVING UNIT	CALORIES (kcal)	PROTEIN (g)	TOTAL CARBOHYDRATES (g)	SODIUM (mg)	POTASSIUM (mg)	PHOSPHORUS (mg)	TOTAL FAT (g)
MUSHROOM									
Shitake, raw	100.00	g	34	2.2	6.8	9.00	304	112.0	
	19.00	g	6	0.4	1.3	1.71	57.76	21.28	
	1.00	pc							
Shitake, dried	100.00	g	296	9.6	75.4	13.00	1,534	294.0	
	32.40	g	96	3.1	24.4	4.21	497	95.26	
	9.00	pcs							
Shitake, cooked	100.00	g	56	1.6	14.4	4.00	117	29.00	
	72.50	g	41	1.1	10.4	2.90	84.83	21.03	
	0.50	c							
Shitake, stir fried	100.00	g	39	3.5	7.7	5.00	326	111.0	
	108.00	g	42	3.7	8.3	5.40	352	119.9	
	1.00	c							
Portabella/Portabello	100.00	g	22	2.1	3.9	9.00	364	108.0	
Portabello, grilled	100.00	g	29	3.3	4.4	11.00	437	135.0	
White, raw	100.00	g	22	3.0	3.3	5.00	318	86.00	
	96.00	g	21	3.0	3.1	4.80	305	82.56	
	1.00	c							
white, sliced, stir-fried	100.00	g	26	3.6	4.0	12.00	396	105.0	
	108.00	g	28	3.9	4.4	12.96	428	113.4	
	1.00	c							
LETTUCE									
romaine, shredded	100.00	g	17	1.2	3.3	8.00	247.0	30.00	
	70.50	g	12	0.9	2.3	5.64	174.1	21.15	
	1.50	c							
butterhead, medium leaves	100.00	g	13	1.4	2.2	5.00	238.0	33.00	
	82.50	g	11	1.1	1.8	4.13	196.3	27.23	
	11.00	pcs							
Red Leaf, shredded	100.00	g	13	1.3	2.3	25	187	28.00	
	28.00	g	4	0.4	0.6	7	52.36	7.84	
	1.00	c							
Iceberg, shredded or chopped	100.00	g	14	0.9	3.0	10	141	20.00	
	108.00	g	15	1.0	3.2	11	152.3	21.60	
	1.50	c							
Iceberg, loose leaves, medium	100.00	g	14	0.9	3.0	10	141.0	20.00	
	80.00	g	11	0.7	2.4	8	112.8	16.00	
	10.00	pcs							

CORN

	SERVING QUANTITY	SERVING UNIT	CALORIES (kcal)	PROTEIN (g)	TOTAL CARBOHYDRATES (g)	SODIUM (mg)	POTASSIUM (mg)	PHOSPHORUS (mg)	TOTAL F...
white, sweet	100.00	g	390	7.8	86.6	956.0	88.00	39.00	
	25.00	g	98	2.0	21.7	239.0	22.00	9.75	
	1.00	c							
white, steamed (Navajo)	100.00	g	386	9.7	75.2	4.00	532.0	312.0	
	85.05	g	328	8.3	64.0	3.40	452.4	265.3	
	3.00	oz							
white, stew, steamed (Navajo)	100.00	g	112	8.8	10.8	104.0	177.0	107.0	
	85.05	g	95	7.5	9.2	88.45	150.5	91.00	
	3.00	oz							
sweet, boiled, drained	100.00	g	94	3.1	22.3	4.00	251.0	75.00	0.74
	82.00	g	77	2.6	18.3	3.28	205.8	61.50	0.6'
	0.50	c							
flour, white, whole grain	100.00	g	361	6.9	76.9	5.00	315.0	272.0	3.8(
	29.25	g	106	2.0	22.5	1.46	92.14	79.56	1.1:
	0.25	c							
yellow, sweet, boiled, drained	100.00	g	96	3.4	21.0	1.00	218.0	77.00	1.5(
	82.00	g	79	2.8	17.2	0.82	178.7	63.14	1.2:
	0.50	c							
yellow, sweet, on the cob	100.00	g	86	3.3	18.7	15.00	270.0	89.00	1.3!
	154.00	g	77	2.9	16.8	13.50	243.0	80.10	1.2:
	1.00	c							
yellow, sweet, creamed, canned	100.00	g	72	1.7	18.1	261.0	134.0	51.00	0.4:
	128.00	g	92	2.2	23.2	334.0	171.5	65.28	0.5
	0.50	c							
yellow, sweet, kernels, frozen	100.00	g	88	3.0	20.7	3.00	213.0	70.00	0.7
	82.00	g	72	2.5	17.0	2.46	174.6	57.40	0.6
	0.50	c							
yellow, sweet, canned with liquid	100.00	g	61	2.0	13.9	195.0	136.0	46.00	0.7:
	128.00	g	78	2.5	17.7	249.6	174.0	58.88	0.9(
	0.50	c							
tortilla, no salt added	100.00	g	222	5.7	46.6	11.00	154.0	314.0	2.5(
	26.00	g	58	1.5	12.1	2.86	40.04	81.64	0.6!
	1.00	pc							

	SERVING QUANTITY	SERVING UNIT	CALORIES (kcal)	PROTEIN (g)	TOTAL CARBOHYDRATES (g)	SODIUM (mg)	POTASSIUM (mg)	PHOSPHORUS (mg)	TOTAL FAT (g)
BROCCOLI									
florets, raw	100.00	g	28	3.0	5.1	27.00	325.0	66.00	0.35
	71.00	g	20	2.1	3.6	19.17	230.7	46.86	0.25
	1.00	c							
Cooked, no salt	100.00	g	35	2.4	7.2	41.00	293.0	67.00	0.41
	78.00	g	27	1.9	5.6	31.98	228.5	52.26	0.32
	0.50	c							
frozen, spears	100.00	g	29	3.1	5.4	17.00	250.0	59.00	0.34
	85.05	g	25	2.6	4.6	14.46	212.6	50.18	0.29
	3.00	oz							
CAULIFLOWER									
green, raw	100.00	g	31	3.0	6.1	23.00	300.0	62.00	0.30
	64.00	g	20	1.9	3.9	14.72	192.0	39.68	0.19
	1.00	c							
cooked, no salt	100.00	g	32	3.0	6.3	23.00	278.0	57.00	0.31
	62.00	g	20	1.9	3.9	14.26	172.3	35.34	0.19
	0.50	c							
CUCUMBER									
sliced, raw	100.00	g	15	0.7	3.6	2.00	147.0	24.00	0.11
	52.00	g	8	0.3	1.9	1.04	76.44	12.48	0.06
	0.50	c							
sliced	100.00	g	15	0.7	3.6	2.00	147.0	24.00	0.11
	78.00	g	12	0.5	2.8	1.56	114.6	18.72	0.09
	0.75	c							
BEETS									
raw	100.00	g	43	1.6	9.6	78.00	325.0	40.00	0.17
	90.67	g	39	1.5	8.7	70.72	294.6	36.27	0.15
	0.67	c							
whole or sliced, boiled, drained, no salt	100.00	g	44	1.7	10.0	77.00	305.0	38.00	0.18
Whole, canned	100.00	g	30	0.7	7.1	143.00	159.0	15.00	0.09
	246.00	g	74	1.8	17.6	351.78	391.1	36.90	0.22
	1.00	c							
sliced, canned, drained	100.00	g	31	0.9	7.2	194.00	148.0	17.00	0.14
	85.00	g	26	0.8	6.1	164.90	125.8	14.45	0.12
	0.50	c							

PEAS

	SERVING QUANTITY	SERVING UNIT	CALORIES (kcal)	PROTEIN (g)	TOTAL CARBOHYDRATES (g)	SODIUM (mg)	POTASSIUM (mg)	PHOSPHORUS (mg)	TOTAL FAT (g)
green	100.00	g	81	5.4	14.5	5.00	244.0	108.0	0.40
	72.50	g	59	3.9	10.5	3.63	176.9	78.30	0.29
	0.50	c							
green, frozen	100.00	g	77	5.2	13.6	108.0	153.0	82.00	0.40
	72.00	g	55	3.8	9.8	77.76	110.1	59.04	0.29
	0.50	c							
green, boiled, drained	100.00	g	84	5.4	15.6	3.00	271.0	117.0	0.22
	80.00	g	67	4.3	12.5	2.40	216.8	93.60	0.18
	0.50	c							
green, canned, drained	100.00	g	68	4.5	11.4	273.0	106.0	67.00	0.80
	87.50	g	60	3.9	9.9	238.8	92.7	58.63	0.70
	0.50	c							
green, frozen, boiled, drained	100.00	g	78	5.2	14.3	72.00	110.0	77.00	0.27
	80.00	g	62	4.1	11.4	57.60	88.00	61.60	0.22
	0.50	c							
split, boiled, no salt added	100.00	g	118	8.3	21.1	2.00	362.0	99.00	0.39
	98.00	g	116	8.2	21.0	1.96	354.7	97.02	0.38
	0.50	c							
sugar or snow peas, whole fresh	100.00	g	42	2.8	7.6	4.00	200.0	53.00	0.20
	78.75	g	33	2.2	6.0	3.15	157.5	41.74	0.16
	1.25	c							
snow/sugar, frozen	100.00	g	42	2.8	7.6	4.00	200.0	53.00	0.20
	78.75	g	33	2.2	6.0	3.15	157.5	41.74	0.16
	1.25	c							
snow/sugar, boiled, drained	100.00	g	42	3.3	7.1	4.00	240.0	55.00	0.23
	80.00	g	34	2.6	5.6	3.20	192.0	44.00	0.18
	0.50	c							
snow/sugar, frozen, boiled, drained	100.00	g	52	3.5	9.0	5.00	217.0	58.00	0.38
	80.00	g	42	2.8	7.2	4.00	173.6	46.40	0.30
	0.50	c							

POTATOES

	SERVING QUANTITY	SERVING UNIT	CALORIES (kcal)	PROTEIN (g)	TOTAL CARBOHYDRATES (g)	SODIUM (mg)	POTASSIUM (mg)	PHOSPHORUS (mg)	TOTAL FAT (g)
russet, flesh and skin	100.00	g	79	2.1	18.1	5.00	417.0	55.00	0.08
russet, flesh and skin, baked	100.00	g	95	2.6	21.4	14.00	550.0	71.00	0.13
	173.00 1.00	g pc	164	4.6	37.1	24.22	951.5	122.8	0.22
white, flesh and skin	100.00	g	69	1.7	15.7	16.00	407.0	62.00	0.10
white, flesh and skin, baked	100.00	g	92	2.1	21.1	7.00	544.0	75.00	0.15
	173.00 1.00	g pcs	159	3.6	36.5	12.11	941.1	129.7	0.26
French fries, frozen	100.00	g	147	2.2	24.8	332.0	408.0	83.00	4.66
	71.50 11.00	g pcs	105	1.6	17.7	237.3	291.7	59.35	3.33
sweet, cubed	100.00	g	86	1.6	20.1	55.00	337.0	47.00	0.05
	99.75 0.75	g c	86	1.6	20.1	54.86	336.1	46.88	0.05
sweet, boiled, mashed	100.00	g	76	1.4	17.7	27.00	230.0	32.00	0.14
	328.00 1.00	g c	249	4.5	58.1	88.56	754.4	105	0.46
sweet, frozen, baked	100.00	g	100	1.7	23.4	8.00	377.0	44.00	0.12
	117.33 0.67	g c	117	2.0	27.5	9.39	442.3	51.63	0.14
sweet, baked, peeled	100.00	g	90	2.0	20.7	36.00	475.0	54.00	0.15
	0.50	c							
chips, unsalted	100.00	g	536	7.0	52.9	8.00	1,275	165.0	34.60
	28.35 1.00	g oz	152	2.0	15.0	2.27	361.4	46.78	9.81
hash browns, frozen	100.00	g	82	2.1	17.7	22.00	285.0	47.00	0.62
	70.00 0.33	g c	57	1.4	12.4	15.40	199.5	32.90	0.43
wedges, frozen	100.00	g	129	2.7	25.5	49.00	394.0	87.00	2.20

ARTI-CHOKES	SERVING QUANTITY	SERVING UNIT	CALORIES (kcal)	PROTEIN (g)	TOTAL CARBOHYDRATES (g)	SODIUM (mg)	POTASSIUM (mg)	PHOSPHORUS (mg)	TOTAL F
whole, boiled, drained	100.00	g	53	2.9	12.0	60.00	286	73.00	0.3
med size	120.00	g	64	3.5	14.3	72.00	343	87.60	0.4
	1.00	pc							
hearts, boiled, drained	100.00	g	53	2.9	11.9	60.00	286	73.00	0.3
	84.00	g	45	2.4	10.0	50.40	240	61.32	0.2
	0.50	c							
Globe or French, frozen	100.00	g	45	3.1	9.2	53.00	264	61.00	0.5
boiled, drained	80.00	g	36	2.5	7.3	42.40	211	48.80	0.4
1 svg = 1/3 of 9oz package	1.00	svg							

ALFALFA

sprouts	100.00	g	23	4.0	2.1	6.00	79.00	70.00	0.6
	33.00	g	8	1.3	0.7	1.98	26.07	23.10	0.2
	1.00	c							

CELERY

stalk	100.00	g	14	0.7	3.0	80.00	260	24.00	0.1
medium 7.5 - 8 in long	80.00	g	11	0.6	2.4	64.00	208	19.20	0.1
	2.00	stalks							
diced, chopped	100.00	g	14	0.7	3.0	80.00	260	24.00	0.1
	101.00	g	14	0.7	3.0	80.80	263	24.24	0.1
	1.00	c							
celeriac or celery root	100.00	g	42	1.5	9.2	100.0	300	115	0.3
	78.00	g	33	1.2	7.2	78.00	234	90	0.2
	0.50	c							
seeds	100.00	g	392	18.1	41.4	160.0	1,400	547	25.2
	2.00	g	8	0.4	0.8	3.20	28.00	10.94	0.5
	1.00	tsp							
flakes, dried	100.00	g	319	11.3	68.7	1,435	4,388	402	2.1
	28.35	g	90	3.2	18.1	406.8	1,244	114	0.6
	1.00	oz							

	SERVING QUANTITY	SERVING UNIT	CALORIES (kcal)	PROTEIN (g)	TOTAL CARBOHYDRATES (g)	SODIUM (mg)	POTASSIUM (mg)	PHOSPHORUS (mg)	TOTAL FAT (g)
COLLARDS									
chopped, raw	100.00	g	32	3.0	5.4	17.00	213.0	25.00	0.61
	90.00	g	29	2.7	4.9	15.30	191.7	22.50	0.55
	2.50	c							
boiled, drained	100.00	g	33	2.7	5.7	15.00	117.0	32.00	0.72
	95.00	g	31	2.6	5.4	14.25	111.1	30.40	0.68
	0.50	c							
frozen, chopped, raw	100.00	g	33	2.7	6.5	48.00	253.0	27.00	0.37
	85.05	g	28	2.3	5.5	40.82	215.1	22.96	0.31
	3.00	oz							
frozen, chopped, boiled/ drained	100.00	g	36	3.0	7.1	50.00	251.0	27.00	0.41
	85.00	g	31	2.5	6.0	42.50	213.3	22.95	0.35
	0.50	c							
EGGPLANT/AUBERGINE									
boiled, drained, no salt	100.00	g	35	0.8	8.7	1.00	123.0	15.00	0.23
	99.00	g	35	0.8	8.6	0.99	121.7	14.85	0.23
cut in 1" cubes	1.00	c							
pickled	100.00	g	49	0.9	9.8	1,674	12.00	9.00	0.70
	136	g	67	1.2	13.3	2,276	16.32	12.24	0.95
	1.00	c							
JICAMA (YAMBEAN)									
raw	100.00	g	38	0.7	8.8	4.00	150.0	18.00	0.09
	86.67	g	33	0.6	7.6	3.47	130.0	15.60	0.08
	0.67	c							
boiled, drained, no salt	100.00	g	38	0.7	8.8	4.00	135.0	16.00	0.09
	85.05	g	32	0.6	7.5	3.40	114.8	13.61	0.08
1 svg = 3oz	3.00	oz							

	SERVING QUANTITY	SERVING UNIT	CALORIES (kcal)	PROTEIN (g)	CARBOHYDRATES (g)	SODIUM (mg)	POTASSIUM (mg)	PHOSPHORUS (mg)	TOTAL FAT (g)
ARUGULA									
raw, leaves	100	g	25	2.6	3.7	27.00	369	52.00	0.66
	80.00	g	20	2.1	2.9	21.60	295	41.60	0.53
	4.00	c							
salad mixed	100	g	18	1.5	3.3	16.94	299	32.15	0.27
baby greens	41.25	g	7	0.6	1.4	6.99	123	13.26	0.11
Arugula, butterhead, endives, Radicchio	1.00	c							
ENDIVE OR ESCAROLE									
raw, chopped	100	g	17	1.3	3.4	22.00	314.0	28.00	0.20
	87.50	g	15	1.1	2.9	19.25	274.7	24.50	0.18
	1.75	c							
Chicory, Witlof	100	g	17	0.9	4.0	2.00	211.0	26.00	0.10
or Belgium	90.00	g	15	0.8	3.6	1.80	189.9	23.40	0.09
	1.00	c							
OKRA									
raw	100	g	33	1.9	7.5	7.00	299.0	61.00	0.19
	75.00	g	25	1.5	5.6	5.25	224.2	45.75	0.14
	0.75	c							
sliced, boiled,	100	g	22	1.9	4.5	6.00	135.0	32.00	0.21
drained, n.s.	80.00	g	18	1.5	3.6	4.80	108.0	25.60	0.17
	0.50	c							
frozen	100	g	30	1.7	6.6	3.00	211.0	42.00	0.25
	85.05	g	26	1.4	5.6	2.55	179.4	35.72	0.21
	3.00	oz							
frozen, boiled,	100	g	29	1.6	6.4	3.00	184.0	37.00	0.24
drained, no salt	92.00	g	27	1.5	5.9	2.76	169.2	34.04	0.22
sliced	0.50	c							
PUMPKIN									
fruit/meat, raw,	100	g	26	1.0	6.5	1.00	340.0	44.00	0.10
cut 1" cube	116	g	30	1.2	7.5	1.16	394.4	51.04	0.12
	1.00	c							
boiled, drained,	100	g	20	0.7	4.9	1.00	230.0	30.00	0.07
mashed, n.s.	122.5	g	25	0.9	6.0	1.23	281.7	36.75	0.09
	0.50	c							
flowers	100	g	15	0.0	3.3	5.00	173.0	49.00	0.07
	33.00	g	1	0.0	0.1	0.20	6.92	1.96	0.00
	1.00	c							
flowers, boiled,	100	g	15	1.1	3.3	6.00	106.0	34.00	0.08
drained	89.33	g	13	1.0	3.0	5.36	5.36	30.37	0.07
	0.67	c							
seeds (squash	100	g	559	30.2	10.7	7.00	809.0	1,233	49.05
kernels), dried	34.50	g	193	10.4	3.7	2.42	279.1	425.4	16.92
	0.25	c							
seeds	100	g	446	18.6	53.8	18.00	919.0	92.00	19.40
(pumpkin/squash),	32.00	g	143	5.9	17.2	5.76	294.0	29.44	6.21
whole, roasted no salt added	0.50	c							

	SERVING QUANTITY	SERVING UNIT	CALORIES (kcal)	PROTEIN (g)	TOTAL CARBOHYDRATES (g)	SODIUM (mg)	POTASSIUM (mg)	PHOSPHORUS (mg)	TOTAL FAT (g)
SQUASH									
winter, all varieties cubes	100.00	g	34	1.0	8.6	4.00	350.0	23.00	0.13
	116.00	g	39	1.1	10.0	4.64	406.0	26.68	0.15
	1.00	c							
butternut cubes	100.00	g	45	1.0	11.7	4.00	352.0	33.00	0.10
	140.00	g	63	1.4	16.4	5.60	492.8	46.20	0.14
	1.00	c							
winter, butternut, frozen	100.00	g	57	1.8	14.4	2.00	212.0	22.00	0.10
	85.05	g	48	1.5	12.3	1.70	180.3	18.71	0.09
	3.00	oz							
summer, all varieties sliced	100.00	g	16	1.2	3.4	2.00	262.0	38.00	0.18
	84.75	g	14	1.0	2.8	1.70	222.0	32.21	0.15
	0.75	c							
KOHLRABI									
raw	100.00	g	27	1.7	6.2	20.00	350.0	46.00	0.10
	135.00	g	36	2.3	8.4	27.00	472.5	62.10	0.14
	1.00	c							
boiled, drained, sliced	100.00	g	29	1.8	6.7	21.00	340.0	45.00	0.11
	165.00	g	48	3.0	11.0	34.65	561.0	74.25	0.18
	1.00	c							
LEEKS									
raw	100.00	g	61	1.5	14.2	20.00	180.0	35.00	0.30
	89.00	g	54	1.3	12.6	17.80	160.2	31.15	0.27
	1.00	c							
boiled, drained, chopped or diced	100.00	g	31	0.8	7.6	10.00	87.00	17.00	0.20
	26.00	g	8	0.2	2.0	2.60	22.62	4.42	0.05
	0.25	c							
CASSAVA/YUCCA/MANIOC									
raw	100.00	g	160	1.4	38.1	14.00	271.0	27.00	0.28
	103.00	g	165	1.4	39.2	14.42	279.1	27.81	0.29
	0.50	c							
RADISH									
oriental (Daikon), 7" long	100.00	g	18	0.6	4.1	21.00	227.0	23.00	0.10
	338.00	g	61	2.0	13.9	70.98	767.2	77.74	0.34
	1.00	pc							
oriental, boiled, drained, no salt sliced	100.00	g	17	0.7	3.4	13.00	285.0	24.00	0.24
	73.50	g	13	0.5	2.5	9.56	209.5	17.64	0.18
	0.50	c							
sprouts	100.00	g	43	3.8	3.6	6.00	86.00	113.0	2.53
	38.00	g	16	1.5	1.4	2.28	32.68	42.94	0.96
	1.00	c							

	SERVING QUANTITY	SERVING UNIT	CALORIES (kcal)	PROTEIN (g)	TOTAL CARBOHYDRATES (g)	SODIUM (mg)	POTASSIUM (mg)	PHOSPHORUS (mg)	TOTAL FAT (g)
SWISS CHARD									
raw	100.00	g	19	1.8	3.7	213.0	379.0	46.00	0.20
	36.00	g	7	0.7	1.4	76.68	136.4	16.56	0.07
	1.00	c							
boiled, drained, no salt	100.00	g	20	1.9	4.1	179.0	549.0	33.00	0.08
	175.00	g	35	3.3	7.2	313.2	960.7	57.75	0.14
	1.00	c							
SPINACH									
raw, chopped	100.00	g	23	2.9	3.6	79.00	558.0	49.00	0.39
	90.00	g	21	2.6	3.3	71.10	502.2	44.10	0.35
	3.00	c							
frozen	100.00	g	29	3.6	4.2	74.00	346.0	49.00	0.57
	78.00	g	23	2.8	3.3	57.72	269.8	38.22	0.44
	0.50	c							
chopped, boiled, drained, no salt	100.00	g	23	3.0	3.8	70.00	466.0	56.00	0.26
	90.00	g	21	2.7	3.4	63.00	419.4	50.40	0.23
	0.50	c							
mustard (Tendergreens)	100.00	g	22	2.2	3.9	21.00	449.0	28.00	0.30
	150.00	g	33	3.3	5.9	31.50	673.5	42.00	0.45
	1.00	c							
mustard, boiled, drained, no salt	100.00	g	16	1.7	2.8	14.00	285.0	18.00	0.20
	180.00	g	29	3.1	5.0	25.20	513.0	32.40	0.36
	1.00	c							
TOMATILLOS									
chopped	100.00	g	32	1.0	5.8	1.00	268.0	39.00	1.02
	132.00	g	42	1.3	7.7	1.32	353.7	51.48	1.35
	1.00	c							
TURNIPS									
raw	100.00	g	28	0.9	6.4	67.00	191.0	27.00	0.10
	130.00	g	34	1.1	7.8	81.74	233.0	32.94	0.12
	1.00	c							
frozen	100.00	g	16	1.0	2.9	25.00	137.0	20.00	0.16
	85.05	g	14	0.9	2.5	21.26	116.5	17.01	0.14
	3.00	oz							
cubed, boiled, drained, no salt	100.00	g	22	0.7	5.1	16.00	177.0	40.56	0.08
	156.00	g	34	1.1	7.9	24.96	276.1	26.00	0.12
	1.00	c							
frozen, boiled, drained, no salt	100.00	g	23	1.5	4.4	36.00	182.0	26.00	0.24
	78.00	g	18	1.2	3.4	28.08	142	20.28	0.19
	0.50	c							

TURNIP GREENS	SERVING QUANTITY	SERVING UNIT	CALORIES (kcal)	PROTEIN (g)	TOTAL CARBOHYDRATES (g)	SODIUM (mg)	POTASSIUM (mg)	PHOSPHORUS (mg)	TOTAL FAT (g)
raw, turnip greens, chopped	100.00	g	32	1.5	7.1	40.00	296.0	42.00	0.30
	82.50	g	26	1.2	5.9	33.00	244.2	34.65	0.25
	1.50	c							
frozen	100.00	g	22	2.5	3.7	12.00	184.0	27.00	0.31
	82.00	g	18	2.0	3.0	9.84	150.8	22.14	0.25
	0.50	c							
canned	100.00	g	14	1.4	2.4	277.0	141.0	21.00	0.30
	78.00	g	11	1.1	1.9	216.0	110.0	16.38	0.23
	0.33	c							
chopped, boiled, drained, no salt	100.00	g	20	1.1	4.4	29.00	203.0	29.00	0.23
	144.00	g	29	1.6	6.3	41.76	292.3	41.76	0.33
	1.00	c							
canned, with no salt	100.00	g	19	1.4	2.8	29.00	141.0	21.00	0.30
	144.00	g	27	2.0	4.1	41.76	203.0	30.24	0.43
	1.00	c							
frozen, chopped, boiled, drained, no salt added	100.00	g	29	3.4	5.0	15.00	224.0	34.00	0.42
	164.00	g	48	5.5	8.2	24.60	367.3	55.76	0.69
	1.00	c							
RUTABAGA									
raw, cubes	100.00	g	37	1.1	8.6	12.00	305.0	53.00	0.16
	93.33	g	35	1.0	8.1	11.20	284.6	49.47	0.15
	0.67	c							
boiled, drained, no salt cubed	100.00	g	30	0.9	6.8	5.00	216.0	41.00	0.18
	170.00	g	51	1.6	11.6	8.50	367.2	69.70	0.31
	1.00	c							
boiled, drained, mashed	100.00	g	30	0.9	6.8	5.00	216.0	41.00	0.18
	160.80	g	48	1.5	11.0	8.04	347.3	65.93	0.29
	0.67	c							
PARSNIPS									
raw, sliced	100.00	g	75	1.2	18.0	10.00	375.0	71.00	0.30
	88.67	g	67	1.1	16.0	8.87	332.5	62.95	0.27
	0.67	c							
boiled, drained, sliced, no salt	100.00	g	71	1.3	17.0	10.00	367.0	69.00	0.30
	78.00	g	55	1.0	13.3	7.80	286.2	53.82	0.23
	0.50	c							

	SERVING QUANTITY	SERVING UNIT	CALORIES (kcal)	PROTEIN (g)	TOTAL CARBOHYDRATES (g)	SODIUM (mg)	POTASSIUM (mg)	PHOSPHORUS (mg)	TOTAL F.
WATER CHESTNUTS									
fresh, raw, Chinese (Matai) slices	100.00	g	97	1.4	23.9	14.00	584.0	63.00	0.1
	62.00	g	60	0.9	14.8	8.68	362.0	39.06	0.0
	0.50	c							
canned with liquid Chinese (Matai)	100.00	g	50	0.9	12.3	8.00	118.0	19.00	0.0
	70.00	g	35	0.6	8.6	5.60	82.60	13.30	0.0
	0.50	c							
WATERCRESS									
raw, chopped	100.00	g	11	2.3	1.3	41.00	330.0	60.00	0.1
	34.00	g	4	0.8	0.4	13.94	112.2	20.40	0.0
	1.00	c							
YAM									
raw, in cubes	100.00	g	118	1.5	28.0	9.00	816.0	55.00	0.1
	112.50	g	133	1.7	31.4	10.13	918.0	61.88	0.1
	0.75	c							
baked or broiled, drained, no salt cubed	100.00	g	116	1.5	27.5	8.00	670.0	49.00	0.1
	68.00	g	79	1.0	18.7	5.44	455.6	33.32	0.1
	0.50	c							
Hawaiian Mountain, raw cubed	100.00	g	67	1.3	16.3	13.00	418.0	34.00	0.1
	68.00	g	46	0.9	11.1	8.84	284.2	23.12	0.0
	0.50	c							
Hawaiian Mountain, steamed cubed	100.00	g	82	1.7	20.0	12.00	495.0	40.00	0.0
	145.00	g	119	2.5	29.0	17.40	717.7	58.00	0.1
	1.00	c							
MIXED VEGETABLES									
frozen	100.00	g	72	3.3	13.5	47.00	212.0	59.00	0.5
	72.00	g	52	2.4	9.7	33.84	152.6	42.48	0.3
	0.50	c							
frozen, boiled, drained, no salt added	100.00	g	65	2.9	13.1	35.00	169.0	51.00	0.1
	91.00	g	59	2.6	11.9	31.85	153.8	46.41	0.1
	0.50	c							
canned, drained	100.00	g	49	2.6	9.3	214.0	291.0	42.00	0.2
	163.00	g	80	4.2	15.1	348.8	474.3	68.46	0.4
	1.00	c							
BRUSSEL SPROUTS									
raw	100.00	g	43	33.4	9.0	25.00	389.0	69.00	0.3(
	88.00	g	38	3.0	7.9	22.00	342.0	60.70	0.2(
	1.00	c							

	SERVING QUANTITY	SERVING UNIT	CALORIES (kcal)	PROTEIN (g)	TOTAL CARBOHYDRATES (g)	SODIUM (mg)	POTASSIUM (mg)	PHOSPHORUS (mg)	TOTAL FAT (g)
KALE									
raw, chopped	100.00	g	35	2.9	4.4	53.00	348.0	55.00	1.49
	83.75	g	29	2.5	3.7	44.39	291.4	46.06	1.25
	1.25	c							
chopped, boiled, drained, no salt	100.00	g	36	2.9	5.3	16.00	144.0	42.00	1.21
	65.00	g	23	1.9	3.5	10.40	93.60	27.30	0.79
	0.50	c							
scotch, raw, chopped	100.00	g	42	2.8	8.3	70.00	450.0	62.00	0.60
	83.75	g	35	2.4	7.0	58.63	376.8	51.93	0.50
	1.25	c							
scotch, boiled, drained, chopped no salt	100.00	g	28	1.9	5.6	45.00	274.0	38.00	0.41
	86.67	g	24	1.7	4.9	39.00	237.4	32.93	0.36
	0.67	c							
frozen, raw 1 pack=10 oz/ 284g	100.00	g	28	2.7	4.9	15.00	333.0	29.00	0.46
	85.05	g	24	2.3	4.2	12.76	283.2	24.66	0.39
	3.00	oz							
frozen, chopped, boiled, drained, no salt	100.00	g	36	2.9	5.3	16.00	144.0	42.00	1.21
	65.00	g	23	1.9	3.5	10.40	93.60	27.30	0.79
	0.50	c							
MUSTARD GREENS									
raw, chopped	100.00	g	27	2.9	4.7	20.00	384.0	58.00	0.42
	84.00	g	23	2.4	3.9	16.80	322.5	48.72	0.35
	1.50	c							
boiled, drained, chopped, no salt	100.00	g	26	2.6	4.5	9.00	162.0	42.00	0.47
	70.00	g	18	1.8	3.2	6.30	113.4	29.40	0.33
	0.50	c							
frozen 1 pack=10oz/284g	100.00	g	20	2.5	3.4	29.00	170.0	30.00	0.27
	73.00	g	15	1.8	2.5	21.17	124.1	21.90	0.20
	0.50	c							
frozen, boiled, drained, no salt 1 pack = 10oz/ 212g	100.00	g	19	2.3	3.1	25.00	139.0	24.00	0.25
	75.00	g	14	1.7	2.3	18.75	104.2	18.00	0.19
	0.50	c							

B. Vegetable Proteins

Hey there!

Do you need to print out this Food List?

You can download a printable version of this chart by scanning the QR code below or copying the link on your computer browser.

https://go.renaltracker.com/printfoodlist

BEANS

	SERVING QUANTITY	SERVING UNIT	CALORIES (kcal)	PROTEIN (g)	TOTAL CARBOHYDRATES (g)	SODIUM (mg)	POTASSIUM (mg)	PHOSPHORUS (mg)	TOTAL FAT (g)
Lentils/Pinto/	100.00	g	131	8.6	23.9	1.67	398.9	165.7	0.49
Navy	92.00	g	121	8.0	22.0	1.54	367.0	152.5	0.45
	0.50	c							
Lima	100.00	g	113	6.8	20.2	8.00	467.0	136.0	0.86
	78.00	g	88	5.3	15.7	6.24	364.2	106.0	0.67
	0.50	c							
Broad or Fava	100.00	g	72	5.6	11.7	50.00	250.0	95.00	0.60
	81.75	g	59	4.6	9.6	40.88	204.3	77.60	0.49
	0.75	c							
Black beans,	100.00	g	132	8.9	23.7	1.00	355.0	140.0	0.54
boiled	86.00	g	114	7.6	20.4	0.86	305.3	120.4	0.46
	0.50	c							
Mungo,	100.00	g	105	7.5	18.3	7.00	231.0	156.0	0.55
boiled	90.00	g	95	6.8	16.5	6.30	207.9	140.4	0.50
	0.50	c							
sprouts, Mung	100.00	g	30	3.0	5.9	6.00	149.0	54.00	0.18
	78.00	g	23	2.4	4.6	4.68	116.2	42.12	0.14
	0.75	c							
Kidney, boiled	100.00	g	127	8.7	22.8	1.00	405.0	138.0	0.50
	88.50	g	112	7.7	20.2	0.89	358.4	122.1	0.44
	0.50	c							
Navy, boiled	100.00	g	140	8.2	26.1	0.00	389.0	144.0	0.62
	91.00	g	127	7.5	23.7	0.00	354.0	131.0	0.56
	0.50	c							
Lupin, boiled	100.00	g	119	15	9.9	4.00	245.0	128.0	2.92
	83.00	g	99	12	8.2	3.32	203.3	106.2	2.42
	0.50	c							
Pinto, frozen	100.00	g	170	9.8	32.5	92.00	755.9	117.0	0.50
	94.49	g	161	9.3	31.0	86.93	714.3	110.5	0.47
	3.33	Oz							
Pinto, boiled	100.00	g	143	9.0	26.2	1.00	436.0	147.0	0.65
	85.50	g	122	7.7	22.4	0.86	372.8	125.7	0.56
	0.50	c							
White	100.00	g	139	9.7	25.1	6.00	561.0	113.0	0.35
(Cannellini), boiled no salt	89.50	g	124	8.7	22.5	5.37	502.1	101.1	0.31
	0.50	c							

BEANS

	SERVING QUANTITY	SERVING UNIT	CALORIES (kcal)	PROTEIN (g)	TOTAL CARBOHYDRATES (g)	SODIUM (mg)	POTASSIUM (mg)	PHOSPHORUS (mg)	TOTAL FAT (g)
White, small, boiled, no salt	100.00	g	142	9.0	25.8	2.00	463.0	169.0	0.64
	89.50	g	127	8.0	23.1	1.79	414.4	151.2	0.57
	0.50	c							
sprouts,	100.00	g	29	4.2	4.1	6.00	187.0	37.00	0.50
Kidney	92.00	g	27	3.9	3.8	5.52	172.0	34.04	0.46
	0.50	c							
Sprouts, Navy	100.00	g	67	6.2	13.1	13.00	307.0	100.0	0.70
	78.00	g	52	4.8	10.2	10.14	239.4	78.00	0.55
	0.75	c							
sprouts, Pinto	100.00	g	62	5.3	11.6	153.0	307.0	94.00	0.90
	85.05	g	53	4.5	9.9	130.1	262.1	79.95	0.77
	3.00	oz							
French, boiled	100.00	g	129	7.1	24.0	6.00	370.0	102.0	0.76
	88.50	g	114	6.2	21.3	5.31	327.4	90.27	0.67
	0.50	c							
baked, prepared	100.00	g	155	5.5	21.6	422.0	358.0	109.0	5.15
	126.50	g	196	7.0	27.4	533.8	452.8	138.0	6.51
	0.50	c							
Refried, canned	100.00	g	90	5.0	13.6	370.0	319.0	92.00	2.01
	119.00	g	107	5.9	16.1	440.3	379.6	109.4	2.39
	0.50	c							

CHICKPEAS

	SERVING QUANTITY	SERVING UNIT	CALORIES	PROTEIN	TOTAL CARBOHYDRATES	SODIUM	POTASSIUM	PHOSPHORUS	TOTAL FAT
garbanzos/ Bengal gram, canned	100.00	g	88	4.9	13.5	278.0	144.0	80.00	1.95
	120.00	g	106	5.9	16.2	333.6	172.8	96.00	2.34
	0.50	c							
garbanzos/ Bengal gram, boiled	100.00	g	164	8.9	27.4	7.00	291.0	168.0	2.59
	82.00	g	134	7.3	22.5	5.74	238.6	137.7	2.12
	0.50	c							
garbanzos/ Bengal gram, canned drained, rinsed in tap water	100.00	g	138	7.0	22.9	212.0	109.0	80.00	2.47
	152.00	g	210	10.7	34.8	322.3	165.6	121.6	3.75
	1.00	c							
garbanzos/ Bengal gram, canned low sodium	100	g	88	4.9	13.5	132.0	144.0	80.00	1.95
	240	g	211	11.8	32.4	316.8	345.6	192.0	4.68
	1	c							
flour	100.00	g	387	22.4	57.8	64.00	846.0	318.0	6.69
	92.00	g	110	6.4	16.4	18.14	239.8	90.15	1.90
	1.00	c							

TOFU

	Serving Quantity	Serving Unit	Calories (kcal)	Protein (g)	Total Carbohydrates (g)	Sodium (mg)	Potassium (mg)	Phosphorus (mg)	Total Fat (g)
soft with calcium sulfate and magnesium chloride (Nigari)	100.00	g	61	7.2	1.2	8.00	120.0	92.00	3.69
	85.05	g	52	6.1	1.0	6.80	102.0	78.25	3.14
	3.00	oz							
firm with calcium sulfate and magnesium chloride (Nigari)	100.00	g	78	9.0	2.9	12.00	148.0	121.0	4.17
	85.05	g	66	7.7	2.4	10.21	125.8	102.9	3.55
	3.00	oz							
silken tofu (Vitasoy USA)	100.00	g	43	4.8	0.6	2.00	Na	na	2.40
	91.00	g	39	4.4	0.5	1.82	Na	na	2.18
	0.20	Package							

TEMPEH

	Serving Quantity	Serving Unit	Calories (kcal)	Protein (g)	Total Carbohydrates (g)	Sodium (mg)	Potassium (mg)	Phosphorus (mg)	Total Fat (g)
raw	100.00	g	192	20.3	7.6	9.00	412.0	266.0	10.80
	83.00	g	159	16.8	6.3	7.47	341.9	220.8	8.96
	0.50	c							
cooked	100.00	g	185	19.8	7.6	14.00	401.0	253.0	11.38

EDAMAME

	Serving Quantity	Serving Unit	Calories (kcal)	Protein (g)	Total Carbohydrates (g)	Sodium (mg)	Potassium (mg)	Phosphorus (mg)	Total Fat (g)
frozen, unprepared	100.00	g	109	11.2	7.6	6.00	482.0	161.0	4.73
	118.00	g	129	13.2	9.0	7.08	568.7	189.9	5.58
	1.00	c							
frozen, prepared	100.00	g	121	11.9	8.9	6.00	436.0	261.9	5.20
	155.00	g	188	18.5	13.8	9.30	676	169	8.06
	1.00	c							

SPIRULINA

	Serving Quantity	Serving Unit	Calories (kcal)	Protein (g)	Total Carbohydrates (g)	Sodium (mg)	Potassium (mg)	Phosphorus (mg)	Total Fat (g)
seaweed, fresh/raw	100.00	g	26	5.9	2.4	98.00	127	11.00	0.39
	28.35	g	7	1.7	0.7	27.78	36.00	3.12	0.11
	1.00	Oz							
seaweed, dried	100.00	g	290	57.5	23.9	1,048	1363	118	7.72
	112.00	g	325	64.4	26.8	1,174	1527	133	8.65
	1.00	c							

C. Fruits

Hey there!

Do you need to print out this Food List?

You can download a printable version of this chart by scanning the QR code below or copying the link on your computer browser.

https://go.renaltracker.com/printfoodlist

	SERVING QUANTITY	SERVING UNIT	CALORIES (kcal)	PROTEIN (g)	TOTAL CARBOHYDRATES (g)	SODIUM (mg)	POTASSIUM (mg)	PHOSPHORUS (mg)	TOTAL FAT (g)
APPLE									
Gala, raw, with skin	100.0	g	57	0.3	13.7	1.00	108.0	11.00	0.12
	172.0	g	98	0.4	23.5	1.72	185.7	18.92	0.21
	1.00	pc, med							
fuji, raw, with skin	100.0	g	63	0.2	15.2	1.00	109.0	13.00	0.18
	192.0	g	121	0.4	29.2	1.92	209.2	24.96	0.35
	1.00	pc, med							
golden delicious, with skin	100.0	g	57	0.3	13.6	2.00	100.0	10.00	0.15
	169.0	g	96	0.5	23.0	3.38	169.0	16.90	0.25
	1.00	pc, med							
granny smith, w/ skin, raw	100.0	g	58	0.4	13.6	1.00	120.0	12.00	0.19
	167.0	g	97	0.7	22.7	1.67	200.4	20.04	0.32
	1.00	pc, med							
juice, frozen concentrate	100.0	g	47	0.1	11.5	7.00	126.0	7.00	0.10
	239.0	g	112	0.3	27.6	16.73	301.1	16.73	0.24
	8.00	fl oz							
applesauce, sweetened, canned	100.0	g	68	0.2	17.5	2.00	75.00	6.00	0.17
	123.0	g	84	0.2	21.5	2.46	92.25	7.38	0.21
	0.50	c							
applesauce, unsweetened, canned	100.0	g	42	0.2	11.3	2.00	74.00	5.00	0.10
	122.0	g	51	0.2	13.8	2.44	90.28	6.10	0.12
	0.50	c							
BLACK BERRIES									
raw	100.0	g	43	1.4	9.6	1.00	162.0	22.00	0.49
	144.0	g	62	2.0	13.8	1.44	233.2	31.68	0.71
	1.00	c							
frozen, unsweetened	100.0	g	64	1.2	15.7	1.00	140.0	30.00	0.43
	151.0	g	97	1.8	23.7	1.51	211.4	45.30	0.65
	1.00	c							
canned, heavy syrup	100.0	g	92	1.3	23.1	3.00	99.00	14.00	0.14
	256.0	g	236	3.4	59.1	7.68	253.4	35.84	0.36
	1.00	c							

RASPBERRIES

	SERVING QUANTITY	SERVING UNIT	CALORIES (kcal)	PROTEIN (g)	TOTAL CARBOHYDRATES (g)	SODIUM (mg)	POTASSIUM (mg)	PHOSPHORUS (mg)	TOTAL FAT (g)
raw	100.0	g	52	1.2	11.9	1.00	151.0	29.00	0.69
	123.0	g	64	1.5	14.7	1.23	185.7	35.67	0.80
	1.00	c							
frozen, unsweetened	100.0	g	56	1.2	12.6	4.00	184.0	30.00	0.81
	140.0	g	78	1.6	17.6	5.60	257.6	42.00	1.13
	1.00	c							
red, frozen, sweetened, unthawed	100.0	g	103	0.7	26.2	1.00	114.0	17.00	0.16
	125.0	g	129	0.9	32.7	1.25	142.5	21.25	0.20
	0.50	c							
puree, with seeds	100.0	g	55	na	11.5	4.00	195.0	30.00	0.97
juice concentrate	100.0	g	221	3.0	53.2	10.0	1,178	100.0	1.34

PEARS

whole, medium (2.5/lb)	100.0	g	57	0.4	15.2	1.00	116.0	16.00	0.14
	166.0	g	95	0.6	25.3	1.66	192.5	19.92	0.23
	1.00	pc							
halves, canned in water	100.0	g	29	0.2	7.8	2.00	53.00	7.00	0.03
	244.0	g	71	0.5	19.1	4.88	129.3	17.08	0.07
	1.00	c							
Asian	100.0	g	42	0.5	10.7	0.00	121.0	11.00	0.23
	122.0	g	51	0.6	13.0	0.00	147.6	13.42	0.28
	1.00	pc							

CRANBERRY

fresh, chopped	100.0	g	46	0.5	12.0	2.00	80.00	11.00	0.13
	55.00	g	25	0.3	6.6	1.10	44.00	6.05	0.07
	0.50	c							
dried, sweetened	100.0	g	308	0.2	82.8	5.00	49.00	8.00	1.09
	40.00	g	123	0.1	33.1	2.00	19.60	3.20	0.44
	0.33	c							
juice, unsweetened	100.0	g	46	0.4	12.2	2.00	77.00	13.00	0.13
	253.0	g	116	1.0	30.9	5.06	194.8	32.89	0.33
	1.00	c							
juice, cran cocktail	100.0	g	54	0.0	13.5	2.00	14.00	1.00	0.10
	253.0	g	137	0.0	34.2	5.06	35.42	2.53	0.25
	8.00	fl oz							
sauce, canned, sweetened	100.0	g	159	0.9	40.4	5.00	28.00	4.00	0.15
	69.25	g	110	0.6	28.0	3.46	19.39	2.77	0.10
	0.25	c							

GRAPE

	SERVING QUANTITY	SERVING UNIT	CALORIES (kcal)	PROTEIN (g)	TOTAL CARBOHYDRATES (g)	SODIUM (mg)	POTASSIUM (mg)	PHOSPHORUS (mg)	TOTAL FAT (g)
red or green, seedless	100.0	g	69	0.7	18.1	2.00	191.0	20.00	0.16
	151.0	g	104	1.1	27.3	3.02	288.4	30.20	0.24
	1.00	c							
juice, unsweetened, plus Vit.C	100.0	g	60	0.4	14.8	5.00	104.0	14.00	0.13
	252.8	g	152	0.9	37.3	12.64	262.9	35.39	0.33
	8.00	fl oz							
fruit mixed/ fruit cocktail, light, drained	100.0	g	55	0.4	14.3	6.00	85.00	13.00	0.08
juice, sweetened, frozen concentrate 6 fl oz can	100.0	g	179	0.7	44.4	7.00	74.00	15.00	0.31
	216.0	g	387	1.4	95.8	15.12	159.8	32.40	0.67
	1.00	can/ item							
seedless, Thompson, canned in water	100.0	g	40	0.5	10.3	6.00	107.0	18.00	0.11
	245.0	g	98	1.2	25.2	14.70	262.1	44.10	0.27
	1.00	c							
jelly 1 packet- 14g (0.5oz)	100.0	g	266	0.2	70.0	30.00	54.00	6.00	0.02
	21.00	g	56	0.0	14.7	6.30	11.34	1.26	0.00
	1	tbsp							

PINE APPLE

	SERVING QUANTITY	SERVING UNIT	CALORIES (kcal)	PROTEIN (g)	TOTAL CARBOHYDRATES (g)	SODIUM (mg)	POTASSIUM (mg)	PHOSPHORUS (mg)	TOTAL F
traditional varieties, diced	100.0	g	45	0.6	18.3	1.00	125.0	9.00	0.1
	155.0	g	70	0.9	11.8	1.55	193.7	13.95	0.2
	1.00	c							
sweetened, frozen, chunks	100.0	g	86	0.4	22.2	2.00	100.0	4.00	0.1
	245.0	g	211	1.0	54.4	4.90	245.0	9.80	0.2
	1.00	c							
canned in water crushed, sliced, or chunks	100.0	g	32	0.4	8.3	1.00	127.0	4.00	0.0
	246.0	g	79	1.1	20.4	2.46	312.4	9.84	0.2
	1.00	c							
canned in juice crushed, sliced, or chunks	100.0	g	60	0.4	15.7	1.00	122.0	6.00	0.0
	249.0	g	149	1.1	39.1	2.49	303.8	14.94	0.2
	1.00	c							
extra sweet variety, diced	100.0	g	51	0.5	13.5	1.00	108.0	8.00	0.1
	155.0	g	79	0.8	20.9	1.55	167.4	12.40	0.1
	1.00	c							
juice, unsweetened, canned	100.0	g	53	0.4	12.9	2.00	130.0	8.00	0.1
	250.0	g	133	0.9	32.2	5.00	325.0	20.00	0.3
	8.00	fl oz							
canned in light syrup crushed, sliced, or chunks	100.0	g	52	0.4	13.5	1.00	105.0	7.00	0.1
	126.0	g	66	0.5	17.0	1.26	132.3	8.82	0.1
	0.50	c							
juice, unsweetened, frozen concentrate	100.0	g	179	1.3	44.3	3.00	472.0	28.00	0.1
	288.0	g	387	2.8	95.7	8.48	1,019	80.48	0.2
	1.00	c							
juice, 45pprox.45ned with Vit A, C & E	100.0	g	50	0.4	12.2	3.00	132.0	9.00	0.1
	250.0	g	125	0.9	30.5	7.50	330.0	22.50	0.3
	1.00	c							

BLUE BERRIES

	SERVING QUANTITY	SERVING UNIT	CALORIES (kcal)	PROTEIN (g)	TOTAL CARBOHYDRATES (g)	SODIUM (mg)	POTASSIUM (mg)	PHOSPHORUS (mg)	TOTAL FAT (g)
fresh	100.0	g	57	0.7	14.5	1.00	77.00	12.00	0.33
	145.0	g	83	1.1	21.0	1.45	111.6	17.40	0.48
	1.00	c							
sweetened, dried	100.0	g	317	2.5	80.0	3.00	214.0	36.00	2.50
	40.00	g	127	1.0	32.0	1.20	85.60	14.40	1.00
	0.25	c							
wild, frozen	100.0	g	57	0.0	13.9	3.00	68.00	13.00	0.16
	140.0	g	80	0.0	19.4	4.20	95.20	18.20	0.22
	1.00	c							
unsweetened, frozen	100.0	g	51	0.4	12.2	1.00	54.00	11.00	0.64
	155.0	g	79	0.7	18.9	1.55	83.70	17.05	0.99
	1.00	c							
canned, light syrup, drained	100.0	g	88	1.0	22.7	3.00	54.00	12.00	0.40
	244.0	g	215	2.5	55.3	7.32	131.7	29.28	0.98
	1.00	c							

STRAWBERRIES

	SERVING QUANTITY	SERVING UNIT	CALORIES (kcal)	PROTEIN (g)	TOTAL CARBOHYDRATES (g)	SODIUM (mg)	POTASSIUM (mg)	PHOSPHORUS (mg)	TOTAL FAT (g)
fresh, whole	100.0	g	32	0.7	7.7	1.00	153.0	24.00	0.30
	144.0	g	46	1.0	11.1	1.44	220.3	34.56	0.43
	1.00	c							
unsweetened, frozen (unthawed)	100.0	g	35	0.4	9.1	2.00	148.0	13.00	0.11
	149.0	g	52	0.6	13.6	2.98	220.5	19.37	
									0.16
	1.00	c							
sweetened, frozen, thawed	100.0	g	78	0.5	21.0	1.00	98.00	12.00	0.14
	127.5	g	99	0.7	26.8	1.28	124.9	15.30	0.18
	0.50	c							
fruit topping	100.0	g	254	0.2	66.3	21.00	51.00	5.00	0.10
	42.00	g	107	0.1	27.9	8.82	21.42	2.10	0.04
	2.00	tbsp							
pastry, 46pprox, enriched	100.0	g	371	5.4	47.8	445.0	83.00	89.00	18.50
	71.00	g	263	3.8	33.9	315.9	58.93	63.19	13.14
	1.00	pc							
Milkshake (fastfood)	100.0	g	113	3.4	18.9	83.00	182.0	100.0	2.80
	226.4	g	256	7.7	42.8	187.9	412.1	226.4	6.34
	8.00	fl oz							
yogurt 46ppro, low fat	100.0	g	105	8.2	12.3	33.00	129.0	109.0	2.57
1 item = 1 container	150.0	g	158	12.3	18.4	49.50	193.5	163.5	3.86
	1.00	item							

	SERVING QUANTITY	SERVING UNIT	CALORIES	PROTEIN (g)	TOTAL CARBOHYDRATES (g)	SODIUM (mg)	POTASSIUM (mg)	PHOSPHORUS (mg)	TOTAL FAT (g)
GRAPEFRUIT									
fresh	100.0	g	32	0.6	8.1	0.00	139.0	8.00	0.10
	153.3	g	49	1.0	12.4	0.00	213.1	12.27	0.15
	0.67	c							
white, fresh, small (3.5 diameter)	100.0	g	33	0.7	8.4	0.00	148.0	8.00	0.10
	118.0	g	39	0.8	9.9	0.00	174.6	9.44	0.12
	0.50	pc							
pink or red	100.0	g	42	0.8	10.7	0.00	135.0	18.00	0.14
	153.3	g	64	1.2	16.4	0.00	207.0	27.60	0.21
	0.67	c							
juice, white	100.0	g	39	0.5	9.2	1.00	162.0	15.00	0.10
	247.0	g	96	1.2	22.7	2.47	400.2	37.05	0.25
	8.00	fl oz							
juice, pink	100.0	g	39	0.5	9.2	1.00	162.0	15.00	0.10
	247.0	g	96	1.2	22.7	2.47	400.2	37.05	0.25
	1.00	c							
juice, unsweetened, pink, canned	100.0	g	37	0.6	7.5	2.00	141.0	17.00	0.66
	247.2	g	91	1.4	18.6	4.94	348.6	42.02	1.63
	8.00	fl oz							
ELDERBERRIES									
fresh	100.0	g	73	7.0	18.4	6.00	280.0	39.00	0.50
	145.0	g	106	1.0	26.7	8.70	406.0	56.55	0.73
	1.00	c							
GOOSEBERRIES									
fresh	100.0	g	44	0.9	10.2	1.00	198.0	27.00	0.58
	150.0	g	66	1.3	15.3	1.50	297.0	40.50	0.87
	1.00	c							
canned in light syrup	100.0	g	73	0.7	18.8	2.00	77.00	7.00	0.20
	252.0	g	184	1.6	47.3	5.04	194.1	17.64	0.50
	1.00	c							
KIWI (Chinese gooseberries)									
fresh, medium, without skin	100.0	g	61	1.1	14.7	3.00	312.0	34.00	0.52
	76.00	g	46	0.9	11.1	2.28	237.1	25.84	0.40
	1.00	pc							
LOGANBERRIES									
frozen	100.0	g	55	1.5	13.0	1.00	145.0	26.00	0.31
	147.0	g	81	2.2	19.1	1.47	213.2	38.22	0.46
	1.00	c							

CHERRIES	SERVING QUANTITY	SERVING UNIT	CALORIES (kcal)	PROTEIN (g)	TOTAL CARBOHYDRATES (g)	SODIUM (mg)	POTASSIUM (mg)	PHOSPHORUS (mg)	TOTAL FAT (g)
sweet, without pits	100.0	g	63	1.1	16.0	0.00	222.0	21.00	0.20
	154.0	g	97	1.6	24.7	0.00	341.9	32.34	0.31
	1.00	c							
sour red, without pits	100.0	g	50	1.0	12.2	3.00	173.0	15.00	0.30
	155.0	g	78	1.6	18.9	4.65	268.2	23.25	0.47
	1.00	c							
juice, tart	100.0	g	59	0.3	13.7	4.00	161.0	17.00	0.54
	269.0	g	159	0.8	36.9	10.76	433.1	45.73	1.45
	1.00	c							
Pitanga or Surinam	100.0	g	33	0.8	7.5	3.00	103.0	11.00	0.40
	173.0	g	57	1.4	13.0	5.19	178.2	19.03	0.69
	1.00	c							
tart, dried, sweetened	100.0	g	333	1.3	80.5	13.00	376.0	36.00	0.73
	40.00	g	133	0.5	32.2	5.20	150.4	14.40	0.29
	0.25	c							
maraschino, canned, drained	100.0	g	165	0.2	42.0	4.00	21.0	3.00	0.21
	5.00	g	8	0.0	2.1	0.20	1.05	0.15	0.01
	1.00	pc/ item							
sweet, canned in juice, pitted	100.0	g	54	0.9	13.8	3.00	131.0	22.00	0.02
	250.0	g	135	2.3	34.5	7.50	327.5	55.00	0.05
	1.00	c							
sweet, canned in water	100.0	g	46	0.8	11.8	1.00	131.0	15.00	0.13
	248.0	g	114	1.9	29.2	2.48	324.9	37.20	0.32
	1.00	c							
sweet, frozen, sweetened thawed	100.0	g	89	1.2	22.4	1.00	199.0	16.00	0.13
	259.0	g	231	3.0	57.9	2.59	515.4	41.44	0.34
	1.00	c							
pie filling, canned 1/8 of 21 oz can	100.0	g	115	0.4	28.0	18.00	105.0	15.00	0.07
	74.00	g	85	0.3	20.7	13.32	77.70	11.10	0.05
	1.00	svg							
pie fillings, low calorie	100.0	g	53	0.8	12.0	12.00	118.0	15.00	0.16
	264.0	g	140	2.2	31.6	31.68	311.5	39.60	0.42
	1.00	c							
sour red, canned in water, drained	100.0	g	42	0.7	10.5	4.00	115.0	16.00	0.21
	168.0	g	71	1.2	17.6	6.72	193.2	26.88	0.35
	1.00	c							
sour red, , frozen unthawed	100.0	g	46	0.9	11.0	1.00	124.0	16.00	0.44
	155.0	g	71	1.4	17.1	1.55	192.2	24.80	0.68
	1.00	c							
sour red, canned in light syrup	100.0	g	75	0.7	19.3	7.00	95.00	10.00	0.10
	126.0	g	95	0.9	24.3	8.82	119.7	12.60	0.13
	0.50	c							

PEACHES	SERVING QUANTITY	SERVING UNIT	CALORIES (kcal)	PROTEIN (g)	TOTAL CARBOHYDRATES (g)	SODIUM (mg)	POTASSIUM (mg)	PHOSPHORUS (mg)	TOTAL
raw, medium	100.0	g	39	0.9	9.5	0.00	190.0	20.00	0.
(approx. 4/lb)	150.0	g	59	1.4	14.3	0.00	285.0	30.00	0.
	1.00	pc/ item							
dried	100.0	g	325	4.9	83.2	10.00	1,351	162.0	1.
	38.67	g	126	1.9	32.2	3.87	522.4	62.64	0.
	0.33	c							
slices	100.0	g	39	0.9	9.5	0.00	190.0	20.00	0.
	154.0	g	60	1.4	14.7	0.00	292.6	30.80	0.
	1.00	c							
nectar, canned	100.0	g	49	0.1	11.6	11.00	30.00	3.00	0.
	249.0	g	122	0.3	28.9	27.39	74.70	7.47	1.
	8.00	fl oz							
pie, prepared	100.0	g	224	1.9	33.0	217.00	125.0	22.00	10
1/6 of 8-in. pie	117.0	g	262	2.2	38.5	253.89	146.3	25.74	11
	1.00	slice							
slices,	100.0	g	94	0.6	24.0	6.00	130.0	11.00	0.
sweetened,	125.0	g	118	0.8	30.0	7.50	162.5	13.75	0.
frozen									
	0.50	c							
halves/ slices,	100.0	g	24	0.4	6.1	3.00	99.00	10.00	0.
canned in	122.0	g	29	0.5	7.5	3.66	120.8	12.20	0.
water									
	0.50	c							
halves/ slices,	100.0	g	44	0.6	11.6	4.00	128.0	17.00	0.
canned in	124.0	g	55	0.8	14.4	4.96	158.7	21.08	0.
juice									
	0.50	c							
canned in	100.0	g	42	0.4	11.1	5.00	74.00	11.00	0.
extra light	123.5	g	52	0.5	13.7	6.18	91.39	13.59	0.
syrup									
	0.50	c							
canned in	100.0	g	75	0.4	20.1	4.00	85.00	9.00	0.
heavy syrup	242.0	g	182	1.0	48.6	9.68	205.7	21.78	0.
	1.00	c							
canned in light syrup, drained	100.0	g	61	0.6	15.7	7.00	87.00	10.00	0.
fruit cocktail, canned light syrup with solids and liquid	100.0	g	55	0.4	14.3	6.00	85.00	13.00	0.

CANTALOUPE MELON	SERVING QUANTITY	SERVING UNIT	CALORIES (kcal)	PROTEIN (g)	TOTAL CARBOHYDRATES (g)	SODIUM (mg)	POTASSIUM (mg)	PHOSPHORUS (mg)	TOTAL FAT (g)
composite, raw	100.0	g	31	0.7	7.5	8.22	202.4	8.67	0.20
	165.5	g	51	1.1	12.5	13.60	334.9	14.34	0.33
	1.00	c							
honeydew, balls 1 slice = 125g	100.0	g	36	0.5	9.1	18.00	228.0	11.00	0.14
	132.7	g	48	0.7	12.1	23.90	302.7	14.60	0.19
	0.75	c							
Navajo	100.0	g	21	0.8	4.1	11.00	140.0	9.00	0.20
	85.05	g	18	0.7	3.5	9.36	119.1	7.65	0.17
	3.00	oz							
melon balls, frozen, unthawed	100.0	g	33	0.8	7.9	31.00	280.0	12.00	0.25
	173.0	g	57	1.5	13.7	53.63	484.4	20.76	0.43
	1.00	c							

BANANA

	SERVING QUANTITY	SERVING UNIT	CALORIES (kcal)	PROTEIN (g)	TOTAL CARBOHYDRATES (g)	SODIUM (mg)	POTASSIUM (mg)	PHOSPHORUS (mg)	TOTAL FAT (g)
medium, 77.8 in long	100.0	g	89	1.1	22.8	1.00	358.0	22.00	0.33
	118.0	g	105	1.3	27.0	1.18	422.5	25.96	0.39
	1.00	pc/item							
dehydrated, powder	100.0	g	346	3.9	88.3	3.00	1,491	74.00	1.81
	6.20	g	21	0.2	5.5	0.19	92.44	4.59	0.11
	1.00	tbsp							
chips, dried	100.0	g	519	2.3	58.4	6.00	536.0	56.00	14.29
	42.53	g	221	1.0	24.8	2.55	227.9	23.81	33.60
	1.50	oz							
pudding, mix mix to make ½ c 1 package= 88g = 3 ⅛ oz	100.0	g	366	0.0	93.0	788.0	17.00	5.00	0.40
	22.00	g	81	0.0	20.5	172.3	3.74	1.10	0.09
	1.00	svg							
pudding, ready to eat 1 can = 5 oz	100.0	g	127	2.4	21.2	196.0	110	69.00	3.60
	142.0	g	180	3.4	30.1	278.3	156.2	97.98	5.11
	5.00	oz							

ORANGE	SERVING QUANTITY	SERVING UNIT	CALORIES	PROTEIN (g)	TOTAL CARBOHYDRATES (g)	SODIUM (mg)	POTASSIUM (mg)	PHOSPHORUS (mg)	TOTAL FAT (g)
whole, 2-5/8" diameter	100.0	g	47	0.9	11.8	0.00	181.0	14.00	0.1
	131.0	g	62	1.2	15.4	0.00	237.1	18.34	0.1
	1.00	pc/ item							
Valencia (California)	100.0	g	49	1.0	11.9	0.00	179.0	17.00	0.3
	135.0	g	66	1.4	16.1	0.00	241.7	22.95	0.4
	0.75	c							
Navel (California)	100.0	g	49	0.9	12.5	1.00	166.0	28.46	0.1
	123.7	g	61	1.1	15.5	1.24	205.4	23.00	0.1
	0.75	c							
Clementines	100.0	g	47	0.9	12.0	1.00	177.0	21.00	0.1
	74.00	g	35	0.6	8.9	0.74	130.9	15.54	0.1
	1.00	pc/ item							
orange sections	100.0	g	47	0.9	11.8	0.00	181.0	14.00	0.1
	135.0	g	63	1.3	15.9	0.00	244.4	18.90	0.1
	0.75	c							
juice	100.0	g	45	0.7	10.4	1.00	200.0	17.00	0.2
	248.0	g	112	1.7	25.8	2.48	496.0	42.16	0.5
	8.00	fl oz							
Florida, sections 1 fruit = 141g	100.0	g	46	0.7	11.5	0.00	169.0	12.00	0.2
	138.7	g	64	1.0	16.0	0.00	234.5	16.65	0.2
	0.75	c							
soda	100.0	g	48	0.0	12.3	12.00	2.00	1.00	0.0
	248.0	g	119	0.0	30.5	29.76	4.96	2.48	0.0
	8.00	fl oz							
marmalade	100.0	g	246	0.3	66.3	56.00	37.00	4.00	0.0
	20.00	g	49	0.1	13.3	11.20	7.40	0.80	0.0
	1.00	tbsp							
juice, frozen	100.0	g	95	0.5	23.2	8.00	100.0	13.00	0.0
	238.4	g	70	0.4	17.2	5.92	74.00	9.62	0.0
	1.00	c							
orange peel zest	100.0	g	97	1.5	25.0	3.00	212.0	21.00	0.2
	2.00	g	2	0.0	0.5	0.06	4.24	0.42	0.0
	1.00	tsp							
juice, unsweetened, canned	100.0	g	47	0.7	11.0	4.00	184.0	17.00	0.15
	249.0	g	117	1.7	27.4	9.96	458.2	42.33	0.37
	8.00	fl oz							
Mandarin, canned in juice	100.0	g	37	0.6		9.6	5.00	133.0	10.0
	249.0	g	92	1.5		23.8	12.45	331.2	24.9
	1.00	c							
juice, light, no pulp	100.0	g	21	0.2		5.4	4.00	188.0	4.00
	240.0	g	50	0.5		13.0	9.60	451.2	9.60
	8.00	fl oz							
Mandarin, canned in light syrup	100.0	g	61	0.5		16.2	6.00	78.00	10.0
	252.0	g	154	1.1		40.8	15.12	196.6	25.2
	1.00	c							

LEMON

	SERVING QUANTITY	SERVING UNIT	CALORIES (kcal)	PROTEIN (g)	TOTAL CARBOHYDRATES (g)	SODIUM (mg)	POTASSIUM (mg)	PHOSPHORUS (mg)	TOTAL FAT (g)
whole, without seeds	100.0	g	20	1.2	10.7	3.00	145.0	15.00	0.30
	108.0	g	22	1.3	11.6	3.24	156.6	16.20	0.32
	1.00	pc/ item							
peeled, 2-1/8" in diameter)	100.0	g	29	1.1	9.3	2.00	138.0	16.00	0.30
	58.00	g	17	0.6	5.4	1.16	80.04	9.28	0.17
	1.00	pc/ item							
juice, fresh	100.0	g	22	0.4	6.9	1.00	103.0	8.00	0.24
	30.50	g	7	0.1	2.1	0.31	31.42	2.44	0.07
	1.00	fl oz							
peel or zest	100.0	g	47	1.5	16.0	6.00	160.0	12.00	0.30
	2.00	g	1	0.0	0.3	0.12	3.20	0.24	0.01
	1.00	tsp							
pudding mix 1 svg = ½ c 1 package = 85g	100.0	g	363	0.1	91.8	506.0	5.00	3.00	0.50
	21.20	g	77	0.0	19.5	107.2	1.06	0.64	0.11
	1.00	svg							
juice, canned	100.0	g	17	0.5	5.6	24.00	109.0	9.00	0.07
	30.50	g	5	0.1	1.7	7.32	33.25	2.75	0.02
	1.00	fl oz							
soda, lemon lime	100.0	g	40	0.1	24.9	9.00	1.00	0.00	0.02
	245.6	g	98	0.1	10.1	22.10	2.46	0.00	0.05
	8.00	fl oz							
juice, unsweetened, frozen	100.0	g	22	0.5	6.5	1.00	89.00	8.00	0.32
	5.08	g	1	0.0	0.3	0.05	4.52	0.41	0.02
	1.00	tsp							
pudding, ready to eat 1 can = 5 oz	100.0	g	125	0.1	25.0	140.0	1.00	5.00	3.00
	142.0	g	178	0.1	35.5	198.8	1.42	7.10	4.26
	1.00	can/ item							
tea, black, sweetened, ready to drink	100.0	g	45	0.0	10.8	3.00	14.00	1.00	0.22
	271.0	g	122	0.0	29.3	8.13	37.94	2.71	0.60
	1.00	c							

	SERVING QUANTITY	SERVING UNIT	CALORIES (kcal)	PROTEIN (g)	TOTAL CARBOHYDRATES (g)	SODIUM (mg)	POTASSIUM (mg)	PHOSPHORUS (mg)	TOTAL FAT (g)
LIME									
whole, 2" in diameter	100.0	g	30	0.7	10.5	2.00	102.0	18.00	0.20
	67.00	g	20	0.5	7.1	1.34	68.34	12.06	0.13
	1.00	pc/ item							
juice, fresh	100.0	g	25	0.4	8.4	2.00	117.0	14.00	0.07
	5.13	g	1	0.0	0.4	0.10	6.01	0.72	0.00
	1.00	tsp							
juice, unsweetened, canned	100.0	g	21	0.3	6.7	16.00	75.00	10.00	0.23
	246.0	g	52	0.6	16.5	39.36	184.5	24.60	0.57
	1.00	c							
frozen ice dessert	100.0	g	128	0.4	32.6	22.00	3.00	1.00	0.00
	99.00	g	127	0.4	32.3	21.78	2.97	0.99	0.00
	0.50	c							
LYCHEE									
whole, fresh	100.0	g	66	0.8	16.5	1.00	171.0	31.00	0.44
	142.5	g	94	1.2	23.6	1.43	243.7	44.18	0.63
	0.75	c							
dried	100.0	g	277	3.8	70.7	3.00	1,110	181.00	1.20
	40.00	g	111	1.5	28.3	1.20	444.0	72.40	0.48
	16.00	pcs/ items							
MANGO									
whole, fresh	100.0	g	60	0.8	15.0	1.00	168.0	14.00	0.38
	207.0	g	124	1.7	31.0	2.07	347.8	28.98	0.79
	1.00	pc/ item							
dried, sweetened	100.0	g	319	2.5	78.6	162.00	279.0	50.00	1.18
nectar, canned	100.0	g	51	0.1	13.1	5.00	24.00	2.00	0.06
	251.0	g	128	0.3	32.9	12.55	60.24	5.02	0.15
	1.00	c							

APRICOT	Serving Quantity	Serving Unit	Calories (kcal)	Protein (g)	Total Carbohydrates (g)	Sodium (mg)	Potassium (mg)	Phosphorus (mg)	Total Fat (g)
whole, fresh	100.0	g	48	1.4	11.1	1.00	259.0	23.00	0.39
	140.0	g	67	2.0	15.6	1.40	362.6	32.20	0.55
	4.00	pcs/ items							
jam or preserves	100.0	g	242	0.7	64.4	40.00	77.00	3.00	0.20
1 packet = 0.5 oz = 14g	20.00	g	48	0.1	12.9	8.00	15.40	0.60	0.04
	1.00	tbsp							
nectar, canned	100.0	g	56	0.2	13.6	8.00	67.00	5.00	0.45
	251.0	g	141	0.4	34.2	20.08	168.2	12.55	1.13
	8.00	fl oz							
sweetened, frozen	100.0	g	98	0.7	25.1	4.00	229.0	19.00	0.10
	242.0	g	237	1.7	60.7	9.68	554.2	45.98	0.24
	1.00	c							
dehydrated, sulfured	100.0	g	320	4.9	82.9	13.00	1,850	157.0	0.62
	30.00	g	96	1.5	24.9	3.90	555.0	47.10	0.19
	0.25	c							
dried, halves, sulfured	100.0	g	241	3.4	62.6	10.00	1,162	71.00	0.51
	43.33	g	104	1.5	27.1	4.33	503.5	30.77	0.22
	0.33	c							
halves w/ skin, canned in juice	100.0	g	48	0.6	12.3	4.00	165.0	20.00	0.04
	244.0	g	117	1.5	30.1	9.76	402.6	48.80	0.10
	1.00	c							
halves with skin, canned in light syrup	100.0	g	63	0.5	16.5	4.00	138.0	32.89	0.05
	253.0	g	159	1.3	41.7	10.12	349.1	13.00	0.13
	1.00	c							

PLUM

	Serving Quantity	Serving Unit	Calories (kcal)	Protein (g)	Total Carbohydrates (g)	Sodium (mg)	Potassium (mg)	Phosphorus (mg)	Total Fat (g)
whole, fresh, sliced	100.0	g	46	0.7	11.4	0.00	157.0	16.00	0.28
	165.0	g	76	1.2	18.8	0.00	259.1	26.40	0.46
	1.00	c							
sauce	100.0	g	184	0.9	42.8	538.0	259.0	22.00	1.04
	19.00	g	35	0.2	8.1	102.2	49.21	4.18	0.20
	1.00	tbsp							
purple, pitted, canned in water	100.0	g	41	0.4	11.0	1.00	126.0	13.00	0.01
	249.0	g	102	1.0	27.5	2.49	313.7	32.37	0.02
	1.00	c							
purple, canned in juice	100.0	g	58	0.5	15.2	1.00	154.0	15.00	0.02
	252.0	g	146	1.3	38.2	2.52	388.1	37.80	0.05
	1.00	c							

	SERVING QUANTITY	SERVING UNIT	CALORIES	PROTEIN (g)	TOTAL CARBOHYDRATES (g)	SODIUM (mg)	POTASSIUM (mg)	PHOSPHORUS (mg)	TOTAL F
PRUNE									
puree	100.0	g	257	2.1	65.1	23.00	852.0	72.00	0.20
	28.35	g	73	0.6	18.5	6.52	241.5	20.41	0.06
	1.00	oz							
dried	100.0	g	240	2.2	63.9	2.00	732.0	69.00	0.35
	42.50	g	102	0.9	27.2	0.85	311.1	29.33	0.16
	0.25	c							
juice, canned	100.0	g	71	0.6	17.5	4.00	276.0	25.00	0.03
	256.0	g	182	1.6	44.7	10.24	706.5	64.00	0.08
	8.00	fl oz							
dehydrated, stewed	100.0	g	113	1.2	29.7	2.00	353.0	37.00	0.24
	36.40	g	41	0.5	10.8	0.73	128.5	13.47	0.09
	0.13	c							
dehydrated, low moisture	100.0	g	339	3.7	89.1	5.00	1,058	112.00	0.73
	33.00	g	112	1.2	29.4	1.65	349.1	36.96	0.24
	0.25	c							
RHUBARB									
whole, fresh, diced	100.0	g	21	0.9	4.5	4.00	288.0	14.00	0.20
	81.33	g	17	0.7	3.7	3.25	234.2	11.39	0.16
	0.67	c							
diced, frozen	100.0	g	21	0.6	5.1	2.00	108.0	12.00	0.11
	137.0	g	29	0.8	7.0	2.74	147.9	16.44	0.15
	1.00	c							
frozen, cooked with sugar	100.0	g	116	0.4	31.2	1.00	96.00	8.00	0.05
	120.0	g	139	0.5	37.4	1.20	115.2	9.60	0.06
	0.50	c							
POMEGRANATE									
whole, fresh, 4" in diameter	100.0	g	83	1.7	18.7	3.00	236.0	36.00	1.17
	282.0	g	234	4.7	52.7	8.46	665.5	101.52	3.30
	1.00	pc/ item							
juice, bottled	100.0	g	54	0.2	13.1	9.00	214.0	11.00	0.29
	251.2	g	136	0.4	33.0	22.61	537.5	27.63	0.73
	8.00	fl oz							

PAPAYA

	Serving Quantity	Serving Unit	Calories (kcal)	Protein (g)	Total Carbohydrates (g)	Sodium (mg)	Potassium (mg)	Phosphorus (mg)	Total Fat (g)
whole, fresh, cubes	100.0	g	43	0.5	10.8	8.00	182.0	10.00	0.26
	140.0	g	60	0.7	15.2	11.20	254.8	14.00	0.36
	1.00	c							
nectar, canned	100.0	g	57	0.2	14.5	5.00	31.00	0.00	0.15
	250.0	g	143	0.4	36.3	12.50	77.50	0.00	0.38
	8.00	fl oz							
canned with heavy syrup, drained	100.0	g	206	0.1	55.8	9.00	67.00	6.00	0.55
	39.00	g	80	0.1	21.8	3.51	26.13	2.34	0.21
	1.00	pc/ chunk							

NECTARINE

	Serving Quantity	Serving Unit	Calories	Protein (g)	Total Carbohydrates (g)	Sodium (mg)	Potassium (mg)	Phosphorus (mg)	Total Fat (g)
whole, fresh, slices	100.0	g	44	1.1	10.6	0.00	201.0	26.00	0.32
	138.0	g	61	1.5	14.7	0.00	277.3	35.88	0.44
	1.00	c							

PERSIMMON

	Serving Quantity	Serving Unit	Calories	Protein (g)	Total Carbohydrates (g)	Sodium (mg)	Potassium (mg)	Phosphorus (mg)	Total Fat (g)
whole, fresh	100.0	g	127	0.8	33.5	1.00	310.0	26.00	0.40
	25.00	g	32	0.2	8.4	0.25	77.50	6.50	0.10
	1.00	pc/ item							
Japanese, fresh, 2-1/2" in diameter	100.0	g	70	0.6	18.6	1.00	161.0	17.00	0.19
	168.0	g	118	1.0	31.2	1.68	270.5	28.56	0.32
	1.00	pc/item							
Japanese, dried	100.0	g	274	1.4	73.4	2.00	802.0	81.00	0.59
	34.00	g	93	0.5	25.0	0.68	272.6	27.54	0.20
	1.00	pc/ item							

PURPLE PASSION FRUIT/ GRANADILLA

	Serving Quantity	Serving Unit	Calories	Protein (g)	Total Carbohydrates (g)	Sodium (mg)	Potassium (mg)	Phosphorus (mg)	Total Fat (g)
whole, fresh - no refuse	100.0	g	97	2.2	23.4	28.00	348.0	68.00	0.70
	18.00	g	18	0.4	4.2	5.04	62.60	12.20	0.13
	1.00	pc/ fruit							
nectar, no ice	100.0	g	67	1.2	17.4	4.00	112.0	5.00	0.06
	31.00	g	21	0.1	5.4	1.24	34.70	1.55	0.02
	1.00	fl oz							
juice, purple passion fruit	100.0	g	51	0.4	13.6	6.00	278.0	13.00	0.05
	30.90	g	16	0.1	4.2	1.85	85.90	4.02	0.02
	1.00	fl oz							
juice, yellow passion fruit	100.0	g	60	0.7	14.5	6.00	278.0	25.00	0.18
	30.90	g	19	0.2	4.5	1.85	85.90	7.72	0.06
	1.00	fl oz							

WATER MELON	SERVING QUANTITY	SERVING UNIT	CALORIES (kcal)	PROTEIN (g)	TOTAL CARBOHYDRATES (g)	SODIUM (mg)	POTASSIUM (mg)	PHOSPHORUS (mg)	TOTAL FAT (g)
raw, balls	100.0	g	30	0.6	7.6	1.00	112.0	11.00	0.15
	154.0	g	46	0.9	11.6	1.54	172.0	16.00	0.23
	1.00	c							
juice,	100.0	g	30	0.6	7.6	1.00	112.0	11.00	0.15
100%, no	30.00	g	9	0.2	2.3	0.30	33.60	3.30	0.05
ice	1.00	fl oz							
seeds,	100.0	g	557	28.3	15.3	99.00	648.0	755.0	47.37
kernels,	28.35	g	158	8.0	4.3	28.10	184.0	214.0	13.40
dried	1.00	oz							

FIG

	SERVING QUANTITY	SERVING UNIT	CALORIES	PROTEIN (g)	TOTAL CARBOHYDRATES (g)	SODIUM (mg)	POTASSIUM (mg)	PHOSPHORUS (mg)	TOTAL FAT (g)
raw	100.0	g	74	0.8	19.2	1.00	232.0	14.00	0.30
	50.00	g	37	0.4	9.6	0.50	116.0	7.00	0.15
	1.00	pc/ item							
dried	100.0	g	249	3.3	63.9	10.00	680.0	67.00	0.92
	8.00	g	20	0.3	5.1	0.80	54.40	5.36	0.07
	1.00	pc							
canned	100.0	g	75	0.6	19.4	1.00	157.0	10.00	0.24
	250.0	g	188	1.4	48.4	2.50	392.0	25.00	0.60
	1.00	c							
dried,	100.0	g	107	1.4	27.6	4.00	294.0	29.00	0.40
stewed	259.0	g	277	3.7	71.4	10.40	761.0	75.10	1.04
	1.00	c							
canned,	100.0	g	53	0.4	14.0	1.00	103.0	10.00	0.10
water pack,	248.0	g	131	1.0	34.7	2.48	255.0	24.80	0.25
solids/liquids	1.00	c							
canned,	100.0	g	69	0.4	18.0	1.00	102.0	10.00	0.10
light syrup	252.0	g	174	1.0	45.2	2.52	257.0	25.20	0.25
pack, solids/liquids	1.00	c							

GUAVA

	SERVING QUANTITY	SERVING UNIT	CALORIES	PROTEIN (g)	TOTAL CARBOHYDRATES (g)	SODIUM (mg)	POTASSIUM (mg)	PHOSPHORUS (mg)	TOTAL FAT (g)
raw	100.0	g	68	2.6	14.3	2.00	417.0	40.00	0.95
	55.00	g	37	1.4	7.9	1.10	229.0	22.00	0.52
	1.00	pc/ item							
nectar	100.0	g	48	0.3	13.3	6.00	33.00	3.00	0.07
no ice	31.00	g	15	0.1	4.1	1.86	10.20	0.93	0.02
	1.00	fl oz							
paste	100.0	g	280	0.1	77.6	2.00	69.00	3.00	0.27
	20.00	g	56	0.0	14.5	0.40	13.80	0.60	0.05
	1.00	tbsp							

	SERVING QUANTITY	SERVING UNIT	CALORIES (kcal)	PROTEIN (g)	TOTAL CARBOHYDRATES (g)	SODIUM (mg)	POTASSIUM (mg)	PHOSPHORUS (mg)	TOTAL FAT (g)
DATES									
whole, dried	100.0	g	282	2.5	75.0	2.00	656.0	62.00	0.39
	8.00	g	23	0.2	6.0	0.16	52.50	4.96	0.03
	1.00	pc/item							
Medjool, pitted	100.0	g	277	1.8	75.0	1.00	696.0	62.00	0.15
	24.00	g	67	0.4	18.0	0.24	167.0	14.90	0.04
	1.00	pc/item							
candy	100.0	g	379	4.2	58.1	22.00	540.0	117.0	18.04
	28.35	g	107	1.2	16.5	6.24	153.0	33.20	5.11
	1.00	oz							
POMELO									
whole, fresh	100.0	g	38	0.8	9.6	1.00	216.0	17.00	0.04
section	190.0	g	72	1.4	18.3	1.90	410.0	32.30	0.08
	1.00	c							
MANGOSTEEN									
canned, syrup pack	100.0	g	73	0.4	17.9	7.00	48.00	8.00	0.58
drained	196.0	g	143	0.8	35.1	13.70	94.10	15.70	1.14
	1.00	c							
JACKFRUIT									
raw, fresh	100.0	g	95	1.7	23.3	2.00	448.0	21.00	0.64
slices	165.0	g	157	2.8	38.4	3.30	739.0	34.60	1.06
	1.00	c							
canned, syrup pack	100.0	g	92	0.4	23.9	11.00	96.00	6.00	0.14
drained	178.0	g	164	0.6	42.6	19.60	171.0	10.70	0.25
	1.00	c							
DURIAN									
raw or frozen	100.0	g	147	1.5	27.1	2.00	436.0	39.00	5.33
chopped or diced	243.0	g	357	3.6	65.8	4.86	1,060	94.80	13.00
	1.00	c							
SOURSOP									
raw, pulp	100.0	g	66	1.0	16.8	14.00	278.0	27.00	0.30
	225.0	g	148	2.3	37.9	31.50	626.0	60.80	0.68
	1.00	c							
nectar	100.0	g	59	0.1	14.9	8.00	25.00	2.00	0.17
no ice, pure	31.00	g	18	0.0	4.6	2.48	7.75	0.62	0.05
	1.00	fl oz							

	SERVING QUANTITY	SERVING UNIT	CALORIES (kcal)	PROTEIN (g)	TOTAL CARBOHYDRATES (g)	SODIUM (mg)	POTASSIUM (mg)	PHOSPHORUS (mg)	TOTAL FAT (g)
PLANTAIN									
ripe, raw, fresh	100.0	g	122	1.3	31.9	4.00	487.0	32.00	0.35
	180.0	g	220	2.3	57.4	7.20	877.0	57.60	0.63
	1.00	pc/item							
green, raw, fresh	100.0	g	152	1.3	36.7	2.00	431.0	31.00	0.07
	267.0	g	406	3.3	97.9	5.34	1,150	82.80	0.19
	1.00	pc/item							
green, boiled	100.0	g	121	1.1	29.2	2.00	289.0	24.00	0.08
	137.0	g	166	1.5	39.9	2.74	396.0	32.90	0.11
	1.00	c							
green, fried	100.0	g	309	1.5	49.2	2.00	482.0	44.00	11.81
	118.0	g	365	1.8	58.0	2.36	569.0	51.90	13.90
	1.00	c							
yellow, raw, fresh	100.0	g	122	1.3	31.9	4.00	487.0	32.00	0.35
	270.0	g	329	3.5	86.1	10.8	1,310	86.40	0.95
	1.00	pc/item							
yellow, baked	100.0	g	155	1.5	41.4	2.00	477.0	37.00	0.16
	139.0	g	215	2.1	57.5	2.78	663.0	51.40	0.22
	1.00	c							
chips	100.0	g	531	2.3	63.8	202	786.0	78.00	29.59
	28.35	g	151	0.6	18.1	57.3	223.0	22.10	8.39
	1.00	oz							
AVOCADO									
fresh, raw mashed/pureed	100.0	g	160	2.0	8.5	7.00	485.0	52.00	14.66
	230.0	g	368	4.6	19.6	16.1	1,120	120.0	33.70
	1.00	c							
oil	100.0	g	884	0.0	0.0	0.00	0.00	0.00	100.0
	14.00	g	124	0.0	0.0	0.00	0.00	0.00	14.00
	1.00	tbsp							
dressing	100.0	g	427	1.9	7.4	867	58.00	31.00	43.33
	15.30	g	65	0.3	1.1	133.	8.87	4.74	6.63
	1.00	tbsp							
California, raw/fresh no seed and skin	100.0	g	167	2.0	8.6	8.00	507.0	54.00	15.41
	136.0	g	227	2.7	11.8	10.9	690.0	73.40	21.00
	1.00	pc/item							
Florida, fresh/raw no seed and skin	100.0	g	120	2.2	7.8	2.00	351.0	40.00	10.06
	304.0	g	365	6.8	23.8	6.08	1,070	122.0	30.60
	1.00	pc/item							
Guacamole	100.0	g	155	2.0	8.5	344	472.0	51.00	14.18
	15.00	g	23	0.3	1.3	51.6	70.80	7.65	2.13
	1.00	tbsp							

	SERVING QUANTITY	SERVING UNIT	CALORIES (kcal)	PROTEIN (g)	TOTAL CARBOHYDRATES (g)	SODIUM (mg)	POTASSIUM (mg)	PHOSPHORUS (mg)	TOTAL FAT (g)
TAMARIND									
fresh, raw	100.0	g	239	2.8	62.5	28.00	628	113	0.60
	2.00	g	5	0.1	1.3	0.56	12.60	2.26	0.01
	1.00	pc/item							
candy	100.0	g	331	0.0	92.0	1,643	309.0	56.00	0.00
	22.00	g	73	0.0	20.2	361.0	68.00	12.30	0.00
	1.00	tbsp							
dried	100.0	g	254	2.5	66.2	25.00	565	102	0.57
	160.0	g	406	4.0	106	40.00	904	163	0.91
	1.00	c							
SAPODILLA									
fresh/raw	100.0	g	83	0.4	20.0	12.00	193	12.00	1.10
	170.0	g	141	0.8	33.9	20.40	328	20.40	1.87
	1.00	pc/item							
SUGARAPPLE (Sweetsop)									
fresh, raw	100.0	g	94	2.1	23.6	9.00	247	32.00	0.29
(2-7/8" in diameter)	155.0	g	146	3.2	36.6	14.00	383	49.60	0.45
	1.00	pc/item							
STARFRUIT									
fresh/raw	100.0	g	31	1.0	6.7	2.00	133	12.00	0.33
	90.00	g	28	0.9	6.1	1.80	120.0	10.80	0.30
	1.00	pc/item							

D. Carbohydrates

(Grains, Breads, Pasta/Noodles, Cereals)

Hey there!

Do you need to print out this Food List?

You can download a printable version of this chart by scanning the QR code below or copying the link on your computer browser.

https://go.renaltracker.com/printfoodlist

BREADS

	SERVING QUANTITY	SERVING UNIT	CALORIES (kcal)	PROTEIN (g)	TOTAL CARBOHYDRATES (g)	SODIUM (mg)	POTASSIUM (mg)	PHOSPHORUS (mg)	TOTAL FAT (g)
whole wheat	100.0	g	252	12.5	42.7	455.0	254	212.0	3.50
	50.00	g	126	6.2	21.4	227.5	127.0	106.0	1.75
	2.00	slices							
white	100.0	g	266	8.9	49.4	490.0	126.0	98.00	490.0
	50.00	g	133	4.4	24.7	245.0	63.00	49.00	245.0
	2.00	slices							
french, small (2"x2.5"x1.75")	100.0	g	272	10.8	51.9	602.0	117.0	105.0	2.42
	32.00	g	87	3.4	16.6	192.6	37.44	33.60	0.77
	1.00	slice							
pita, 6.5"	100.0	g	275	9.1	55.7	536.0	120.0	97.00	1.20
	60.00	g	165	5.5	33.4	321.6	72.00	58.20	0.72
	1.00	pc							
sourdough	100.0	g	272	10.8	51.9	602.0	117.0	105.0	2.42
	50.00	g	136	5.4	25.9	301.0	58.50	52.50	1.21
	2.00	slices							
rye	100.0	g	259	8.5	48.3	603.0	166.0	125.0	33.00
	32.00	g	83	2.7	15.5	192.9	53.12	40.00	1.06
	1.00	slice							
bagels, wheat	100.0	g	250	10.2	48.9	439.0	165.0	142.0	1.53
	105.0	g	262	10.7	51.3	461.0	173.0	149.0	1.61
	1.00	reg pc							
biscuits	100.0	g	362	7.5	43.9	930.0	184.0	501.0	18.19
	45.00	g	163	3.4	19.8	418.0	82.80	225.0	8.19
	1.00	pc							
sprouted, wheat	100.0	g	188	13.2	33.9	474.0	198.0	176.0	0.00
	26.00	g	49	3.4	8.8	123.0	51.50	45.80	0.00
	1.00	slice							
cracked, wheat	100.0	g	274	10.7	47.5	473.0	141.0	129.0	4.53
	28.00	g	77	3.0	13.3	132.0	39.50	36.10	1.27
	1.00	reg slice							
tortillas, corn ready-to-bake or fry	100.0	g	218	5.7	44.6	45.00	186.0	314.0	2.85
	24.00	g	52	1.4	10.7	10.80	44.60	75.40	0.68
	1.00	Pc							
tortillas, flour approx. 6" diameter ready-to-bake or fry, refrigerated	100.0	g	306	8.2	49.4	736.0	125.0	206.0	7.99
	30.00	g	92	2.5	14.8	221.0	37.50	61.80	2.40
	1.00	pc							

BREADS

	SERVING QUANTITY	SERVING UNIT	CALORIES (kcal)	PROTEIN (g)	TOTAL CARBOHYDRATES (g)	SODIUM (mg)	POTASSIUM (mg)	PHOSPHORUS (mg)	TOTAL FAT (g)
tortilla, whole wheat	100.0	g	310	9.8	45.9	617.0	262.0	346.0	9.76
ready-to-bake or fry	41.00	g	127	4.0	18.8	253.0	107.0	142.0	4.00
	1.00	pc							
ciabatta	100.0	g	259	9.5	48.1	618.0	124.0	95.00	2.73
(yeast bread)	43.00	g	111	4.1	20.7	266.0	53.30	40.80	1.17
italian, Grecian, Armenian thick slice	1.00	pc							
focaccia, plain	100.0	g	249	8.8	35.8	561.0	114.0	128.0	7.89
(italian flatbread)	57.00	g	142	5.0	20.4	320.0	65.00	73.00	4.50
	1.00	pc							
Pita, medium	100.0	g	275	9.1	55.7	536.0	120.0	97.00	1.20
	57.00	g	157	5.2	31.7	306.0	68.40	55.30	0.68
	1.00	pc							
Naan, plain	100.0	g	291	9.6	50.4	465.0	125.0	100.0	5.65
	90.00	g	262	8.7	45.4	418.0	112.0	90.00	5.08
	1.00	pc							
Paratha, whole wheat, frozen	100.0	g	326	6.4	45.4	467.0	185.0	188.0	6.70
	79.00	g	258	5.0	35.9	495.0	196.0	199.0	7.10
	1.00	pc							
brioche	100.0	g	418	8.8	35.8	452.0	139.0	120.0	13.20
	77.00	g	322	6.7	27.6	357.0	110.0	94.80	10.40
	1.00	pc							
croissants, plain medium	100.0	g	406	8.2	45.8	440.0	120.0	125.0	26.80
	57.00	g	231	4.7	26.1	339.0	92.40	96.20	20.60
	1.00	pc							
croissants, chocolate	100.0	g	421	7.4	49.4	384.0	118.0	105.0	21.00
	57.00	g	240	4.2	28.2	219.0	67.30	59.80	12.00
	1.00	pc							
croissants, cheese	100.0	g	414	9.2	47.0	361.0	132.0	130.0	20.90
	57.00	g	236	5.2	26.8	206.0	75.22	74.10	11.90
	1.00	pc							
muffins, english, whole grain white	100.0	g	245	7.0	50.2	386.0	130.0	127.0	1.75
	57.00	g	140	4.0	28.6	220.0	74.10	72.40	1.00
	1.00	pc							
muffins, english, whole wheat	100.0	g	203	8.8	40.4	364.0	210.0	282.0	2.10
	66.00	g	134	5.8	26.7	240.0	139.0	186.0	1.39
	1.00	pc							

BREADS

	SERVING QUANTITY	SERVING UNIT	CALORIES (kcal)	PROTEIN (g)	TOTAL CARBOHYDRATES (g)	SODIUM (mg)	POTASSIUM (mg)	PHOSPHORUS (mg)	TOTAL FAT (g)
muffins, english, mixed-grain includes granola	100.0	g	235	9.1	46.3	298.0	156.0	81.00	1.80
	66.00	g	155	6.0	30.6	197.0	103.0	53.40	1.19
	1.00	pc							
pumpernickle, med or regular slice	100.0	g	250	8.7	47.5	596.0	208.0	178.0	3.10
	32.00	g	80	2.8	15.2	191.0	66.60	57.00	0.99
	1.00	pc							
cinammon, medium or regular slice	100.0	g	253	7.1	44.4	388.0	74.00	57.00	5.29
	28.00	g	71	2.0	12.4	109.0	20.70	16.00	1.48
	1.00	pc							
raisin, med or regular slice	100.0	g	273	8.8	52.2	432.0	180.0	112.0	3.26
	28.00	g	76	2.5	14.6	121.0	50.40	31.40	0.91
	1.00	pc							
roll, multigrain med, reg, sandwich size	100.0	g	263	9.6	44.6	458.0	160.0	122.0	6.00
	43.00	g	113	4.1	19.2	197.0	68.80	52.50	2.58
	1.00	pc							
bread stuffing, homemade dry mix, prepared	100.0	g	177	3.1	21.7	471.0	72.00	41.00	8.51
	228.0	g	404	7.2	49.5	1,070	164.0	93.50	19.40
	1.00	pc							

GRITS

	SERVING QUANTITY	SERVING UNIT	CALORIES (kcal)	PROTEIN (g)	TOTAL CARBOHYDRATES (g)	SODIUM (mg)	POTASSIUM (mg)	PHOSPHORUS (mg)	TOTAL FAT (g)
corn, yellow, quick, unenriched cooked with water, no salt	100.0	g	59	1.4	12.9	2.00	21.00	11.00	0.19
	242.0	g	143	3.4	31.2	4.84	50.82	26.62	0.46
	1.00	c							
corn, white, quick, unenriched cooked with water	100.0	g	59	1.4	12.9	2.00	21.00	11.00	0.19
	242.0	g	143	3.4	31.2	4.84	50.82	26.62	0.46
	1.00	c							

POLENTA

	SERVING QUANTITY	SERVING UNIT	CALORIES (kcal)	PROTEIN (g)	TOTAL CARBOHYDRATES (g)	SODIUM (mg)	POTASSIUM (mg)	PHOSPHORUS (mg)	TOTAL FAT (g)
(cornmeal)	100.0	g							
	240.0	g	139	2.7	30.	170.0	50.40	36.00	0.67
	1	c							

PASTA

	SERVING QUANTITY	SERVING UNIT	CALORIES (kcal)	PROTEIN (g)	TOTAL CARBOHYDRATES (g)	SODIUM (mg)	POTASSIUM (mg)	PHOSPHORUS (mg)	TOTAL F… (g…
spaghetti, unenriched, cooked	100.0	g	158	5.8	30.9	1.00	44.00	58.00	0.93
	70.00	g	111	4.1	21.6	0.70	30.80	40.60	0.65
	0.50	c							
spaghetti, enriched, cooked	100.0	g	158	5.8	30.9	1.00	44.00	58.00	0.93
	140.0	g	221	8.1	43.2	1.40	61.60	81.20	1.30
	1.00	c							
spaghetti, whole wheat, cooked	100.0	g	149	6.0	30.1	4.00	96.00	127.0	1.71
	140.0	g	209	8.4	42.1	5.60	134.4	177.8	2.39
	1.00	c							
bowtie/farfalle, enriched, cooked	100.0	g	136	4.8	27.4	1.10	24.51	-na-	0.55
	154.8	g	210	7.4	42.3	0.16	37.93	-na-	0.86
	1.00	c							
fusilli, enriched, cooked	100.0	g	161	5.7	32.5	1.30	29.09	-na-	0.66
	130.4	g	210	7.4	42.3	1.70	37.93	-na-	0.86
	1.00	c							
penne, enriched, cooked	100.0	g	169	6.0	34.1	1.37	30.55	-na-	0.69
	124.1	g	210	7.4	42.3	1.70	37.93	-na-	0.86
	1.00	c							
macaroni, enriched, cooked	100.0	g	133	4.7	26.8	1.08	24.04	-na-	0.54
	157.8	g	210	7.4	42.3	1.70	37.93	-na-	0.86
	1.00	c							
lasagna, enriched, boiled/drained	100.0	g	150	5.3	30.1	1.21	26.98	-na-	0.61
	140.6	g	210	7.4	42.3	1.70	37.93	-na-	0.86
	1.00	c							
whole grain, 51%whole wheat rest enriched semolina, cooked spaghetti, unenriched, cooked	100.0	g	156	5.7	30.9	4.00	71.00	97.00	1.48

CRACKERS	SERVING QUANTITY	SERVING UNIT	CALORIES (kcal)	PROTEIN (g)	TOTAL CARBOHYDRATES (g)	SODIUM (mg)	POTASSIUM (mg)	PHOSPHORUS (mg)	TOTAL FAT (g)
melba toast, rye 3 3/4" x 1 3/4" x 1/8"	100.0	g	389	11.6	77.3	899.0	193.0	183.0	3.40
	15.00 3.00	g pcs	58	1.7	11.6	134.8	28.95	27.45	0.51
melba toast, wheat	100.0	g	374	12.9	76.4	837.0	148.0	165.0	2.30
	15.00 3.00	g pcs	56	1.9	11.5	125.5	22.20	24.75	0.35
saltine, low salt (square)	100.0	g	421	9.5	74.3	198.0	724.0	111.0	8.85
	15.00 5.00	g pcs	63	1.4	11.2	29.70	108.6	16.65	1.33
saltine, fat-free, low sodium	100.0	g	393	10.5	82.3	849.0	115.0	113.0	1.60
	15.00 3.00	g pcs	59	1.6	12.4	127.3	17.25	16.95	0.24
saltines, whole wheat/multi-grain	100.0	g	398	7.1	68.3	1,214	221.0	196.0	10.71
	14.00 1.00	g svg	56	1.0	9.6	169.9	30.94	27.44	1.50
whole wheat, low salt	100.0	g	443	8.8	68.6	186.0	297.0	295.0	17.20
	28.00 7.00	g pcs	124	2.5	19.2	52.08	83.16	82.60	4.82
whole wheat, reduced fat 1 svg = 29g	100.0	g	416	11.3	75.5	745.0	373.0	364.0	7.59
	4.20 1.00	g pcs	17	0.5	3.2	31.29	15.67	15.29	0.32
graham, plain or honey, low fat	100.0	g	386	5.7	78.0	629.0	171.0	163.0	5.71
	35.00 1.00	g svg	135	2.0	27.3	220.1	59.85	57.05	2.00
goldfish (fish-shaped), flavored	100.0	g	463	10.2	65.7	970.0	224.0	167.0	17.71
	5.20 10.00	g pcs	24	0.5	3.4	50.44	11.65	8.68	0.92
toast thins, low sodium	100.0	g	442	6.5	67.7	177.0	306.0	266.0	16.13
	31.00 1.00	g svg	137	2.0	21.0	54.87	94.86	82.46	5.00

RICE

	SERVING QUANTITY	SERVING UNIT	CALORIES (kcal)	PROTEIN (g)	TOTAL CARBOHYDRATES (g)	SODIUM (mg)	POTASSIUM (mg)	PHOSPHORUS (mg)	TOTAL FAT (g)
white, unenriched	100.0	g	359	6.9	79.8	5.00	75.00	94.00	1.30
white, cooked, glutinous	100.0	g	96	2.0	21.0	5.00	20.00	33.00	0.27
	174.0	g	167	3.5	36.5	8.60	26.40	43.60	0.36
	1.00	c							
white, long-grain,	100.0	g	123	2.9	26.1	0.00	29.00	37.00	0.21
parboiled enriched, cooked	158.0	g	194	4.6	41.2	0.00	53.90	68.80	0.39
	1.00	c							
flour, white, unenriched	100.0	g	359	6.9	79.8	0.00	26.00	33.00	0.19
white, steamed, Chinese	100.0	g	151	3.2	33.9	0.00	53.30	67.60	0.39
restaurant cup, loosely packed	132.0	g	199	4.2	44.7	1.00	265.0	319.0	3.85
	1.00	c							
white, medium-grain, cooked	100.0	g	130	2.4	28.6	201.0	86.00	102.0	0.96
unenriched	186.0	g	242	4.4	53.2	394.0	169.0	200.0	1.88
	1.00	c							
white, short-grain, cooked	100.0	g	130	2.4	28.7	3.00	101.0	82.00	0.34
unenriched	205.0	g	266	4.8	58.8	4.92	166.0	134.0	0.56
	1.00	c							
flour, brown,	100.0	g	365	7.2	75.5	7.00	427.0	433.0	1.08
brown, cooked, no salt, no fat	100.0	g	122	2.7	25.5	11.20	683.0	693.0	1.73
	196.0	g	239	5.4	49.9	5.00	75.00	94.00	1.30
	1.00	c							
wild, cooked	100.0	g	101	4.0	21.3	5.00	20.00	33.00	0.27
	164.0	g	166	6.5	35.0	8.60	26.40	43.60	0.36
	1.00	c							
wild, raw	100.0	g	357	14.7	74.9	0.00	29.00	37.00	0.21
	160.0	g	571	23.6	120	0.00	53.90	68.80	0.39
	1.00	c							

OATS

	Serving Quantity	Serving Unit	Calories (kcal)	Protein (g)	Total Carbohydrates (g)	Sodium (mg)	Potassium (mg)	Phosphorus (mg)	Total Fat (g)
raw	100.0	g	379	12.2	67.7	6.00	362.0	410.0	6.52
	81.00	g	307	10.7	54.8	4.86	293.0	332.0	5.28
	1.00	c							
cereal, oat,	100.0	g	372	12.4	73.2	497.0	633.0	357.0	6.60
	33.00	g	123	4.1	24.2	164.0	209.0	118.0	2.18
	1.00	c							
steel cut	100.0	g	378	13.3	66.7	0.00	356.0	na	6.67
Brand: ARROWHEAD MILLS	45.00	g	170	6.0	30.0	0.00	160.0	na	3.00
	1.00	svg							
rolled	100.0	g	350	12.5	67.5	0.00	350.0	na	6.25
Brand: MILLVILLE by Aldi	40.00	g	140	5.0	27.0	0.00	140.0	na	2.50
	1.00	svg							
bran, cooked	100.0	g	40	3.2	11.4	1.00	92.00	119.0	0.86
	219.0	g	88	7.0	25.1	2.19	201.0	261.0	1.88
	1.00	c							
bran, uncooked (raw)	100.0	g	246	17.3	66.2	4.00	566.0	734.0	7.03
	94.00	g	231	16.3	62.2	3.76	532.0	690.0	6.61
	1.00	c							
flour, partially debranned	100.0	g	404	14.7	65.7	19.00	371.0	452.0	9.12
	104.0	g	420	15.2	68.3	19.80	386.0	470.0	9.48
	1.00	c							
regular, rolled, not fortified, dry	100.0	g	379	13.2	67.7	6.00	362.0	410.0	6.52
	81.00	g	307	10.7	54.8	4.86	293.0	332.0	5.28
	1.00	c							

WHEAT

	SERVING QUANTITY	SERVING UNIT	CALORIES (kcal)	PROTEIN (g)	TOTAL CARBOHYDRATES (g)	SODIUM (mg)	POTASSIUM (mg)	PHOSPHORUS (mg)	TOTAL FAT (g)
durum	100.0	g	399	13.7	71.1	2.00	431.0	508.0	2.4
	192.0	g	651	26.3	137	3.84	828.0	975.0	4.7
	1.00	c							
sprouted	100.0	g	198	7.5	42.5	16.00	169.0	200.0	1.2
	108.0	g	214	8.1	45.9	17.30	183.0	216.0	1.3
	1.00	c							
germ	100.0	g	360	23.2	51.8	12.00	892.0	842.0	9.7
	115.0	g	414	26.7	59.6	13.80	1,030	968	11.2
	1.00	c							
bran	100.0	g	216	15.6	64.5	2.00	1,180	1,010	4.2
	58.00	g	125	9.1	37.4	1.16	684.0	586.0	2.4
	1.00	c							
cream of wheat, instant, dry	100.0	g	366	10.6	75.5	571.0	115.0	103.0	1.4
	11.50	g	42	1.2	8.7	65.70	13.20	11.80	0.1
	1.00	tbsp							
flour, whole wheat, unenriched	100.0	g	370	15.1	71.2	3.00	376.0	352.0	2.7
whole grain, soft wheat	100.0	g	332	9.6	74.5	3.00	394.0	323.0	1.9
bread flour, unenriched	100.0	g	361	12.0	72.5	2.00	100.0	97.00	1.6
unsifted	137.0	g	495	16.4	99.4	2.74	137.0	133.0	2.2
	1.00	c							
flour, bread, white, enriched	100.0	g	361	12.0	72.5	2.00	100.0	97.00	1.6
	137.0	g	495	16.4	99.4	2.74	137.0	133.0	2.2
	1.00	c							
flour, cake, enriched	100.0	g	362	8.2	78.0	2.00	105.0	85.00	0.8
unsifted	137.0	g	496	11.2	107	2.74	144.0	116.0	1.1
	1.00	c							

CUOSCUOS

	SERVING QUANTITY	SERVING UNIT	CALORIES (kcal)	PROTEIN (g)	TOTAL CARBOHYDRATES (g)	SODIUM (mg)	POTASSIUM (mg)	PHOSPHORUS (mg)	TOTAL FAT (g)
dry	100.0	g	376	12.8	77.4	10.00	166.0	170.0	0.64
	173.0	g	680	22.1	134	17.30	287.0	294.0	1.11
	1.00	c							
cooked	100.0	g	112	3.8	23.2	5.00	58.00	22.00	0.16
	157.0	g	176	6.0	36.4	7.85	91.10	34.50	0.25
	1.00	c							

BARLEY

	SERVING QUANTITY	SERVING UNIT	CALORIES	PROTEIN	TOTAL CARBOHYDRATES	SODIUM	POTASSIUM	PHOSPHORUS	TOTAL FAT
pearled, cooked	100.0	g	123	2.3	28.2	3.00	93.00	54.00	0.44
	157.0	g	193	3.6	44.3	4.71	146.0	84.80	0.69
	1.00	c							
flour or meal	100.0	g	345	10.5	74.5	4.00	309.0	296.0	1.60
	148.0	g	511	15.5	110.	5.92	457.0	438.0	2.37
	1.00	c							

QUINOA

	SERVING QUANTITY	SERVING UNIT	CALORIES	PROTEIN	TOTAL CARBOHYDRATES	SODIUM	POTASSIUM	PHOSPHORUS	TOTAL FAT
cooked	100.0	g	120	4.4	21.3	7.00	172.0	152.0	1.92
	185.0	g	222	8.1	39.4	13.00	318.0	281.0	3.55
	1.00	c							
uncooked	100.0	g	368	14.1	64.2	5.00	563.0	457.0	6.07
	170.0	g	626	24.0	109	8.50	957.0	777.0	10.30
	1.00	c							
pasta from quinoa flour (gluten-free) not packed	100.0	g	152	3.2	31.1	4.00	63.00	91.00	2.07
	132.0	g	201	4.3	41.1	5.28	83.20	120.0	2.73
	1.00	c							

AMARANTH

	SERVING QUANTITY	SERVING UNIT	CALORIES	PROTEIN	TOTAL CARBOHYDRATES	SODIUM	POTASSIUM	PHOSPHORUS	TOTAL FAT
Grain	100.0	g	102	3.8	18.7	6.00	135.0	148.0	1.58
cooked	246.0	g	251	9.4	46.0	14.80	332.0	364.0	3.89
	1.00	c							

CEREALS	SERVING QUANTITY	SERVING UNIT	CALORIES (kcal)	PROTEIN (g)	TOTAL CARBOHYDRATES (g)	SODIUM (mg)	POTASSIUM (mg)	PHOSPHORUS (mg)	TOTAL FAT (g)
corn flakes, plain (store brands)	100.0	g	357	7.5	84.1	729.0	168.0	102.0	0.4
	25.00	g	89	1.9	21.0	182.0	42.00	25.50	0.1
	1.00	c							
corn flakes, frosted (store brands)	100.0	g	389	4.3	90.2	451.0	82.00	46.00	0.8
	40.00	g	156	1.7	36.1	180.0	32.80	18.40	0.3
	1.00	c							
crispy rice	100.0	g	383	6.7	86.2	545.0	106.0	98.00	1.2
	26.00	g	100	1.7	22.4	142.0	27.60	25.50	0.3
	1.00	c							
cocoa puffs (General Mills)	100.0	g	383	5.6	83.7	564.0	272.0	222.0	5.2
	36.00	g	138	2.0	30.1	203.0	97.90	79.90	1.8
	1.00	c							
muesli, with fruits & nuts	100.0	g	335	8.6	74.9	239.0	324.0	225.0	5.4
	85.00	g	302	7.3	63.7	203.0	275.0	191.0	4.5
	1.00	c							
muesli Brand: Safeway	100.0	g	386	8.8	73.7	228.0	474.0	175.0	5.2
	57.00	g	220	5.0	42.0	130.0	270.0	99.80	3.0
	1.00	svg							
granola, homemade, ready-to-eat	100.0	g	489	13.7	53.9	26.00	539.0	431.0	24.3
	122.0	g	597	16.7	65.8	31.70	658.0	526.0	29.6
	1.00	c							
granola bars, plain	100.0	g	471	10.1	64.4	294.0	336.0	277.0	19.8
	28.00	g	132	2.8	18.0	82.30	94.10	77.60	5.5
	1.00	bar/ oz							
granola bars, almond	100.0	g	495	7.7	62.0	256.0	273.0	228.0	25.5
	28.35	g	140	2.2	17.6	72.60	77.40	64.60	7.2
	1.00	oz							

PANCAKE	SERVING QUANTITY	SERVING UNIT	CALORIES (kcal)	PROTEIN (g)	TOTAL CARBOHYDRATES (g)	SODIUM (mg)	POTASSIUM (mg)	PHOSPHORUS (mg)	TOTAL FAT (g)
buttermilk (from recipe)	100.0	g	227	6.8	28.7	522.0	145.0	139.0	9.30
	38.00	g	86	2.6	10.9	198.0	55.10	52.80	3.53
	1-4" diameter	pc							
plain, (prepared from recipe)	100.0	g	227	6.4	28.3	439.0	132.0	159.0	9.70
	38.00	g	86	2.4	10.8	167.0	50.20	60.40	3.69
	1-4" diameter	pc							
plain, reduced fat	100.0	g	269	5.7	57.3	429.0	97.00	190.0	1.90
	105.0	g	282	6.0	60.2	450.0	102.0	200.0	2.00
	3.00	pcs							
plain, frozen, ready to heat includes buttermilk	100.0	g	233	5.2	37.8	461.0	90.00	215.0	6.83
	40.00	g	93	2.1	15.1	184.0	36.00	86.00	2.73
	1 (4")	pc							
gluten-free, frozen, ready to heat	100.0	g	215	3.3	40.3	331.0	127.0	306.0	4.55
	48.00	g	103	1.6	19.3	159.0	61.00	147.0	2.18
	1.00	pc							
WAFFLE									
plain, prepared from recipe	100.0	g	291	7.9	32.9	511.0	159.0	190.0	14.10
	75.00	g	218	5.9	24.7	383.0	119.0	142.0	10.60
	1 (7")	pc							

E. Milk and Cheeses

(Dairy and Non-Dairy)

Hey there!

Do you need to print out this Food List?

You can download a printable version of this chart by scanning the QR code below or copying the link on your computer browser.

https://go.renaltracker.com/printfoodlist

MILK

	SERVING QUANTITY	SERVING UNIT	CALORIES (kcal)	PROTEIN (g)	TOTAL CARBOHYDRATES (g)	SODIUM (mg)	POTASSIUM (mg)	PHOSPHORUS (mg)	TOTAL FAT (g)
(cow) whole	100.0	g	60	3.3	4.7	38.0	150.0	101.0	3.20
	244.0	g	146	8.0	11.4	92.7	366.0	246.0	7.81
	1	c							
2% reduced fat	100.0	g	50	3.4	4.9	39.0	159.0	103.0	1.90
	244.0	g	122	8.2	12.0	95.2	388.0	251.0	4.64
	1	c							
low fat (1%)	100.0	g	43	3.4	5.2	39.0	159.0	103.0	0.95
	244.0	g	105	8.3	12.7	95.2	388.0	251.0	2.32
	1	c							
skim, fat free	100.0	g	34	3.4	4.9	41.0	167.0	107.0	0.08
	244.0	g	83	8.4	11.9	100.0	407.0	261.0	0.20
	1	c							
lactose free, from whole milk	100.0	g	60	3.3	4.7	38.0	150.0	101.0	3.20
	244.0	g	146	8.0	11.4	92.7	366.0	246.0	7.81
	1	c							
Buttermilk, dried	100.0	g	387	34.3	49.0	517.0	1592	933	5.78
	6.5	g	25	2.2	3.2	33.6	103.0	60.60	0.38
	1	tbsp							
buttermilk, fluid, whole	100.0	g	62	3.2	4.9	105.0	135.0	85.00	3.31
	245.0	g	152	7.9	12.0	257.0	331.0	208.0	8.11
	1	c							
condensed, sweetened	100.0	g	321	7.9	54.4	127.0	371.0	253.0	8.70
	38.0	g	122	3.0	20.7	48.3	141.0	96.10	3.31
	1	fl oz							
evaporated, whole	100.0	g	134	6.8	10.0	106.0	303.0	203.0	7.56
	31.5	g	42	2.1	3.2	33.4	95.40	63.90	2.38
	1	fl oz							
malted	100.0	g	64	3.2	8.7	60.0	150.0	98.00	1.91
	256.0	g	164	8.2	22.2	154.0	384.0	251.0	4.89
	1	c							
chocolate	100.0	g	67	3.4	13.5	79.0	182.0	101.0	0.00
	248.0	g	166	8.4	33.4	196.0	451.0	250.0	0.00
	1	c							
strawberry (whole milk)	100.0	g	85	3.0	11.8	38.0	139.0	94.00	2.97
	248.0	g	211	7.5	29.3	94.2	345.0	233.0	7.37
	1	c							

MILK

	SERVING QUANTITY	SERVING UNIT	CALORIES (kcal)	PROTEIN (g)	TOTAL CARBOHYDRATES (g)	SODIUM (mg)	POTASSIUM (mg)	PHOSPHORUS (mg)	TOTAL F
SOY	100.0	g	43	2.6	4.9	47.0	122.0	43.00	1.47
	244.0	g	105	6.3	12.0	115.0	298.0	105.0	3.59
	1	c							
soy, light	100.0	g	30	2.4	3.5	48.0	117.0	87.00	0.77
	244.0	g	73	5.8	8.6	117.0	285.0	212.0	1.88
	1	c							
soy, chocolate	100.0	g	63	2.3	10.0	53.0	143.0	51.00	1.53
	244.0	g	154	5.5	24.3	129.0	349.0	124.0	3.73
	1	c							
soy, non-fat	100.0	g	28	2.5	4.1	57.0	105.0	87.00	0.04
	244.0	g	68	6.0	10.1	139.0	256.0	212.0	0.10
	1	c							
RICE	100.0	g	47	0.3	9.2	39.0	27.00	56.00	0.97
	244.0	g	115	0.7	22.4	95.2	65.90	137.0	2.37
	1	c							
rice milk, unsweetened	100.0	g	47	0.3	9.2	39.0	27.00	56.00	0.97
	240.0	g	113	0.7	22.0	93.6	64.80	134.0	2.33
	8	fl oz							
ALMOND, unsweetened	100.0	g	15	0.4	1.3	72.0	67.00	9.00	0.96
	244.0	g	37	1.0	3.2	176.0	163.0	22.00	2.34
	1	c							
almond, unsweetened, chocolate	100.0	g	16	0.5	1.5	72.0	71.00	11.00	1.00
	244.0	g	39	1.1	3.6	176.0	173.0	26.80	2.44
	1	c							
almond milk, sweetened	100.0	g	30	0.4	5.2	69.0	64.00	9.00	0.93
	244.0	g	73	0.9	12.8	168.0	156.0	22.00	2.27
	1	c							
almond, sweetened, chocolate	100.0	g	41	0.4	8.3	67.0	67.00	11.00	0.95
	244.0	g	100	1.1	20.4	163.0	163.0	26.80	2.32
	1	c							
COCONUT	100.0	g	31	0.2	2.9	19.0	19.00	0.00	2.08
	244.0	g	76	0.5	7.1	46.4	46.40	0.00	5.08
	1	c							
GOAT, whole	100.0	g	69	3.6	4.5	50.0	204.0	111.0	4.14
	244.0	g	168	8.7	10.9	122.0	498.0	271.0	10.1
	1	c							

MILK SUBSTITUTE

	SERVING QUANTITY	SERVING UNIT	CALORIES (kcal)	PROTEIN (g)	TOTAL CARBOHYDRATES (g)	SODIUM (mg)	POTASSIUM (mg)	PHOSPHORUS (mg)	TOTAL FAT (g)
Non-dairy milk/creamer	100.0	g	29	1.0	3.8	60.0	80.00	19.00	1.17
	30.5	g	9	0.3	1.1	18.3	24.40	5.80	0.36
	1	fl oz							
imitation, non-soy	100.0	g	46	1.6	5.3	55.0	150.0	100.0	2.00
	244.0	g	112	3.9	12.9	134.0	366.0	244.0	4.88
	1	cup							
Kefir	100.0	g	52	3.6	7.5	38.0	159.0	100.0	0.96
	244.0	g	127	8.8	18.3	92.7	388.0	244	2.34
	1	c							
Sorbet	100.0	g	110	0.8	27.1	13.0	28.00	3.00	0.05
	80.0	g	88	0.6	21.7	10.4	22.40	2.40	0.04
	1	bar							

YOGURT

	SERVING QUANTITY	SERVING UNIT	CALORIES (kcal)	PROTEIN (g)	TOTAL CARBOHYDRATES (g)	SODIUM (mg)	POTASSIUM (mg)	PHOSPHORUS (mg)	TOTAL FAT (g)
coconut milk, yogurt	100.0	g	64	0.3	8.0	21.0	27.00	2.00	3.50
	170.0	g	109	0.5	13.5	35.7	45.90	3.40	5.95
	6	oz							
dressing	100.0	g	220	3.5	11.8	43.0	146.0	85.00	18.27
	15.4	g	34	0.5	1.8	6.6	22.50	13.10	2.81
	1	tbsp							
liquid	100.0	g	72	3.7	11.8	53.0	171.0	103.0	1.09
	245.0	g	176	9.1	28.9	130.0	419.0	252.0	2.67
	1	c							
plain, whole milk	100.0	g	61	3.5	4.7	46.0	155.0	95.00	3.25
	227.0	g	138	7.9	10.6	104.0	352.0	216.0	7.38
	8	oz							
Whole milk with fruit	100.0	g	87	3.1	12.4	44.0	146.0	86.00	2.87
	170.0	g	148	5.3	21.0	74.8	248.0	146.0	4.88
	6	oz							

YOGURT	SERVING QUANTITY	SERVING UNIT	CALORIES (kcal)	PROTEIN (g)	TOTAL CARBOHYDRATES (g)	SODIUM (mg)	POTASSIUM (mg)	PHOSPHORUS (mg)	TOTAL FAT (g)
whole milk, flavored (non-fruit)	100.0	g	77	3.3	9.4	44.0	147.0	90.00	3.10
	170.0	g	131	5.6	16.0	74.8	250.0	153.0	5.27
	6	oz							
non-fat milk, plain, vanilla	100.0	g	78	2.9	17.0	47.0	141.0	88.00	0.00
	227.0	g	177	6.7	38.7	107.0	320.0	200.0	0.00
	8	oz							
non-fat milk, fruit	100.0	g	83	5.1	15.0	72.0	234.0	140.0	0.17
	170.0	g	141	8.7	25.5	122.0	398.0	238.0	0.29
	6	oz							
Soy, yogurt, plain	100.0	g	94	3.5	16.0	35.0	47.00	38.00	1.80
	170.0	g	160	6.0	27.1	59.5	79.90	64.60	3.06
	6	oz							
Greek, plain, whole milk	100.0	g	97	9.0	4.0	35.0	141.0	135.0	5.00
	170.0	g	165	15.3	6.8	59.5	240.0	230.0	8.50
	6	oz							
Greek, fruit, whole milk	100.0	g	106	7.3	12.3	37.0	113.0	109.0	3.00
	170.0	g	180	12.5	20.9	62.9	192.0	185.0	5.10
	6	oz							
Greek, flavored, other than fruit	100.0	g	111	8.5	9.4	39.0	121.0	117.0	4.44
	170.0	g	189	14.4	15.9	66.3	206.0	199.0	7.55
	6	oz							
Greek, plain, low fat	100.0	g	73	10.0	3.9	34.0	141.0	137.0	1.92
	170.0	g	124	16.9	6.7	57.8	240.0	233.0	3.26
	6	oz							
Greek, LF, flavors other than fruit	100.0	g	95	8.6	9.5	40.0	123.0	119.0	2.50
	170.0	g	162	14.7	16.2	68.0	209.0	202.0	4.25
	6	oz							
Greek, non-fat (NF), plain	100.0	g	59	10.2	3.6	36.0	141.0	135.0	0.39
	170.0	g	100	17.3	6.1	61.2	240.0	230.0	0.66
	6	oz							
Greek, NF, flavors other than fruit	100.0	g	78	8.6	10.4	34.0	123.0	119.0	0.18
	170.0	g	133	14.7	17.6	57.8	209.0	202.0	0.31
	6	oz							
Frozen yogurt, chocolate 1 scoop = small cup	100.0	g	131	3.0	21.6	63.0	234.0	89.00	3.60
	160.0	g	210	4.8	34.6	101.0	374.0	142.0	5.76
	1	scoop							

YOGURT	SERVING QUANTITY	SERVING UNIT	CALORIES (kcal)	PROTEIN (g)	TOTAL CARBOHYDRATES (g)	SODIUM (mg)	POTASSIUM (mg)	PHOSPHORUS (mg)	TOTAL FAT (g)
Frozen yogurt, vanilla	100.0	g	127	3.0	21.6	63.0	156.0	89.00	3.60
	160.0	g	203	4.8	34.6	101.0	250.0	142.0	5.76
1 scoop= small cup	1	scoop							
Frozen yogurt, soft serve, chocolate	100.0	g	160	4.3	24.9	86.0	237.0	141.0	5.76
	175.0	g	280	7.5	43.5	150.0	415.0	247.0	10.10
	1	c							
Frozn yogurt, soft serve, vanilla	100.0	g	159	4.0	24.2	87.0	211.0	129.0	5.60
	175.0	g	278	7.0	42.4	152.0	369.0	226.0	9.80
	1	c							
Frozn yogurt bar, vanilla	100.0	g	127	3.0	21.6	63.0	156.0	89.00	3.60
	65.0	g	83	2.0	14.0	41.0	101.0	57.80	2.34
	1	bar							
Frozn yogurt bar, chocolate	100.0	g	131	3.0	21.6	63.0	234.0	89.00	3.60
	65.0	g	85	2.0	14.0	41.0	152.0	57.80	2.34
	1	bar							
Frozn yogurt cone, vanilla	100.0	g	139	3.2	23.9	71.0	154.0	89.00	3.73
	125.0	g	174	4.0	29.9	88.8	192.0	111.0	4.66
	1	cone							
Frozn yogurt cone, chocolate	100.0	g	142	3.2	23.9	71.0	229.0	89.00	3.73
	125.0	g	178	4.0	29.9	88.8	286.0	111.0	4.66
	1	cone							
Frozn yogurt, waffle cone, vanilla	100.0	g	143	3.3	25.3	77.0	155.0	90.00	3.61
	255.0	g	365	8.4	64.5	196.0	395.0	230.0	9.20
	1	cone							
Frozn yogurt, waffle cone, choco	100.0	g	147	3.3	25.3	77.0	229.0	90.00	3.61
	255.0	g	375	8.4	64.5	196.0	584.0	230.0	9.20
	1	cone							

CHEESE

	SERVING QUANTITY	SERVING UNIT	CALORIES (kcal)	PROTEIN (g)	TOTAL CARBOHYDRATES (g)	SODIUM (mg)	POTASSIUM (mg)	PHOSPHORUS (mg)	TOTAL FAT (g)
mozzarella, from whole milk shredded	100.0	g	299	22.2	2.4	486.0	76.00	354.0	22.1
	112.0	g	335	24.8	2.7	544.0	85.10	396.0	24.8
	1	c							
mozzarella, part skim milk	100.0	g	254	24.3	2.8	619.0	84.00	463.0	15.9
	28.35	g	72	6.9	0.8	175.0	23.80	131.0	4.51
	1	oz							
Mozzarella, reduced sodium (shredded)	100.0	g	280	27.5	3.1	16.0	95.00	524.0	17.1
	113.0	g	316	31.1	3.5	18.1	107.0	592.0	19.3
	1	cup							
ricotta, from whole milk	100.0	g	158	7.8	6.9	105.0	230.0	162.0	11.0
	129.0	g	204	10.1	8.9	135.0	297.0	209.0	14.2
	0.5	c							
riccota, part skim milk	100.0	g	138	11.4	5.1	99.0	125.0	183.0	7.91
	124.0	g	171	14.1	6.4	123.0	155.0	227.0	9.81
	0.5	c							
cream cheese, regular	100.0	g	295	7.1	3.5	436.0	112.0	91.00	28.6
	28.35	g	84	2.0	1.0	124.0	31.80	25.80	8.11
	1	oz							
cream cheese, light	100.0	g	201	7.9	8.1	359.0	247.0	152.0	15.2
	28.35	g	57	2.2	2.3	102.0	70.00	43.10	4.33
	1	oz							
processed cheese food	100.0	g	307	16.1	8.9	1279.0	295.0	768.0	23.0
	21.0	g	65	3.4	1.9	269.0	62.00	161.0	4.84
	1	slice							
Cottage cheese	100.0	g	84	11.0	4.3	321.0	120.0	148.0	2.30
	210.0	g	176	23.1	9.1	674.0	252.0	311.0	4.83
	1	cup							
cottage cheese, low fat	100.0	g	84	11.0	4.3	321.0	120.0	148.0	2.30
	226.0	g	190	24.9	9.7	725.0	271.0	334.0	5.20
	1	cup							
Monterey shredded	100.0	g	373	24.5	0.7	600.0	81.00	444.0	30.2
	113.0	g	421	27.7	0.8	678.0	91.50	502.0	34.2
	1	cup							
Cheddar	100.0	g	408	23.3	2.4	654.0	77.00	458.0	34.0
	21.0	g	86	4.9	0.5	137.0	16.20	96.20	7.14
	1	slice							

CHEESE

	SERVING QUANTITY	SERVING UNIT	CALORIES (kcal)	PROTEIN (g)	TOTAL CARBOHYDRATES (g)	SODIUM (mg)	POTASSIUM (mg)	PHOSPHORUS (mg)	TOTAL FAT (g)
Cheddar, reduced sodium	100.0 21.0 1	g g slice	398 84	24.4 5.1	1.9 0.4	21.0 4.4	112.0 23.50	484.0 102.0	32.62 6.85
Cheddar, sharp sliced	100.0 28.0 1	g g oz	410 115	24.3 6.8	2.1 0.6	644.0 180.0	76.00 21.30	460.0 129.0	33.82 9.47
Cheddar/American cheese spread	100.0 21.0 1	g g wedge	290 61	16.4 3.5	8.7 1.8	1625 341.0	242.0 50.80	875.0 184.0	21.23 4.46
American	100.0 21.0 1	g g slice	307 65	16.1 3.4	8.9 1.9	1279. 269.0	295.0 62.00	768.0 161.0	23.06 4.84
Brick	100.0 17.2 1	g g cubic inch	371 64	23.2 4.0	2.8 0.5	560.0 96.3	136.0 23.40	451.0 77.60	29.68 5.10
Brie	100.0 17.0 1	g g cubic inch	334 57	20.8 3.5	0.5 0.1	629.0 107.0	152.0 25.80	188.0 32.00	27.68 4.71
blue	100.0 28.35 1	g g oz	353 100	21.4 6.1	2.3 0.7	1146 325.0	256.0 72.60	387.0 110.0	28.74 8.15
Camembert 1 wedge = 1.33 oz	100.0 38.0 1	g g wedge	300 114	19.8 7.5	0.5 0.2	842.0 320.0	187.0 71.10	347.0 132.0	24.26 9.22
Colby	100.0 21.0 1	g g slice	394 83	23.8 5.0	2.6 0.5	604.0 127.0	127.0 26.70	457.0 96.00	32.11 6.74
Caraway	100.0 28.35 1	g g oz	376 107	25.2 7.1	1.1 0.9	690.0 196.0	93.00 26.40	490.0 139.0	29.20 8.28
Edam	100.0 21.0 1	g g slice	356 75	24.9 5.2	2.2 0.5	819.0 172.0	121.0 25.40	546.0 115.0	27.44 5.76
Feta	100.0 17.0 1	g g cubic inch	265 45	14.2 2.4	3.9 0.7	1139. 194.0	62.00 10.50	337.0 57.30	21.49 3.62
Fontina	100.0 21.0 1	g g Slice	389 82	25.6 5.4	1.6 0.3	800.0 168.0	64.00 13.40	346.0 72.70	31.14 6.54
goat	100.0 25.0 1	g g cubic inch	364 91	21.6 5.4	0.1 0.0	415.0 104.0	158.0 39.50	375.0 93.80	29.84 7.46

CHEESE

	SERVING QUANTITY	SERVING UNIT	CALORIES (kcal)	PROTEIN (g)	TOTAL CARBOHYDRATES (g)	SODIUM (mg)	POTASSIUM (mg)	PHOSPHORUS (mg)	TOTAL F
Gouda	100.0	g	356	24.9	2.2	819.0	121.0	546.0	27.4
	28.35	g	101	7.0	0.6	232.0	34.30	155.0	7.78
	1	oz							
Gruyere	100.0	g	413	29.8	0.4	714.0	81.00	605.0	32.3
	21.0	g	87	6.3	0.1	150.0	17.00	127.0	6.70
	1	slice							
Blue or Roquefort	100.0	g	353	21.4	2.3	1146.0	256.0	387.0	28.7
	17.3	g	61	3.7	0.4	198.0	44.30	67.00	4.97
	1	cubic inch							
Colby Jack	100.0	g	384	24.1	1.6	602.0	104.0	450.0	31.2
	21.0	g	81	5.1	0.3	126.0	21.80	94.50	6.55
	1	slice							
Parmesan, grated	100.0	g	420	29.6	12.4	1750.0	184.0	834.0	28.0
	7.6	g	32	2.3	0.9	133.0	14.00	48.20	1.82
	1	tbsp							
Parmesan, hard	100.0	g	421	29.6	12.4	1750.0	184.0	834.0	28.0
	10.3	g	43	3.1	1.3	180.0	19.00	65.30	2.88
	1	cubic inch							
Mexican blend shredded	100.0	g	358	23.5	1.8	607.0	85.00	438.0	28.5
	113.0	g	405	26.6	2.0	686.0	96.00	495.0	32.2
	1	cup							
Mexican blend, reduced fat shredded	100.0	g	282	24.7	3.4	776.0	93.00	583.0	19.4
	113.0	g	319	27.9	3.9	877.0	105.0	659.0	21.9
	1	cup							
Muenster	100.0	g	368	23.4	1.1	628.0	134.0	468.0	30.0
	21.0	g	77	5.0	0.2	132.0	28.10	98.30	6.31
	1	slice							
Neufchatel	100.0	g	253	9.2	3.6	334.0	152.0	138.0	22.7
	28.35	g	72	2.6	1.0	94.7	43.10	39.10	6.46
	1	oz							
Provolone	100.0	g	351	25.6	2.1	727.0	138.0	496.0	26.6
	21.0	g	74	5.4	0.4	153.0	29.00	104.0	5.59
	1	slice							
Romano	100.0	g	387	31.8	3.6	1433.0	86.00	760.0	26.9
	28.35	g	110	9.0	1.0	406.0	24.40	215.0	7.64
	1	oz							
Swiss	100.0	g	393	27.0	1.4	185.0	71.00	574.0	31.0
	21.0	g	83	5.7	0.3	38.8	14.90	121.0	6.51
	1	slice							
Tilsiter/Tilsit	100.0	g	340	24.4	1.9	753.0	65.00	500.0	25.9
	28.35	g	96	6.9	0.5	213.0	18.40	142.0	7.36
	1	oz							

CREAM

	SERVING QUANTITY	SERVING UNIT	CALORIES (kcal)	PROTEIN (g)	TOTAL CARBOHYDRATES (g)	SODIUM (mg)	POTASSIUM (mg)	PHOSPHORUS (mg)	TOTAL FAT (g)
sour cream, regular	100.0	g	198	2.4	4.6	31.0	125.0	76.00	19.35
	30.0 1	g container	59	0.7	1.4	9.3	37.50	22.80	5.80
sour cream, light	100.0	g	136	3.5	7.1	83.0	212.0	71.00	10.60
	240.0 1	g cup	326	8.4	17.0	199.0	509.0	170.0	25.40
sour cream, imitation	100.0	g	208	2.4	6.6	102.0	161.0	45.00	19.52
	240.0 1	g cup	499	5.8	15.9	245.0	386.0	108.0	46.80
sour cream, fat free	100.0	g	74	3.1	15.6	141.0	129.0	95.00	0.00
	240.0 1	g cup	178	7.4	37.4	338.0	310.0	228.0	0.00
heavy full cream	100.0	g	340	2.8	2.8	27.0	95.00	58.00	36.08
	30.0 1	g fl oz	102	0.9	1.0	8.1	28.50	17.40	10.80
whipped	100.0	g	343	2.7	8.6	26.0	89.00	55.00	33.94
	40.0 1	g cup	137	1.1	3.4	10.4	35.60	22.00	13.60
half and half	100.0	g	131	3.1	4.3	61.0	132.0	95.00	11.50
	30.0 1	g fl oz	39	0.9	1.3	18.3	39.60	28.50	3.45
coffee, light cream	100.0	g	195	3.0	3.7	72.0	136.0	92.00	19.10
	11.0 1	g ind. container	21	0.3	0.4	7.9	15.00	10.10	2.10

F. Fats

(Oils, Nuts, & Seeds)

Hey there!

Do you need to print out this Food List?

You can download a printable version of this chart by scanning the QR code below or copying the link on your computer browser.

ALMOND

	SERVING QUANTITY	SERVING UNIT	CALORIES (kcal)	PROTEIN (g)	TOTAL CARBOHYDRATES (g)	SODIUM (mg)	POTASSIUM (mg)	PHOSPHORUS (mg)	TOTAL FAT (g)
whole	100.0	g	579	21.2	21.6	1.00	733.0	481.0	49.9
	35.75	g	207	7.6	7.7	0.36	262.0	171.9	17.9
	0.25	c							
slivered	100.0	g	579	21.2	21.6	1.00	733.0	481.0	49.9
	27.0	g	156	5.7	5.8	0.27	197.9	129.8	13.5
	0.25	c							
ground	100.0	g	579	21.2	21.6	1.00	733.0	481.0	49.9
	23.75	g	138	5.0	5.1	0.24	174.1	114.4	11.9
	0.25	c							
paste (marzipan)	100.0	g	458	9.0	47.8	9.00	314.0	258.0	27.7
	28.38	g	130	2.6	13.6	2.55	89.10	73.21	7.9
	2	tbsp							
oil	100.0	g	884	0.0	0.0	0.00	0.00	0.00	100.0
	13.6	g	120	0.0	0.0	0.00	0.00	0.00	13.6
	1	tbsp							
butter, without salt added	100.0	g	614	21.0	18.8	227.0	748.0	508.0	55.5
	16.0	g	98	3.4	3.0	1.12	119.6	81.28	8.9
	1	tbsp							
dry roasted, without salt added	100.0	g	598	3.0	21.0	3.00	713.0	471.0	52.5
	34.5	g	206	7.2	7.3	1.04	246.0	162.5	18.1
	0.25	c							
oil roasted, without salt	100.0	g	607	21.2	17.7	1.00	699.0	466.0	55.2
	39.25	g	238	8.3	6.9	0.39	274.3	182.9	21.7
	0.25	c							
milk, unsweetened, shelf stable	100.0	g	15	0.4	1.3	72.00	67.00	9.00	1.0
	262.0	g	39	1.1	3.4	188.6	175.5	23.58	2.5
	1	c							
milk, sweetened, vanilla flavor ready-to-drink	100.0	g	38	0.4	6.6	63.00	50.00	8.00	1.0
	240.0	g	91	1.0	15.8	151.2	120.0	19.20	2.5
	1	c							
milk, chocolate flavor, unsweetened fortified Vit. D2 and E	100.0	g	21	0.8	1.3	75.00	96.00	17.00	1.5
	240.0	g	50	2.0	3.0	180.0	130.4	40.80	3.5
	1	c							

WALNUT

	SERVING QUANTITY	SERVING UNIT	CALORIES (kcal)	PROTEIN (g)	TOTAL CARBOHYDRATES (g)	SODIUM (mg)	POTASSIUM (mg)	PHOSPHORUS (mg)	TOTAL FAT (g)
english, halves	100.0	g	654	15.2	13.7	2.00	441.0	346.0	65.2
	25.0	g	164	3.8	3.4	0.50	110.2	86.50	16.3
	0.25	c							
english, ground	100.0	g	654	15.2	13.7	2.00	441.0	346.0	65.2
	20.0	g	131	3.1	2.7	0.40	88.20	69.20	13.0
	0.25	c							
english, chopped	100.0	g	654	15.2	13.7	2.00	441.0	346.0	65.2
	29.25	g	191	4.5	4.0	0.59	129.0	101.2	19.1
	0.25	c							
butternut or white walnut, dried	100.0	g	612	24.9	12.1	1.00	421.0	446.0	57.0
	120.0	g	734	29.9	14.5	1.20	505.2	535.2	68.4
	1	c							
black or american, dried, chopped	100.0	g	619	24.1	9.6	2.00	523.0	513.0	59.3
	31.25	g	193	7.5	3.0	0.63	163.4	160.3	18.5
	0.25	c							
black or american, dried, ground	100.0	g	604	23.5	9.3	1.95	509.9	500.2	57.9
	26.67	g	161	6.3	2.5	0.52	135.9	133.4	15.4
	0.33	c							
glazed	100.0	g	500	8.3	47.6	446.0	232.0	na	35.7
	28.35	g	142	2.4	13.5	126.5	65.77	na	10.1
	1	oz							
oil	100.0	g	884	0.0	0.0	0.0	0.00	0.00	100.0
	13.6	g	120	0.0	0.0	0.0	0.00	0.00	13.6
	1	tbsp							

	SERVING QUANTITY	SERVING UNIT	CALORIES (kcal)	PROTEIN (g)	TOTAL CARBOHYDRATES (g)	SODIUM (mg)	POTASSIUM (mg)	PHOSPHORUS (mg)	TOTAL FAT (g)
PECANS									
chopped	100.0	g	691	9.2	13.9	0.00	410.0	277.0	72.0
	109.0	g	753	10.0	15.1	0.00	446.9	410.0	78.5
	1	c							
halves	100.0	g	691	9.2	13.9	0.00	410.0	277.0	72.0
	24.75	g	171	2.3	3.4	0.00	101.4	68.56	17.8
	0.25	c							
halves, oil roasted	100.0	g	715	9.2	13.0	1.00	392.0	263.0	75.2
	110.0	g	787	10.1	14.3	1.10	431.2	289.3	82.8
	1	c							
dry roasted, without salt added	100.0	g	710	9.5	13.6	1.00	424.0	293.0	74.3
	28.35	g	201	2.7	3.8	0.28	120.2	83.07	21.1
	1	oz							
PISTACHIO									
raw	100.0	g	560	20.2	27.2	1.00	1,025	490.0	45.3
(1 oz = 49 kernels)	123.0	g	689	24.8	33.4	1.23	1,261	602.7	55.7
	1	c							
dry roasted, no salt added	100.0	g	572	21.1	28.3	6.00	1,007	469.0	45.8
	123.0	g	704	25.9	34.8	7.38	1,239	576.8	56.4
	1	c							
MACADAMIA									
whole or halves	100.0	g	718	7.9	13.8	5.00	368.0	188.0	75.8
(1 oz = 10-12 kernels)	134.0	g	962	10.6	18.5	6.70	493.1	251.9	101.5
	1	c							
dry roasted, without salt added	100.0	g	718	7.8	13.4	4.00	363.0	198.0	76.1
	33.5.0	g	241	2.6	4.5	1.34	121.6	66.33	25.5
	0.25	c							

	SERVING QUANTITY	SERVING UNIT	CALORIES (kcal)	PROTEIN (g)	TOTAL CARBOHYDRATES (g)	SODIUM (mg)	POTASSIUM (mg)	PHOSPHORUS (mg)	TOTAL
CASHEW									
raw	100.0	g	553	18.2	30.2	12.00	660.0	593.0	43.(
	28.35	g	157	5.2	8.6	3.40	187.1	168.1	12.4
	1	oz							
oil roasted, no salt added	100.0	g	580	16.8	29.9	13.00	632.0	531.0	47.(
	129.0	g	748	21.7	38.5	16.77	815.2	685	61.(
	1	c							
dry roasted, no salt added (halves and whole)	100.0	g	574	15.3	32.7	16.00	565.0	490.0	46.4
	137.0	g	786	21.0	44.8	21.92	774.0	671.3	63.5
	1	c							
butter, without salt added	100.0	g	587	17.6	27.6	15.00	546.0	457.0	49.4
	32.0	g	188	5.6	8.8	4.80	174.7	146.3	15.(
	2	tbsp							
HAZELNUT									
oil	100.0	g	884	0.0	0.0	0.00	0.00	0.00	100
	13.6	g	120	0.0	0.0	0.00	0.00	0.00	13.(
	1	tbsp							
whole (1 oz = 21 kernels)	100.0	g	628	15.0	16.7	0.00	680.0	290.0	60.(
	33.75	g	212	5.1	5.6	0.00	229.5	97.88	20.5
	0.25	c							
blanched	100.0	g	629	13.7	17.0	0.00	658.0	310.0	61.2
	28.35	g	178	3.9	4.8	0.00	186.5	87.89	17.3
	1	oz							
chopped	100.0	g	628	15.0	16.7	0.00	680.0	290.0	60.(
	28.75	g	181	4.3	4.8	0.00	195.5	83.38	17.5
	0.25	c							
ground	100.0	g	628	15.0	16.7	0.00	680.0	290.0	60.(
	18.75	g	118	2.8	3.1	0.00	127.5	54.38	11.4
	0.25	c							
dry roasted, without salt added	100.0	g	646	15.0	17.6	0.00	755.0	310.0	62.4
	28.35	g	183	4.3	5.0	0.00	214.0	87.89	17.7
	1	oz							
spread, chocolate flavored	100.0	g	539	5.4	62.4	41.00	407.0	152.0	29.7

PEANUT

	SERVING QUANTITY	SERVING UNIT	CALORIES (kcal)	PROTEIN (g)	TOTAL CARBOHYDRATES (g)	SODIUM (mg)	POTASSIUM (mg)	PHOSPHORUS (mg)	TOTAL FAT (g)
oil	100.0	g	884	0.0	0.0	0.00	0.00	0.00	100.0
	13.5	g	119	0.0	0.0	0.00	0.00	0.00	13.5
	1	tbsp							
all types	100.0	g	567	25.8	16.1	18.00	705.0	376.0	49.2
	36.5	g	207	9.4	5.9	6.57	257.3	137.2	18.0
	0.25	c							
all types, dry roasted, no salt added (1 0z = 28.35g)	100.0	g	587	24.4	21.4	6.00	634.0	363.0	49.7
	36.5	g	214	8.9	7.8	2.19	231.4	132.5	18.1
	0.25	c							
all types, oil roasted, no salt	100.0	g	599	28.0	15.3	6.00	726.0	397.0	52.5
	133.0	g	797	37.3	20.3	7.98	965.5	528.0	69.8
	1	c							
butter, smooth, reduced fat	100.0	g	520	25.9	36.7	540.0	669.0	369.0	34.0
	36.0	g	187	9.3	12.8	194.4	240.8	132.8	12.2
	2	tbsp							
butter, smooth, no salt added	100.0	g	598	22.2	22.3	17.00	558.0	335.0	51.4
	32.0	g	191	7.1	7.1	5.44	178.5	107.2	16.4
	2	tbsp							
butter, chunky, no salt added	100.0	g	589	24.1	21.6	17.00	745.0	319.0	49.9
	32.0	g	188	7.7	6.9	5.44	238.4	102.0	16.0
	2	tbsp							
butter, reduced sodium	100.0	g	590	24.0	21.8	203.0	747.0	317.0	49.9
	16.0	g	94	3.8	3.5	32.48	119.5	50.72	8.0
	1	tbsp							
sauce, made with PB, water & soy sauce	100.0	g	257	6.3	22.0	1338	235.0	107.0	16.0
	18.0	g	46	1.1	4.0	240.8	42.30	19.26	2.9
	1	tbsp							
brittle	100.0	g	486	7.6	71.2	445.0	168.0	106.0	19.0
	42.53	g	207	3.2	30.3	189.2	71.44	45.08	8.1
	1.5	oz							
flour, defatted	100.0	g	327	52.2	34.7	180.0	1,290	760.0	0.6
	30.0	g	98	15.7	10.4	54.00	387.0	228.0	0.2
	0.5	c							

PINE

	SERVING QUANTITY	SERVING UNIT	CALORIES	PROTEIN (g)	TOTAL CARBOHYDRATES (g)	SODIUM (mg)	POTASSIUM (mg)	PHOSPHORUS (mg)	TOTAL
(Pinyon), dried	100.0	g	629	11.6	19.3	72.00	628.0	35.00	61.0
	28.35	g	178	3.3	5.5	20.41	178.0	9.92	17.3
	1	oz							
(Pignolia),	100.0	g	673	13.7	13.1	2.00	597.0	575.0	68.4
dried	8.6	g	58	1.2	1.1	0.17	51.34	49.45	5.9
	1	tbsp							

CHESTNUT

	SERVING QUANTITY	SERVING UNIT	CALORIES	PROTEIN (g)	TOTAL CARBOHYDRATES (g)	SODIUM (mg)	POTASSIUM (mg)	PHOSPHORUS (mg)	TOTAL
Japanese	100.0	g	154	2.3	34.9	14.00	329.0	72.00	0.5
	28.35	g	44	0.6	9.9	3.97	93.27	20.41	0.2
	1	oz							
Chinese	100.0	g	224	4.2	49.1	3.00	447.0	96.00	1.1
	28.35	g	64	1.2	13.9	0.85	126.7	27.22	0.3
	1	oz							
European,	100.0	g	213	2.4	45.5	3.00	518.0	93.00	2.3
unpeeled	36.25	g	77	0.9	16.5	1.09	187.7	33.71	0.8
	0.25	c							
European,	100.0	g	196	1.6	44.2	2.00	484.0	38.00	1.3
peeled	28.35	g	56	0.5	12.5	0.57	137.2	10.77	0.4
	1	oz							
European,	100.0	g	245	3.2	53.0	2.00	592.0	107.0	2.2
roasted	28.35	g	69	0.9	15.0	0.57	167.8	30.33	0.6
	1	oz							
Japanese,	100.0	g	201	3.0	45.1	19.00	427.0	93.00	0.8
roasted	28.35	g	57	0.8	12.8	5.39	121.0	26.37	0.2
	1	oz							
Chinese,	100.0	g	239	4.5	52.4	4.00	477.0	102.0	1.2
roasted	28.35	g	68	1.3	14.8	1.13	135.2	28.92	0.3
	1	oz							
Chinese,	100.0	g	153	2.9	33.6	2.00	306.0	66.00	0.8
boiled and steamed	28.35	g	43	0.8	9.5	0.57	86.75	18.71	0.2
	1	oz							
European,	100.0	g	131	2.0	27.8	27.00	715.0	99.00	1.4
boiled and steamed	28.35	g	37	0.6	7.9	7.65	202.7	15.31	0.4
	1	oz							
Japanese,	100.0	g	56	0.8	12.6	5.00	119.0	26.00	0.2
boiled and steamed	28.35	g	16	0.2	3.6	1.42	33.74	7.37	0.1
	1	oz							

ACORN

	SERVING QUANTITY	SERVING UNIT	CALORIES (kcal)	PROTEIN (g)	TOTAL CARBOHYDRATES (g)	SODIUM (mg)	POTASSIUM (mg)	PHOSPHORUS (mg)	TOTAL FAT (g)
Nuts	100.0	g	387	6.2	40.8	0.00	539.0	79.00	23.9
	28.35	g	110	1.7	11.6	0.00	152.8	22.40	6.8
	1	oz							
flour	100.0	g	501	7.5	54.7	0.00	712.0	103.0	30.2
	28.35	g	142	2.1	15.5	0.00	201.8	29.20	8.6
	1	oz							
nuts, dried	100.0	g	509	8.1	53.7	0.00	709.0	103.0	31.4
	28.35	g	144	2.3	15.2	0.00	201.0	29.20	8.9
	1	oz							

CHIA

seeds, dried	100.0	g	486	16.5	42.1	16.00	407.0	860.0	30.7
	28.35	g	138	4.7	11.9	4.54	115.3	243.8	8.7
	1	oz							

HEMP

seeds, hulled	100.0	g	553	31.6	8.7	5.00	1,200	1,650	48.8
	30.0	g	166	9.5	2.6	1.50	360.0	495.0	14.6
	3	tbsp							

FLAXSEED

seeds, whole	100.0	g	534	18.3	28.9	30.00	813.0	642.0	42.2
	10.3	g	55	1.9	3.0	3.09	83.70	66.10	4.3
	1	tbsp							
seeds, ground	7.0	g	37	1.3	2.0	2.10	56.90	44.90	3.0
	1	tbsp							
oil	100.0	g	884	0.1	0.0	0.00	0.00	1.00	100.0
	14.0	g	124	0.0	0.0	0.00	0.00	0.14	14.0
	1	tbsp							
oil with added sliced flaxseed	100.0	g	878	0.4	0.4	6.00	31.00	27.00	99.0
	13.7	g	120	0.1	0.1	0.82	4.25	3.70	13.6
	1	tbsp							
oil, cold pressed	100.0	g	884	0.1	0.0	0.00	0.00	1.00	100.0
	13.6	g	120	0.0	0.0	0.00	0.00	0.14	13.6
	1	tbsp							

	SERVING QUANTITY	SERVING UNIT	CALORIES (kcal)	PROTEIN (g)	TOTAL CARBOHYDRATES (g)	SODIUM (mg)	POTASSIUM (mg)	PHOSPHORUS (mg)	TOTAL FAT (g)
SESAME									
seeds, kernels, toasted	100	g	567	17.0	26.0	39.00	406.0	774.0	48.0
	128	g	726	21.7	33.3	49.92	519.6	990.7	61.4
	1	c							
butter or Tahini	100	g	592	17.4	21.5	35.00	459.0	790.0	53.0
	30	g	178	5.2	6.5	10.50	137.7	237.0	15.9
	2	tbsp							
seeds, whole, dried	100	g	573	17.7	23.5	11.00	468.0	629.0	49.7
	9	g	52	1.6	2.1	0.99	42.12	56.61	4.5
	1	tbsp							
butter or Tahini, from roasted/toasted kernels	100	g	595	17.0	21.2	115.0	414.0	732.0	53.8
	30	g	179	5.1	6.4	34.50	124.2	219.6	16.1
	2	tbsp							
SUNFLOWER									
seeds, kernels, toasted	100	g	619	17.2	20.6	3.00	491.0	1,158	56.8
	33.5	g	207	5.8	6.9	1.01	164.5	387.9	19.0
	0.25	c							
seeds, kernels, dried	100	g	584	20.8	20.0	9.00	645.0	660.0	51.5
	36	g	210	7.5	7.2	3.24	232.2	237.6	18.5
	0.25	c							
seeds, kernels, oil roasted	100	g	592	20.1	22.9	3.00	483.0	1,139	51.3
	135	g	799	27.1	31.0	4.05	652.0	1,538	69.3
	1	c							
seeds, kernel, dry roasted	100	g	582	19.3	24.1	3.00	850.0	1,155	49.8
	32	g	186	6.2	7.7	0.96	272.0	369.6	15.9
	0.25	c							
butter, without salt added	100	g	617	17.3	23.3	3.00	576.0	666.0	55.2
	16	g	99	2.8	3.7	0.48	92.16	106.5	8.8
	1	tbsp							
oil, <60% / >60% / >70% Linoleic	100	g	884	0.0	0.0	0.00	0.00	0.00	100.0
	13.6	g	120	0.0	0.0	0.00	0.00	0.00	13.6
	1	tbsp							
oil, industrial, mid-oleic for frying and salad dressings	100	g	884	0.0	0.0	0.00	0.00	0.00	100.0
	13.6	g	120	0.0	0.0	0.00	0.00	0.00	13.6
	1	tbsp							

PUMPKIN

	SERVING QUANTITY	SERVING UNIT	CALORIES (kcal)	PROTEIN (g)	TOTAL CARBOHYDRATES (g)	SODIUM (mg)	POTASSIUM (mg)	PHOSPHORUS (mg)	TOTAL FAT (g)
meat, 1" cubes	100.0	g	26	1.0	6.5	1.00	340.0	44.00	0.1
	116.0	g	30	1.2	7.5	1.16	394.4	51.04	0.1
	1	c							
flowers	100.0	g	15	1.0	3.3	5.00	173.0	49.00	0.1
	33.0	g	1	0.0	0.1	0.20	6.92	1.96	0.0
	1	c							
meat, boiled, drained, no salt added	100.0	g	20	0.7	4.9	1.00	230.0	30.00	0.1
	122.5	g	25	0.9	6.0	1.23	281.7	36.75	0.1
	0.5	c							
pumpkin pie spice powder	100.0	g	342	5.8	69.3	52.00	663.0	118.0	12.6
	1.7	g	6	0.1	1.2	0.88	11.27	2.01	0.2
	1	tsp							
seed sunfish, cooked dry heat	100.0	g	114	24.9	0.0	103.0	449.0	231.0	0.9
	85.05	g	97	21.2	0.0	87.60	381.8	196.4	0.8
	3	oz							
seeds, kernels, whole, roasted without salt added	100.0	g	446	18.6	53.8	18.00	919.0	92.00	19.4
	32.0	g	143	5.9	17.2	5.76	294.0	29.44	6.2
	0.5	c							

POPPYSEED

	SERVING QUANTITY	SERVING UNIT	CALORIES (kcal)	PROTEIN (g)	TOTAL CARBOHYDRATES (g)	SODIUM (mg)	POTASSIUM (mg)	PHOSPHORUS (mg)	TOTAL FAT (g)
oil	100.0	g	884	0.0	0.0	0.00	0.00	0.00	100.0
	13.6	g	120	0.0	0.0	0.00	0.00	0.00	13.6
	1	tbsp							
salad dressing, creamy	100.0	g	399	0.9	23.7	933.0	61.00	49.00	33.3
	33.0	g	132	0.3	7.8	307.9	20.13	16.17	11.0
	2	tbsp							

OLIVE	SERVING QUANTITY	SERVING UNIT	CALORIES (kcal)	PROTEIN (g)	TOTAL CARBOHYDRATES (g)	SODIUM (mg)	POTASSIUM (mg)	PHOSPHORUS (mg)	TOTAL FAT (g)
oil, extra virgin,	100.0	g	884	0.0	0.0	2.00	1.00	0.00	100.0
virgin	14.0	g	124	0.0	0.0	0.28	0.14	0.00	14.0
	1	Tbsp							
black, kalamata	100.0	g	116	0.8	6.0	735.0	8.00	3.00	10.9
	15.0	g	17	0.1	0.9	110.0	1.20	0.45	1.6
	3	pcs							
green	100.0	g	145	1.0	3.8	1556	42.00	4.00	15.3
	15.0	g	22	0.2	0.6	233.0	6.30	0.60	2.3
	3	pcs							
spread (tapenade)	100.0	g	278	0.7	4.2	835.0	17.00	3.00	30.1
	16.0	g	45	0.1	0.7	134.0	2.72	0.48	4.8
	1	tbsp							
stuffed	100.0	g	128	1.0	4.0	1340	58.00	6.00	13.2
	15.0	g	19	0.2	0.6	201.0	8.70	0.90	2.0
	3	pcs							

COCONUT

	SERVING QUANTITY	SERVING UNIT	CALORIES (kcal)	PROTEIN (g)	TOTAL CARBOHYDRATES (g)	SODIUM (mg)	POTASSIUM (mg)	PHOSPHORUS (mg)	TOTAL FAT (g)
fresh	100.0	g	354	3.3	15.2	20.00	356.0	113.0	33.5
	85.0	g	301	2.8	12.9	17.00	303.0	96.00	28.5
	1	c							
water, unsweetened	100.0	g	18	0.2	4.2	26.00	165.0	5.00	0.0
	240.0	g	43	0.5	10.2	62.40	396.0	12.00	0.0
	1	c							
milk	100.0	g	31	0.2	2.9	19.00	19.00	0.00	2.1
	244.0	g	76	0.5	7.1	46.40	46.40	0.00	5.1
	1	c							
milk/cream for cooking	100.0	g	230	2.3	5.5	15.00	263.0	100.0	23.8
	240.0	g	552	5.5	13.3	36.00	631.0	240.0	57.2
	1	c							
yogurt	100.0	g	64	0.3	8.0	21.00	27.00	2.00	3.5
	170.0	g	109	0.5	13.5	35.70	45.90	3.40	6.0
	6	oz							
cream, canned, sweetened	100.0	g	357	1.2	53.2	36.00	101.0	22.00	16.3
	37.0	g	132	0.4	19.7	13.30	37.40	8.14	6.0
	¼	c							
oil	100.0	g	833	0.0	0.0	0.00	0.00	0.00	99.1
	14.0	g	117	0.0	0.0	0.00	0.00	0.00	13.9
	1	tbsp							
flaked, shredded, packed	100.0	g	456	3.1	51.9	285.0	361.0	100.0	28.0
	28.0	g	128	1.0	14.5	79.80	101.0	28.00	7.8
	2	tbsp							

	Serving Quantity	Serving Unit	Calories (kcal)	Protein (g)	Total Carbohydrates (g)	Sodium (mg)	Potassium (mg)	Phosphorus (mg)	Total Fat (g)
SAFFLOWER									
oil	100.0	g	884	0.0	0.0	0.00	0.00	0.00	100.0
	14.0	g	124	0.0	0.0	0.00	0.00	0.00	14.0
	1	tbsp							
CANOLA									
oil	100.0	g	884	0.0	0.0	0.00	0.00	0.00	100.0
	14.0	g	124	0.0	0.0	0.00	0.00	0.00	14.0
	1	tbsp							
SOYBEAN									
oil	100.0	g	884	0.0	0.0	0.00	0.00	0.00	100.0
	14.0	g	124	0.0	0.0	0.00	0.00	0.00	14.0
	1	tbsp							
BUTTER									
stick	100.0	g	717	0.9	0.1	643.00	24.00	24.00	81.1
	14.0	g	100	0.1	0.0	90.00	3.36	3.36	11.4
	1	tbsp							
light, stick or tub	100.0	g	499	3.3	0.0	450.00	71.00	34.00	55.1
	14.0	g	70	0.5	0.0	63.00	9.94	4.76	7.7
	1	tbsp							
unsalted	100.0	g	717	0.9	0.1	11.00	24.00	24.00	81.1
	14.0	g	102	0.1	0.0	1.56	3.41	3.41	11.5
	1	tbsp							
GHEE									
clarified butter	100.0	g	876	0.3	0.0	2.00	5.00	3.00	99.5
	14.0	g	123	0.0	0.0	0.28	0.70	0.42	13.9
	1	tbsp							
MARGARINE									
stick	100.0	g	717	0.2	0.7	751.00	18.00	5.00	80.7
	14.0	g	100	0.0	0.1	105.00	2.52	0.70	11.3
	1	tbsp							

G. Animal Protein

(Meats, Poultry, and Seafood)

Hey there!

Do you need to print out this Food List?

You can download a printable version of this chart by scanning the QR code below or copying the link on your computer browser.

https://go.renaltracker.com/printfoodlist

SALMON	SERVING QUANTITY	SERVING UNIT	CALORIES (kcal)	PROTEIN (g)	TOTAL CARBOHYDRATES (g)	SODIUM (mg)	POTASSIUM (mg)	PHOSPHORUS (mg)	TOTAL FAT (g)
pink, raw	100.0	g	127	20.5	0.0	74.99	365.9	260.9	4.40
	113.4	g	144	23.2	0.0	85.04	415.0	295.9	4.99
	4.00	oz							
atlantic, wild, raw	100.0	g	142	19.8	0.0	44.00	489.9	199.9	0.98
	113.4	g	161	22.5	0.0	49.89	555.6	226.7	1.11
	4.00	oz							
atlantic, farmed, raw	100.0	g	208	20.4	0.0	58.99	362.9	239.9	13.4
	113.4	g	236	23.2	0.0	66.90	411.6	272.1	15.2
	4.00	oz							
pink, canned, drained solids, w/ bone	100.0	g	138	23.1	0.0	380.78	332.8	378.7	5.02
	85.05	g	117	19.6	0.0	323.85	283.0	322.1	4.27
	3.00	oz							
pink, canned, with bone and liquid no salt	100.0	g	139	19.8	0.0	75.00	326.0	329.0	6.05
	56.70	g	79	11.2	0.0	42.52	184.8	186.5	3.43
	2.00	oz							
pink, canned, drained solids without skin and bones	100.0	g	136	24.6	0.0	378.00	326.0	253.0	4.21
	85.05	g	116	20.9	0.0	321.49	277.2	215.1	3.58
	3.00	oz							
chum, canned, drained, with bone no salt	100.0	g	141	21.4	0.0	75.00	300.0	354.0	5.50
	56.70	g	80	12.2	0.0	42.52	170.1	200.7	3.12
	2.00	oz							
nuggets, breaded, frozen, heated	100.0	g	212	12.7	14	173.00	165.0	176.0	11.7

TUNA

bluefin, raw	100.0	g	144	23.3	0.0	39.00	251.9	253.9	4.90
	113.4	g	163	26.5	0.0	44.22	285.7	288.0	5.56
	4.00	oz							
yellowfin or Ahi, raw	100.0	g	109	24.4	0.0	45.00	440.9	277.9	0.49
	113.4	g	124	27.7	0.0	51.03	500.0	315.2	0.56
	4.00	oz							
canned in oil, drained, light no salt	100.0	g	198	29.1	0.0	50.00	207.0	311.0	8.21
	56.70	g	112	16.5	0.0	28.35	117.3	176.3	4.65
	2.00	oz							
white, canned in water, drained no salt	100.0	g	128	23.6	0.0	50.00	237.0	217.0	2.97
	56.70	g	73	13.4	0.0	28.35	134.3	123.0	1.68
	2.00	oz							
canned in water, drained, light no salt	100.0	g	116	25.5	0.0	50.00	237.0	163.0	0.82
	56.70	g	66	14.5	0.0	28.35	134.3	92.42	0.46
	2.00	oz							
white, canned in oil, drained, no salt	100.0	g	186	26.5	0.0	50.00	333.0	267.0	8.08
	56.70	g	105	15.0	0.0	28.35	188.8	151.4	4.58
	2.00	oz							

SARDINES	SERVING QUANTITY	SERVING UNIT	CALORIES (kcal)	PROTEIN (g)	TOTAL CARBOHYDRATES (g)	SODIUM (mg)	POTASSIUM (mg)	PHOSPHORUS (mg)	TOTAL FAT (g)
Spanish	100.0	g	212	6.2	14.2	310.0	0.00	na	14.
	113.0	g	240	7.0	16.0	350.0	0.00	na	16.
	4.00	oz							
atlantic,	100.0	g	208	24.6	0.0	307.0	397.0	490.0	11.
canned in oil, with bones	24.00	g	50	5.9	0.0	73.68	95.28	117.6	2.7
	2.00	oz							
portuguese	100.0	g	236	25.5	0.0	500.0	na	na	12.
	55.00	g	130	14.0	0.0	275.0	na	na	7.0
	0.50	c							
fillets, canned	100.0	g	338	18.2	7.3	364.0	na	na	26.
	55.00	g	186	10.0	4.0	200.0	na	na	14.
	0.25	c							

TILAPIA

	SERVING QUANTITY	SERVING UNIT	CALORIES	PROTEIN	TOTAL CARBS	SODIUM	POTASSIUM	PHOSPHORUS	TOTAL FAT
raw	100.0	g	96	20.1	0.0	52.00	302.0	170.0	1.7
	113.4	g	107	22.8	0.0	58.97	342.5	192.8	1.9
	4.00	oz							
cooked, dry heat	100.0	g	128	26.2	0.0	55.97	379.8	203.9	2.6
	85.05	g	109	22.2	0.0	47.60	323.0	173.4	2.2
	3.00	oz							

POLLOCK

atlantic, raw	100.0	g	92	19.4	0.0	85.99	355.9	220.9	0.9
	113.4	g	104	22.0	0.0	97.51	403.7	250.6	1.
	4.00	oz							
atlantic, cooked, dry heat	100.0	g	118	24.9	0.0	110.0	456.0	283.0	1.2
	85.05	g	100	21.2	0.0	93.55	387.8	240.7	1.0
	3.00	oz							
alaska, untreated, cooked	100.0	g	87	19.4	0.0	166.0	364.0	206.0	1.0
	85.05	g	74	16.5	0.0	141.1	309.6	175.2	0.8
	3.00	oz							

PANGASIUS (CREAM DORY/SWAI)

fillets, boneless	100.0	g	71	14.2	0.0	186.0	na	na	1.77
	113.0	g	80	16.0	0.0	210.0	na	na	2.00
	4.00	oz							
fillets, skinless, boneless	100.0	g	177	20.4	0.0	52.00	na	na	1.77
	113.0	g	200	23.0	0.0	58.80	na	na	2.00
	4.00	oz							

	SERVING QUANTITY	SERVING UNIT	CALORIES (kcal)	PROTEIN (g)	TOTAL CARBOHYDRATES (g)	SODIUM (mg)	POTASSIUM (mg)	PHOSPHORUS (mg)	TOTAL FAT (g)
COD									
atlantic, raw	100.0	g	82	17.8	0.0	54.00	412.9	202.9	0.67
	113.4	g	93	20.2	0.0	61.23	468.3	230.1	0.76
	4.00	oz							
atlantic, canned	100.0	g	105	22.8	0.0	218.0	528.0	260.0	0.86
	56.70	g	60	12.9	0.0	123.6	299.3	147.4	0.49
	2.00	oz							
atlantic, cooked, dry heat	100.0	g	105	22.8	0.0	78.00	244.0	138.0	0.86
	85.05	g	89	19.4	0.0	66.34	207.5	117.3	0.73
	3.00	oz							
pacific, raw	100.0	g	69	15.3	0.0	302.9	234.9	280.9	0.41
	113.4	g	78	17.3	0.0	343.5	266.4	318.6	0.46
	4.00	oz							
pacific, cooked, dry heat	100.0	g	85	18.7	0.0	372.0	289.0	345.0	0.50
	85.05	g	72	15.9	0.0	316.3	245.8	293.4	0.43
	3.00	oz							
ANCHOVIES									
Raw	100.0	g	131	20.4	0.0	104.0	382.9	173.9	4.84
	113.4	g	149	23.1	0.0	117.9	434.2	197.3	5.49
	4.00	oz							
canned, in oil, drained	100.0	g	210	28.9	0.0	3,668	544.0	252.0	9.71
	16.00	g	34	4.6	0.0	586.8	87.04	40.32	1.55
	4.00	pcs							
SHRIMP									
mixed species, raw	100.0	g	71	13.6	0.9	566.0	113.0	244.0	1.01
	113.4	g	81	15.4	1.0	641.8	128.1	276.4	1.15
	4.00	oz							
mixed species, breaded, fried	100.0	g	242	21.4	12	343.8	224.8	217.8	12.27
	85.05	g	206	18.2	9.8	292.4	191.2	185.3	10.44
	3.00	oz							
mixed species, cooked, moist heat	100.0	g	119	22.8	1.5	947.0	170.0	306.0	1.70
	85.05	g	101	19.4	1.3	805.4	144.5	260.2	1.45
	3.00	oz							
cracker	100.0	g	426	7.1	59	571.0	193.0	191.0	17.86

CLAMS

	Serving Quantity	Serving Unit	Calories (kcal)	Protein (g)	Total Carbohydrates (g)	Sodium (mg)	Potassium (mg)	Phosphorus (mg)	Total Fat (g)
mixed species, raw	100.0	g	86	14.7	3.6	601.0	46.00	198.0	0.96
	85.05	g	73	12.5	3.0	511.1	39.12	168.4	0.82
	3.00	oz							
mixed species, breaded, fried	100.0	g	202	14.2	10.3	364.0	326.0	188.0	11.15
	85.05	g	172	12.1	8.8	309.5	277.2	159.9	9.48
	3.00	oz							
mixed species, canned, with liquid	100.0	g	2	0.4	0.1	215.0	149.0	114.0	0.02
	28.35	g	1	0.1	0.0	60.95	42.24	32.32	0.01
	1.00	oz							
mixed species, canned, drained	100.0	g	142	24.3	5.9	112.0	628.0	327.0	1.59
	56.70	g	81	13.8	3.4	63.50	356.0	185.4	0.90
	2.00	oz							

OYSTERS

	Serving Quantity	Serving Unit	Calories (kcal)	Protein (g)	Total Carbohydrates (g)	Sodium (mg)	Potassium (mg)	Phosphorus (mg)	Total Fat (g)
ostrich, raw	100.0	g	125	21.6	0.0	83.00	297.0	204.0	3.67
	85.05	g	106	18.3	0.0	70.59	252.6	173.5	3.12
	3.00	oz							
ostrich, cooked	100.0	g	159	28.8	0.0	81.00	409.0	281.0	3.97
	85.05	g	135	24.5	0.0	68.89	347.8	239.0	3.38
	3.00	oz							
pacific, raw	100.0	g	81	9.5	5.0	106.0	168.0	162.0	2.30
	113.4	g	92	10.7	5.6	120.2	190.5	183.7	2.61
	4.00	oz							
pacific, cooked, moist heat	100.0	g	163	18.9	9.9	212.0	302.0	243.0	4.60
	85.05	g	139	16.1	8.4	180.3	256.8	206.6	3.91
	3.00	oz							
eastern, canned	100.0	g	68	7.1	3.9	112.0	229.0	139.0	2.47
	56.70	g	39	4.0	2.2	63.50	129.8	78.81	1.40
	2.00	oz							
eastern, farmed, raw	100.0	g	59	5.2	5.5	178.0	124.0	93.00	1.55
	85.05	g	50	4.4	4.7	151.4	105.4	79.10	1.32
	3.00	oz							
eastern, wild, raw	100.0	g	51	5.7	2.7	85.00	156.0	97.00	1.71
	113.4	g	58	6.5	3.1	96.39	176.9	110.0	1.94
	4.00	oz							
eastern, wild, breaded, fried	100.0	g	199	8.8	11.6	417.0	244.0	159.0	12.58
	85.05	g	169	7.5	9.9	354.6	207.5	135.2	10.70
	3.00	oz							
battered, breaded, fried, fast food	100.0	g	265	9.0	28.7	487.0	131.0	141.0	12.90
	85.05	g	225	7.7	24.4	414.1	111.4	119.9	10.97
	3.00	oz							

CRAB

	SERVING QUANTITY	SERVING UNIT	CALORIES (kcal)	PROTEIN (g)	TOTAL CARBOHYDRATES (g)	SODIUM (mg)	POTASSIUM (mg)	PHOSPHORUS (mg)	TOTAL FAT (g)
blue, raw	100.0	g	87	18.1	0.0	293.0	329.0	229.0	1.08
	113.4	g	99	20.5	0.5	332.2	373.1	259.7	1.22
	4.00	oz							
blue, canned	100.0	g	83	17.9	0.0	563.0	259.0	234.0	0.74
	56.70	g	47	10.1	0.0	319.2	146.8	132.6	0.42
	2.00	oz							
dungeness, raw	100.0	g	86	17.4	0.7	295.0	354.0	182.0	0.97
	113.4	g	98	19.7	0.8	334.5	401.4	206.4	1.10
	4.00	oz							
dungeness, cooked, moist heat	100.0	g	110	22.3	1.0	378.0	408.0	175.0	1.24
	85.05	g	94	19.0	0.8	321.5	347.0	148.8	1.05
	3.00	oz							
alaska king, raw	100.0	g	84	18.3	0.0	836.0	204.0	219.0	0.60
	113.4	g	95	20.7	0.0	948.0	231.3	248.3	0.68
	4.00	oz							
alaska king, cooked, moist heat	100.0	g	97	19.4	0.0	1,072	262.0	280.0	1.54
	85.05	g	83	16.5	0.0	911.7	222.8	238.1	1.31
	3.00	oz							
imitation, crabmeat (Kani)	100.0	g	95	7.6	15.0	529.0	90.00	282.0	0.46
	85.05	g	81	6.5	12.8	449.9	76.54	239.8	0.39
	3.00	oz							
cakes	100.0	g	266	18.8	8.5	819.0	270.0	378.0	17.25
	60.00	g	160	11.3	5.1	491.0	162.0	226.8	10.35
	1.00	pc							

CATFISH

channel, wild, raw	100.0	g	95	16.4	0.0	43.00	405.9	208.9	2.82
	113.4	g	108	18.6	0.0	48.76	357.9	236.9	3.20
	4.00	oz							
channel, farmed, raw	100.0	g	119	15.2	0.0	97.94	301.8	203.8	5.94
	85.05	g	101	13.0	0.0	83.30	256.7	173.4	5.05
	3.00	oz							
breaded, fried	100.0	g	229	18.1	8.0	280.0	340.0	216.0	13.33
	85.05	g	195	15.4	6.8	238.1	289.1	183.7	11.34
	3.00	oz							
wild, cooked, dry heat	100.0	g	105	18.5	0.0	50.00	419.0	304.0	2.85
	85.05	g	89	15.7	0.0	42.52	356.3	258.5	2.42
	3.00	oz							
farmed, cooked, dry heat	100.0	g	144	18.4	0.0	119.0	366.0	247.0	7.19
	85.05	g	122	15.7	0.0	101.2	311.2	210.0	6.12
	3.00	oz							

	SERVING QUANTITY	SERVING UNIT	CALORIES (kcal)	PROTEIN (g)	TOTAL CARBOHYDRATES (g)	SODIUM (mg)	POTASSIUM (mg)	PHOSPHORUS (mg)	TOTAL FAT (g)
MUSSELS									
blue, raw	100.0	g	86	11.9	3.7	286.0	320.0	197.0	2.24
	113.4	g	98	13.5	4.2	324.3	362.8	223.4	2.54
	4.00	oz							
blue, cooked, moist heat	100.0	g	172	23.8	7.4	369.0	268.0	285.0	4.48
	85.05	g	146	20.2	6.3	313.8	227.9	242.4	3.81
	3.00	oz							
atlantic or pacific, meat only	100.0	g	197	8.8	11.6	415.2	243.8	159.0	12.56
	85.05	g	167	7.5	9.9	353.1	207.4	1,315	10.69
	3.00	oz							
MACKEREL									
Atlantic or Boston, raw fillet	100.0	g	205	18.6	0.0	89.99	313.9	216.9	13.89
	113.4	g	232	21.1	0.0	102.0	356.0	246.0	15.75
	4.00	oz							
pacific and Jack, raw fillet	100.0	g	158	20.1	0.0	85.99	405.9	125.0	7.89
	113.4	g	179	22.8	0.0	97.51	460.3	141.7	8.95
	4.00	oz							
Atlantic Spanish, raw fillet	100.0	g	139	19.3	0.0	58.99	445.9	204.9	6.30
	113.4	g	158	21.9	0.0	66.90	505.7	232.4	7.14
	4.00	oz							
Jack, canned, solids, drained	100.0	g	156	23.2	0.0	379.0	194.0	301.0	6.30
	56.70	g	88	13.2	0.0	214.8	110.0	170.6	3.57
	2.00	oz							
Atlantic or Boston, cooked, dry heat	100.0	g	262	23.9	0.0	83.00	401.0	278.0	17.81
	85.05	g	223	20.3	0.0	70.59	341.0	236.4	15.15
	3.00	oz							
Atlantic, Spanish, cooked, dry heat	100.0	g	158	23.6	0.0	66.00	554.0	271.0	6.32
	85.05	g	134	20.1	0.0	56.13	471.1	230.4	5.38
	3.00	oz							
Pacific and Jack, mixed species, cooked	100.0	g	201	25.7	0.0	110.0	521.0	160.0	10.12
	85.05	g	171	21.9	0.0	93.55	443.1	136.0	8.61
	3.00	oz							

TROUT	SERVING QUANTITY	SERVING UNIT	CALORIES (kcal)	PROTEIN (g)	TOTAL CARBOHYDRATES (g)	SODIUM (mg)	POTASSIUM (mg)	PHOSPHORUS (mg)	TOTAL FAT (g)
rainbow, wild, raw, fillet	100.0	g	119	20.5	0.0	31.00	481.0	271.0	3.46
	113.4	g	135	23.2	0.0	35.15	545.4	307.3	3.92
	4.00	oz							
rainbow, farmed, raw, fillet	100.0	g	141	19.9	0.0	51.00	376.9	225.9	6.18
	113.4	g	160	22.6	0.0	57.83	427.4	256.2	7.01
	4.00	oz							
mixed species, raw fillet	100.0	g	148	20.8	0.0	52.00	360.9	244.9	6.61
	113.4	g	168	23.6	0.0	58.96	409.3	277.8	7.50
	4.00	oz							
sea trout, mixed species, raw	100.0	g	104	16.7	0.0	57.99	340.9	249.9	3.61
	113.4	g	118	19.0	0.0	65.77	386.6	283.4	4.09
	4.00	oz							
rainbow, wild, cooked, dry heat	100.0	g	150	22.9	0.0	56.00	448.0	269.0	5.82
	85.05	g	128	19.5	0.0	47.63	381.0	228.7	4.95
	3.00	oz							
rainbow, farmed, cooked, dry heat	100.0	g	168	23.8	0.0	61.00	450.0	270.0	7.38
	85.05	g	143	20.2	0.0	51.88	382.7	229.6	6.28
	3.00	oz							
mixed species, cooked, dry heat	100.0	g	190	26.6	0.0	67.00	463.0	314.0	8.47
	85.05	g	162	22.7	0.0	56.98	393.7	267.0	7.20
	3.00	oz							
sea trout, mixed species, cooked, dry heat	100.0	g	133	21.5	0.0	74.00	437.0	321.0	4.63
	85.05	g	113	18.3	0.0	62.94	371.6	273.0	3.94
	3.00	oz							

CARP

raw	100.0	g	127	17.8	0.0	49.00	332.9	414.9	5.60
	113.4	g	144	20.2	0.0	55.56	377.6	470.5	6.35
	4.00	oz							
cooked, dry heat	100.0	g	162	22.9	0.0	63.00	427.0	531.0	7.17
	85.05	g	138	19.4	0.0	53.58	363.1	451.6	6.10
	3.00	oz							

MAHI-MAHI

Dorado or Dolphinfish, raw	100.0	g	85	18.5	0.0	87.99	415.9	143.0	0.70
	113.4	g	96	21.0	0.0	99.78	471.7	162.1	0.79
	4.00	oz							
Doradao or Dolphinfish, cooked, dry heat	100.0	g	109	23.7	0.0	113.0	533.0	183.0	0.90
	85.05	g	93	20.2	0.0	96.11	452.3	155.6	0.77
	3.00	oz							

FLATFISH	SERVING QUANTITY	SERVING UNIT	CALORIES (kcal)	PROTEIN (g)	TOTAL CARBOHYDRATES (g)	SODIUM (mg)	POTASSIUM (mg)	PHOSPHORUS (mg)	TOTAL F. (g)
raw	100.0	g	70	12.4	0.0	295.9	159.9	251.9	1.9
	113.4	g	79	14.1	0.0	335.6	181.4	285.7	2.1
	4.00	oz							
cooked, dry	100.0	g	86	15.2	0.0	363.0	197.0	309.0	2.3
heat	85.05	g	73	13.0	0.0	308.7	167.5	262.8	2.0
	3.00	oz							

HALIBUT

	SERVING QUANTITY	SERVING UNIT	CALORIES	PROTEIN	TOTAL CARB	SODIUM	POTASSIUM	PHOSPHORUS	TOTAL F.
greenland, raw	100.0	g	186	14.4	0.0	80.0	267.9	163.9	13.
	113.4	g	211	16.3	0.0	90.7	303.8	185.9	15.
	4.00	oz							
atlantic and	100.0	g	91	18.6	0.0	68.0	434.9	235.9	1.3
pacific, raw	113.4	g	103	21.0	0.0	77.10	493.2	267.6	1.5
	4.00	oz							
greenland, cooked, dry heat	100.0	g	239	18.4	0.0	103.0	344.0	210.0	17.
	85.05	g	203	15.7	0.0	87.60	292.5	178.6	15.
	3.00	oz							
atlantic and pacific, cooked, dry heat	100.0	g	111	22.5	0.0	82.00	528.0	287.0	1.6
	85.05	g	94	19.2	0.0	69.74	449.0	244.1	1.3
	3.00	oz							

LOBSTER

	SERVING QUANTITY	SERVING UNIT	CALORIES	PROTEIN	TOTAL CARB	SODIUM	POTASSIUM	PHOSPHORUS	TOTAL F.
Northern, raw (Langoustine)	100.0	g	77	16.5	0.0	423.0	200.0	161.0	0.7
	113.4	g	87	18.7	0.0	479.6	226.8	182.5	0.8
	4.00	oz							
Spiny, mixed species, raw	100.0	g	112	20.6	2.4	177.0	180.0	238.0	1.5
	113.4	g	127	23.4	2.8	200.7	104.1	269.9	1.7
	4.00	oz							
Northern, cooked, moist heat (Langoustine)	100.0	g	89	19.0	0.0	486.0	230.0	185.0	0.8
	85.05	g	76	16.2	0.0	413.3	195.6	157.3	0.7
	3.00	oz							
Spiny, mixed species, cooked, moist heat	100.0	g	143	26.4	3.1	227.0	208.0	229.0	1.9
	85.05	g	122	22.5	2.7	193.0	176.9	194.7	1.6
	3.00	oz							

SCALLOPS	SERVING QUANTITY	SERVING UNIT	CALORIES (kcal)	PROTEIN (g)	TOTAL CARBOHYDRATES (g)	SODIUM (mg)	POTASSIUM (mg)	PHOSPHORUS (mg)	TOTAL FAT (g)
Mixed species, raw	100.0	g	69	12.1	3.2	392.0	205.0	12.80	0.49
	113.4	g	78	13.7	3.6	444.5	232.4	14.52	0.56
	4.00	oz							
Bay and Sea, steamed	100.0	g	111	20.5	5.4	667.0	314.0	426.0	0.84
	85.05	g	94	17.5	4.6	567.2	267.0	362.3	0.71
	3.00	oz							
mixed species, breaded and fried	100.0	g	216	18.1	10.1	464.0	333.0	236.0	10.94
	46.50	g	100	8.4	4.7	215.7	15.85	109.7	5.09
	3.00	pcs							
breaded, fried, fast food	100.0	g	268	10.9	26.7	638.0	204.0	203.0	13.47
	85.05	g	228	9.3	22.7	542.6	173.5	172.6	11.46
	3.00	oz							
HERRING									
Pacific, raw	100.0	g	195	16.4	0.0	73.99	422.9	227.9	13.88
	113.4	g	221	18.6	0.0	83.91	479.6	258.5	15.74
	4.00	oz							
Atlantic, raw	100.0	g	158	18.0	0.0	89.99	326.9	235.9	9.04
	113.4	g	179	20.4	0.0	102.0	370.7	267.6	10.25
	4.00	oz							
Pacific, cooked, dry heat	100.0	g	250	21.0	0.0	95.00	542.0	292.0	17.79
	85.05	g	213	17.9	0.0	80.80	460.9	248.3	15.13
	3.00	oz							
Atlantic, cooked, dry heat	100.0	g	203	23.0	0.0	115.0	419.0	303.0	11.49
	85.05	g	173	19.6	0.0	97.81	356.3	257.7	9.86
	3.00	oz							
Roe or eggs, Pacific (Alaska Native)	100.0	g	74	9.6	4.5	61.00	na	na	1.93
	85.05	g	63	8.2	3.8	51.88	na	na	1.64
	3.00	oz							

CRAYFISH/ CRAWFISH	SERVING QUANTITY	SERVING UNIT	CALORIES (kcal)	PROTEIN (g)	TOTAL CARBOHYDRATES (g)	SODIUM (mg)	POTASSIUM (mg)	PHOSPHORUS (mg)	TOTAL FAT (g)
Mixed species, farmed, raw	100.0	g	72	14.9	0.0	62.00	261.0	218.0	0.9
	113.4	g	82	16.8	0.0	70.31	295.9	247.2	1.1
	4.00	oz							
Mixed species, wild, raw	100.0	g	77	16.0	0.0	58.00	302.0	256.0	0.9
	113.4	g	87	18.1	0.0	65.77	342.4	290.3	1.0
	4.00	oz							
Mixed species, farmed, cooked, moist heat	100.0	g	87	17.5	0.0	97.00	238.0	241.0	0.2
	85.05	g	74	14.9	0.0	82.50	202.4	204.9	0.1
	3.00	oz							
mixed species, wild, cooked, moist heat	100.0	g	82	16.8	0.0	94.00	296.0	270.0	1.2
	85.05	g	70	14.3	0.0	79.95	251.7	229.6	1.0
	3.00	oz							
SQUID (CALAMARI)									
mixed species, fried	100.0	g	175	17.9	7.8	306.0	279.0	251.0	7.48
	85.05	g	149	15.3	6.6	260.3	237.3	213.4	6.36
	3.00	oz							
mixed species, raw boneless	100.0	g	92	15.6	3.1	44.00	246.0	221.0	1.38
	113.4	g	104	17.7	3.5	49.90	278.9	250.6	1.56
	4.00	oz							

EGG

	SERVING QUANTITY	SERVING UNIT	CALORIES (kcal)	PROTEIN (g)	TOTAL CARBOHYDRATES (g)	SODIUM (mg)	POTASSIUM (mg)	PHOSPHORUS (mg)	TOTAL FAT (g)
chicken, raw, large	100.0	g	143	12.6	0.7	142.0	138.0	198.0	9.51
	50.00	g	72	6.3	0.4	71.00	69.00	99.00	4.76
	1.00	pc							
chicken, fried, large	100.0	g	196	13.6	0.8	207.0	152.0	215.0	14.84
	46.00	g	90	6.3	0.4	95.22	69.92	98.90	6.83
	1.00	pc							
chicken, poached, large	100.0	g	143	12.5	0.7	297.0	138.0	197.0	9.47
	50.00	g	72	6.3	0.4	148.5	69.00	98.50	4.74
	1.00	pc							
chicken, hard boiled, large	100.0	g	155	12.6	1.1	124.0	126.0	172.0	10.61
	50.00	g	78	6.3	0.6	62.00	63.00	86.00	5.31
	1.00	pc							
scrambled, fast food	100.0	g	212	13.8	2.1	187.0	147.0	242.0	16.18
	94.00	g	199	13.0	2.0	175.7	138.1	227.4	15.21
	2.00	pc							
substitute, liquid	100.0	g	84	12.0	0.6	177.0	330.0	121.0	3.31
	251.0	g	211	30.1	1.6	444.2	828.3	303.7	8.31
	1.00	c							
substitute, powder	100.0	g	443	55.8	22	798.2	742.3	476.9	12.97
	9.92	g	44	5.5	2.2	79.20	73.66	47.32	1.29
	0.35	oz							
substitute, frozen	100.0	g	160	11.3	3.2	199.0	213.0	72.00	11.11
	60.00	g	96	6.8	1.9	119.4	127.8	43.20	6.67
	0.25	c							
chicken, egg whites only, raw large egg	100.0	g	52	10.9	0.7	166.0	163.0	15.00	0.17
	33.00	g	17	3.6	0.2	54.78	53.79	4.95	0.06
	1.00	pc							
chicken, yolk only, raw large egg	100.0	g	322	15.9	3.6	48.00	109.0	390.0	26.54
	17.00	g	55	2.7	0.6	8.16	18.53	66.30	4.51
	1.00	pc							
chicken, whole, raw, frozen	100.0	g	147	12.3	1.0	128.0	135.0	193.0	9.95
	56.70	g	83	7.0	0.6	72.57	76.54	109.4	5.64
	2.00	oz							
yolk only, frozen, raw	100.0	g	296	15.5	0.8	67.00	121.0	420.0	25.60
	56.70	g	168	8.8	0.5	37.99	68.61	238.1	14.51
	2.00	oz							
whites, frozen, raw	100.0	g	48	10.2	1.0	169.0	169.0	13.00	0.00
	56.70	g	27	5.8	0.6	95.82	95.82	7.37	0.00
	2.00	oz							
duck, raw	100.0	g	185	12.8	1.5	146.0	222.0	220.0	13.77
	70.00	g	130	9.0	1.0	102.2	155.4	154.0	9.64
	1.00	pc							
quail, raw	100.0	g	158	13.1	0.4	141.0	132.0	226.0	11.09
	9.00	g	14	1.2	0.0	12.69	11.88	20.34	1.00
	1.00	pc							

CHICKEN	SERVING QUANTITY	SERVING UNIT	CALORIES (kcal)	PROTEIN (g)	TOTAL CARBOHYDRATES (g)	SODIUM (mg)	POTASSIUM (mg)	PHOSPHORUS (mg)	TOTAL
ground, raw	100.0	g	143	17.4	0.0	60.00	522.0	178.0	8.10
meat and skin,	100.0	g	215	18.6	0.0	70.00	189.0	147.0	15.0
raw	113.4	g	244	21.1	0.0	79.38	214.3	166.7	17.0
	4.00	oz							
meat and skin,	100.0	g	239	27.3	0.0	82.00	223.0	182.0	13.6
roasted	85.05	g	203	23.2	0.0	69.74	189.6	154.8	11.5
	3.00	oz							
thigh meat	100.0	g	218	28.2	1.2	95.00	259.0	199.0	10.3
only, fried	85.05	g	185	24.0	1.0	80.80	220.2	169.2	8.76
	3.00	oz							
thigh meat	100.0	g	179	24.8	0.0	106.0	269.0	230.0	8.15
only, roasted	85.05	g	152	21.1	0.0	90.15	228.7	195.6	6.93
	3.00	oz							
wing meat	100.0	g	211	30.2	0.0	91.00	208.0	164.0	9.15
only, fried	85.05	g	179	25.6	0.0	77.39	176.9	139.4	7.78
	3.00	oz							
wing meat	100.0	g	203	30.5	0.0	92.00	210.0	166.0	8.13
only, roasted	85.05	g	173	26.0	0.0	78.25	178.6	141.1	6.91
	3.00	oz							
wing meat	100.0	g	181	27.2	0.0	73.00	153.0	134.0	7.18
only, stewed	85.05	g	154	23.1	0.0	62.09	130.1	113.9	6.11
	3.00	oz							
back meat	100.0	g	288	30.0	5.7	99.00	251.0	176.0	4.12
only, fried	85.05	g	245	25.5	4.8	84.20	213.4	149.7	3.50
	3.00	oz							
back meat	100.0	g	239	28.2	0.0	96.00	237.0	165.0	13.1
only, roasted	85.05	g	203	24.0	0.0	81.65	201.5	140.3	11.1
	3.00	oz							
back meat	100.0	g	209	25.3	0.0	67.00	158.0	130.0	11.1
only, stewed	85.05	g	178	21.5	0.0	56.98	134.3	110.5	9.52
	3.00	oz							
drumstick	100.0	g	195	28.6	0.0	96.00	249.0	186.0	8.08
meat only, fried	85.05	g	166	24.3	0.0	81.65	211.7	158.2	6.87
	3.00	oz							
drumstick	100.0	g	155	24.2	0.0	128.0	256.0	200.0	5.70
meat only, roasted	85.05	g	132	20.6	0.0	108.8	217.7	170.1	4.85
	3	oz							

CHICKEN

	SERVING QUANTITY	SERVING UNIT	CALORIES (kcal)	PROTEIN (g)	TOTAL CARBOHYDRATES (g)	SODIUM (mg)	POTASSIUM (mg)	PHOSPHORUS (mg)	TOTAL FAT (g)
drumstick meat only, stewed	100.0	g	169	27.5	0.0	80.00	199.0	150.0	5.71
	85.05 3.00	g oz	144	23.4	0.0	68.04	169.2	127.5	4.86
leg meat only, fried	100.0	g	208	28.4	0.7	96.00	254.0	193.0	9.32
	85.05 3.00	g oz	177	24.1	0.6	81.65	216.0	164.1	7.93
leg meat only, roasted	100.0	g	174	24.2	0.0	99.00	269.0	205.0	7.80
	85.05 3.00	g oz	148	20.6	0.0	84.20	228.7	174.3	6.63
leg meat only, stewed	100.0	g	185	26.3	0.0	78.00	190.0	149.0	8.06
	85.05 3.00	g oz	157	22.3	0.0	66.34	161.6	126.7	6.85
pate, chicken liver, canned	100.0	g	201	13.5	6.6	386.0	95.00	175.0	13.10
	52.00 4.00	g tbsp	105	7.0	3.4	200.7	49.40	91.00	6.81
chicken tenders, fast food	100.0	g	271	19.2	17.3	769.0	373.0	282.0	13.95
	62.00 4.00	g pcs	168	11.9	10.7	476.8	231.2	174.8	8.65
chicken patty, frozen, cooked	100.0	g	287	14.9	12.8	532.0	261.0	208.0	19.58
bratwurst, chicken, cooked	100.0	g	176	19.4	0.0	72.00	211.0	160.0	10.30
	83.92 2.96	g oz	148	16.3	0.0	60.42	177.0	134.2	8.69
sausage, chicken/beef, smoked	100.0	g	295	18.5	0.0	1,020	139.0	111.0	244.0
	138.0 1.00	g c	251	15.7	0.0	867.5	118.2	94.41	20.41

TURKEY	SERVING QUANTITY	SERVING UNIT	CALORIES (kcal)	PROTEIN (g)	TOTAL CARBOHYDRATES (g)	SODIUM (mg)	POTASSIUM (mg)	PHOSPHORUS (mg)	TOTAL F
breast, meat & skin, raw	100.0	g	144	21.6	0.1	112.0	224.0	183.0	5.64
	113.4	g	163	24.5	0.2	127.0	254.0	207.5	6.40
	4.00	oz							
breast, meat & skin, roasted	100.0	g	189	28.6	0.1	103.0	239.0	223.0	7.39
	85.05	g	161	24.3	0.1	87.60	203.2	189.6	6.29
	3.00	oz							
breast, meat only, raw	100.0	g	114	23.3	0.0	74.00	267.0	185.0	2.33
	85.05	g	97	19.9	0.0	62.94	227.0	157.3	1.98
	3.00	oz							
breast, meat only, roasted	100.0	g	136	29.5	0.0	114.0	297.0	253.0	1.97
	85.05	g	116	25.1	0.0	96.96	252.6	215.1	1.68
	3.00	oz							
ground, raw	100.0	g	148	20.0	0.0	58.00	237.0	200.0	7.66
	113.4	g	168	22.3	0.0	65.77	268.7	226.8	8.69
	4.00	oz							
ground, cooked	100.0	g	203	27.4	0.0	78.00	294.0	254.0	10.4
	85.05	g	173	23.3	0.0	66.34	250.0	216.0	8.85
	3.00	oz							
white rotisserie, deli cut	100.0	g	112	13.5	7.7	1,200	349.0	158.0	3.00
	56.70	g	64	7.7	4.4	680.4	197.8	89.59	1.70
	2.00	oz							
ham, extra lean, sliced	100.0	g	134	19.6	0.9	1,038	299.0	304.0	5.80
	20.00	g	27	3.9	0.2	207.6	59.80	60.80	1.16
	1.00	pc							
pastrami, sliced	100.0	g	139	16.3	3.3	1,123	345.0	200.0	6.21
	56.70	g	79	9.2	1.9	636.7	195.6	113.4	3.52
	2.00	slices							
bologna	100.0	g	209	11.4	4.7	1,071	135.0	114.0	16.0
	56.70	g	119	6.5	2.7	607.2	76.55	64.64	9.10
	2.00	slices							
salami	100.0	g	172	19.2	1.6	1,107	216.0	266.0	9.21
	56.70	g	98	10.9	0.9	627.6	122.4	150.8	5.22
	2.00	slices							
bacon, turkey, cooked	100.0	g	382	29.6	3.1	2,285	395.0	460.0	27.9
	28.35	g	108	8.4	0.9	647.8	111.9	130.4	7.91
	1.00	oz							
bacon, turkey, low sodium	100.0	g	253	13.3	4.8	900.0	156.0	145.0	20.0
	15.00	g	38	2.0	0.7	135.0	23.40	21.75	3.00
	1.00	svg							
sausage, turkey, cooked	100.0	g	196	23.9	0.0	665.0	298.0	202.0	10.4
	56.70	g	111	13.6	0.0	377.0	168.9	114.5	5.92
	2.00	oz							

PORK

	Serving Quantity	Serving Unit	Calories (kcal)	Protein (g)	Total Carbohydrates (g)	Sodium (mg)	Potassium (mg)	Phosphorus (mg)	Total Fat (g)
ground, cooked	100.0	g	297	25.7	0.0	73.00	362.0	226.0	20.77
	85.05	g	253	21.9	0.0	62.09	307.8	192.2	17.66
	3.00	oz							
ground, raw	100.0	g	263	16.9	0.0	56.00	287.0	175.0	21.19
	113.4	g	298	19.1	0.0	63.50	325.4	198.4	24.03
	4.00	oz							
loin, sirloin, roasts, separable lean roasted	100.0	g	204	27.8	0.0	59.00	352.0	235.0	9.44
	85.05	g	174	23.6	0.0	50.18	299.3	199.8	8.03
	3.00	oz							
loin, center rib, separable lean, roasted	100.0	g	206	28.8	0.0	95.00	287.0	244.0	9.21
	85.05	g	175	24.5	0.0	80.80	244.1	207.5	7.83
	3.00	oz							
loin, sirloin, boneless, separable lean roasted	100.0	g	178	30.4	0.0	66.00	408.0	311.0	5.31
	85.05	g	151	25.9	0.0	56.13	347.0	264.5	4.52
	3.00	oz							
loin, center rib, boneless roasted	100.0	g	214	28.8	0.0	50.00	363.0	222.0	10.13
	85.05	g	182	24.5	0.0	42.52	308.7	188.8	8.62
	3.00	oz							
shoulder blade, boston roasts roasted turkey, salt.	100.0	g	232	24.2	0.0	88.00	427.0	235.0	14.30
	85.05	g	197	20.6	0.0	74.84	363.1	199.8	12.16
	3.00	oz							
shoulder, whole, roasted	100.0	g	230	25.3	0.0	74.96	345.8	220.8	13.53
	85.05	g	196	21.5	0.0	63.75	294.1	187.8	11.51
	3.00	oz							
loin, whole, roasted	100.0	g	209	28.6	0.0	58.00	425.0	249.0	9.63
	85.05	g	178	24.3	0.0	49.33	361.4	211.7	8.19
	3.00	oz							
leg or ham, whole, roasted	100.0	g	211	29.4	0.0	64.00	373.0	281.0	9.44
	85.05	g	179	25.0	0.0	54.43	317.2	239.0	8.03
	3.00	oz							
loin, tenderloin, separable lean & fat roasted	100.0	g	147	26.0	0.0	57.00	419.0	265.0	3.96
	85.05	g	125	22.2	0.0	48.48	356.3	225.3	3.37
	3.00	oz							
ground, cooked	100.0	g	297	25.7	0.0	73.00	362.0	226.0	20.77
	85.05	g	253	21.9	0.0	62.09	307.8	192.2	17.66
	3.00	oz							

PORK

	SERVING QUANTITY	SERVING UNIT	CALORIES (kcal)	PROTEIN (g)	TOTAL CARBOHYDRATES (g)	SODIUM (mg)	POTASSIUM (mg)	PHOSPHORUS (mg)	TOTAL F
bacon, cured, broiled, panfried or roasted	100.0	g	541	37.0	1.4	1,717	565.0	533.0	41.7
	8.00	g	43	3.0	0.1	137.3	45.20	42.64	3.34
	1.00	slice							
bacon, reduced sodium, cured, broiled, panfried or roasted	100.0	g	541	37.0	1.4	1,030	565.0	533.0	41.7
	56.70	g	307	21.0	0.8	584.0	320.4	302.2	23.6
	2.00	oz							
country style ribs, separable lean & fat roasted	100.0	g	359	21.8	0.0	52.00	322.0	214.0	29.4
	85.05	g	305	18.5	0.0	44.23	273.9	182.0	25.0
	3.00	oz							
sirloin, chops or roasts, boneless, raw	100.0	g	121	22.8	0.0	63.00	354.0	251.0	2.59
	113.4	g	137	25.9	0.0	71.44	401.4	284.6	2.94
	4.00	oz							
kidney, braised	100.0	g	151	25.4	0.0	80.00	143.0	240.0	4.70
	85.05	g	128	21.6	0.0	68.04	121.6	204.1	4.00
	3.00	oz							
liver, braised	100.0	g	165	26.0	3.8	49.00	150.0	241.0	4.40
	85.05	g	140	22.1	3.2	41.67	127.6	205.0	3.74
	3.00	oz							
ham, minced, sliced	100.0	g	263	16.3	1.8	1,245	311.0	157.0	20.6
	21.00	g	55	3.4	0.4	261.4	65.31	32.97	4.34
	1.00	slice							
ham, extra lean, 5% fat	100.0	g	107	16.9	0.7	945.0	463.0	252.0	4.04
	85.05	g	91	14.3	0.6	803.7	393.8	214.3	3.44
	3.00	oz							
ham, low sodium, cured, cooked	100.0	g	165	22.0	0.5	969.0	362.0	248.0	7.70
	85.05	g	140	18.7	0.4	824.1	307.9	210.9	6.55
	3.00	oz							
sausages, Kielbasa, grilled	100.0	g	337	12.5	5.0	1,062	306.0	204.0	29.6
	85.05	g	287	10.6	4.3	903.2	260.3	173.5	25.2
	3.00	oz							
Kielbasa, panfried	100.0	g	333	12.4	4.8	1,046	304.0	199.0	29.4
	85.05	g	283	10.5	4.1	889.6	258.6	169.3	25.0
	3.00	oz							
Beerwurst, pork/beef	100.0	g	276	14.0	4.3	732.0	244.0	135.0	22.5
	56.70	g	156	7.9	2.4	415.0	138.4	76.6	12.7
	2.00	oz							

PORK

	SERVING QUANTITY	SERVING UNIT	CALORIES (kcal)	PROTEIN (g)	TOTAL CARBOHYDRATES	SODIUM (mg)	POTASSIUM (mg)	PHOSPHORUS (mg)	TOTAL FAT (g)
Italian Sweet, links	100.0	g	149	16.1	2.1	570.0	194.0	103.0	8.42
	85.053	g oz	127	13.7	1.8	484.8	165.0	87.60	7.16
Polish, pork, cooked	100.0	g	326	14.1	1.6	876.0	237.0	136.0	28.72
	56.702	g oz	185	8.0	0.9	496.6	134.3	77.11	16.28
Bratwurst, pork, cooked	100.0	g	333	13.7	2.9	846.0	348.0	208.0	29.18
	56.702	g oz	189	7.8	1.6	479.6	197.3	117.9	16.54
meatloaf/ luncheon meat pork/beef	100.0	g	260	15.4	1.6	1,182	245.0	122.0	20.90
	2.01	g slice	60	3.5	0.4	271.8	56.35	28.06	4.81
peperoni, beef/pork	100.0	g	504	19.3	1.2	1,582	274.0	158.0	46.28
	56.702	g oz	286	11.0	0.7	896.9	155.3	89.58	26.24
salami, italian, pork	100.0	g	425	21.7	1.2	1,890	340.0	229.0	37.00
	28.351	g oz	120	6.2	0.3	535.8	96.39	64.92	10.49

BEEF

	SERVING QUANTITY	SERVING UNIT	CALORIES (kcal)	PROTEIN (g)	TOTAL CARBOHYDRATES (g)	SODIUM (mg)	POTASSIUM (mg)	PHOSPHORUS (mg)	TOTAL
chuck eyeroast, boneless, all grades 0" fat, separable lean only, roasted	3.0 85.05 3.00	g g oz	183 156	26.7 22.7	0.0 0.0	68.04 80.00	344.0 292.5	210.0 178.6	8.4(7.2(
chuck eyeroast, boneless, all grades separable lean only, 0", raw	100.0 85.05 3.00	g g oz	137 117	20.6 17.5	0.0 0.0	85.00 72.29	357.0 303.6	204.0 173.5	6.0 5.1
chuck eyeroast, boneless, all grades sep lean & fat, 0" fat, roasted	100.0 85.05 3.00	g g oz	236 201	24.6 21.0	0.0 0.0	76.00 64.64	308.0 261.9	187.0 159.0	15.: 13.(
chuck eyeroast, boneless, all grades sep lean & fat, 0" fat, raw	100.0 85.05 3.00	g g oz	173 147	19.3 16.4	0.0 0.0	82.00 69.74	367.0 312.1	187.0 159.0	10.(9.0
jerky	100.0 28.35 1.00	g g oz	410 116	33.2 9.4	11 3.1	1,785 506.0	597.0 169.2	407.0 115.3	25.(7.2(
corned beef, brisket, raw	100.0 113.4 4.00	g g oz	198 225	14.7 16.7	0.1 0.2	1,217 1,380	297.0 336.8	117.0 132.6	14.(16.(
corned beef, brisket, cooked	100.0 85.05 3.00	g g oz	251 213	18.2 15.5	0.5 0.4	928.0 827.5	145.0 123.3	125.0 106.3	18.(16.
broth cube 1 cube, 6 fl. oz prepared	100.0 3.60 1.00	g g cube	170 6	17.3 0.6	16 0.6	24,000 864.0	403.0 14.51	225.0 8.10	4.0(0.1-
liver, pan fried	100.0 81.00 1.00	g g slice	175 142	26.5 21.5	5.2 4.2	77.00 62.37	351.0 284.3	485.0 392.8	4.6(3.7(
liver, braised	100.0 85.05 3.00	g g oz	191 162	29.1 24.7	5.1 4.4	79.00 67.19	352.0 299.3	497.0 422.7	5.2(4.4
tongue, simmered	100.0 85.05 3.00	g g oz	284 242	19.3 16.4	0.0 0.0	65.00 55.28	184.0 156.5	145.0 123.3	22.: 18.(
kidney simmered	100.0 85.05 3.00	g g oz	158 134	27.3 23.2	0.0 0.0	94.00 79.95	135.0 114.8	304.0 258.5	4.6(3.9(
tripe, simmered	100.0 85.05 3.00	g g oz	94 80	11.7 10.0	2.0 1.7	68.00 57.83	42.00 35.72	66.00 56.13	4.0(3.4-

LAMB

	SERVING QUANTITY	SERVING UNIT	CALORIES (kcal)	PROTEIN (g)	TOTAL CARBOHYDRATES (g)	SODIUM (mg)	POTASSIUM (mg)	PHOSPHORUS (mg)	TOTAL FAT (g)
tenderloin, New Zealand, separable lean only, raw	100.0	g	116	20.5	0.0	49.00	381.0	222.0	3.81
	85.05	g	99	17.5	0.0	41.67	324.0	188.8	3.24
	3.00	oz							
loin, NZ, separable lean, frozen, broiled	100.0	g	199	29.3	0.0	55.00	189.0	240.0	8.24
	85.05	g	169	24.9	0.0	46.78	160.7	204.1	7.01
	3.00	oz							
australian, separable lean, 1/8" fat, cooked	100.0	g	201	26.7	0.0	80.00	318.0	207.0	9.63
	85.05	g	171	22.7	0.0	68.04	270.4	176.0	8.19
	3.00	oz							
Australian, separable lean, 1/8" fat, raw	100.0	g	142	20.3	0.0	83.00	320.0	188.0	6.18
	113.4	g	161	23.0	0.0	94.12	362.8	213.2	7.01
	4.00	oz							
Australian, ground, 85%Lean/15%fat, raw	100.0	g	255	17.1	0.0	65.49	Na	Na	20.17
	85.05	g	217	14.6	0.0	77.00	Na	Na	17.61
	3.00	oz							
NZ, rib, separable lean, frozen, raw	100.0	g	160	20.7	0.0	67.00	309.0	185.0	8.61
	113.4	g	181	23.4	0.0	75.98	350.4	209.8	9.76
	4.00	oz							
NZ, rib, separable lean, frozen, roasted	100.0	g	193	24.4	0.0	72.00	323.0	209.0	10.63
	85.05	g	164	20.8	0.0	61.24	274.7	177.7	9.04
	3.00	oz							

VEAL

	SERVING QUANTITY	SERVING UNIT	CALORIES (kcal)	PROTEIN (g)	TOTAL CARBOHYDRATES (g)	SODIUM (mg)	POTASSIUM (mg)	PHOSPHORUS (mg)	TOTAL FAT (g)
separable lean, cooked	100.0	g	196	32.0	0.0	89.00	338.0	250.0	6.58
	85.05	g	167	27.1	0.0	75.69	287.4	212.6	5.60
	3.00	oz							
liver, pan fried	100.0	g	193	27.4	4.5	85.00	353.0	483.0	6.51
	85.05	g	164	23.3	3.8	72.29	300.2	410.8	5.54
	3.00	oz							
sausage, bratwurst, veal, cooked	100.0	g	341	14.0	0.0	60.00	231.0	150.0	31.70
	83.92	g	286	11.7	0.0	50.35	193.8	125.8	26.60
	2.96	oz							
ground, pan fried	100.0	g	503	8.9	0.9	89.00	107.0	133.0	51.60
	85.05	g	428	7.5	0.8	75.69	91.00	113.1	43.89
	3.00	oz							

VEAL

	SERVING QUANTITY	SERVING UNIT	CALORIES (kcal)	PROTEIN (g)	TOTAL CARBOHYDRATES (g)	SODIUM (mg)	POTASSIUM (mg)	PHOSPHORUS (mg)	TOTAL FAT (g)
sirloin, separable, lean, braised	100.0	g	204	34.0	0.0	81.00	339.0	259.0	6.51
	85.05	g	174	28.9	0.0	68.89	288.3	220.2	5.54
	3.00	oz							
sirloin separable lean, roasted	100.0	g	168	26.3	0.0	85.00	365.0	231.0	6.22
	85.05	g	143	22.4	0.0	72.29	310.4	196.4	5.29
	3.00	oz							
sirloin, lean, raw	100.0	g	110	20.2	0.0	80.00	348.0	220.0	2.59
	113.4	g	125	22.9	0.0	90.72	394.6	249.4	2.94
	4.00	oz							
loin, lean and fat, braised	100.0	g	284	30.2	0.0	80.00	280.0	220.0	17.21
	85.05	g	242	25.7	0.0	68.04	238.1	187.1	14.64
	3.00	oz							
loin, lean and fat, roasted	100.0	g	217	25.0	0.0	93.00	325.0	212.0	12.32
	85.05	g	185	21.1	0.0	79.10	276.4	180.3	10.48
	3.00	oz							
loin, lean, braised	100.0	g	226	33.6	0.0	84.00	297.0	237.0	9.15
	85.05	g	192	28.6	0.0	71.44	252.6	201.5	7.78
	3.00	oz							
loin, lean, roasted	100.0	g	175	26.3	0.0	96.00	340.0	222.0	6.94
	85.05	g	149	22.4	0.0	81.65	289.1	188.8	5.90
	3.00	oz							
loin, lean, raw	100.0	g	114	21.9	0.0	99.00	260.0	237.0	2.90
	113.4	g	129	24.8	0.0	112.2	294.8	268.7	3.29
	4.00	oz							
loin, chop, lean and fat, grilled	100.0	g	198	28.0	0.2	86.00	229.0	208.0	9.48
	85.05	g	168	23.9	0.1	73.14	194.7	176.9	8.06
	3.00	oz							
bratwwurst, veal, cooked	100.0	g	341	14.0	0.0	60.00	231.0	150.0	31.70
	83.92	g	286	11.7	0.0	50.35	193.8	125.8	26.60
	2.96	oz							

H. Herbs and Spices

Hey there!

Do you need to print out this Food List?

You can download a printable version of this chart by scanning the QR code below or copying the link on your computer browser.

https://go.renaltracker.com/printfoodlist

	SERVING QUANTITY	SERVING UNIT	CALORIES (kcal)	PROTEIN (g)	TOTAL CARBOHYDRATES (g)	SODIUM (mg)	POTASSIUM (mg)	PHOSPHORUS (mg)	TOTAL FAT (g)
ONION									
red, raw	100.0	g	44	0.94	9.93	1	197	41	0.1
1 onion	197.0	g	86.7	1.85	19.6	1.97	388	80.8	0.19
white, raw	100.0	g	36	0.89	7.68	2	141	29	0.13
yellow, raw	100.0	g	38	0.83	8.61	1	182	34	0.05
1 onion	143.0	g	54.3	1.19	12.3	1.43	260	48.6	0.07
GARLIC									
raw	100.0	g	149	6.36	33.1	17	401	153	0.5
3 cloves	9.0	g	13.4	0.572	2.98	1.53	36.1	13.8	0.04
GINGER									
raw	100.0	g	80	1.82	17.8	13	415	34	0.75
SPRING ONIONS									
raw	100.0	g	32	1.83	7.34	16	276	37	0.19
1 large	25.0	g	8	0.458	1.84	4	69	9.25	0.04
CHIVES									
raw	100.0	g	30	3.27	4.35	3	296	58	0.73
BASIL									
fresh	100.0	g	23	3.15	2.65	4	295	56	0.64
dried	100.0	g	233	23	47.8	76	2630	274	4.07
OREGANO									
dried	100.0	g	265	9	68.9	25	1260	148	4.28
ROSEMARY									
fresh	100.0	g	131	3.31	20.7	26	668	66	5.86
dried	100.0	g	331	4.88	64.1	50	995	70	15.2
MARJORAM									
dried	100.0	g	271	12.7	60.6	77	1520	306	7.04

	SERVING QUANTITY	SERVING UNIT	CALORIES (kcal)	PROTEIN (g)	TOTAL CARBOHYDRATES (g)	SODIUM (mg)	POTASSIUM (mg)	PHOSPHORUS (mg)	TOTAL FAT (g)
SAGE									
ground	100.0	g	315	10.6	60.7	11	1070	91	12.8
1 Tbsp	2.0	g	6.3	0.21	1.21	0.22	21.4	1.82	0.25
CINNAMON									
ground	100.0	g	247	3.99	80.6	10	431	64	1.24
1 Tbsp	7.8.0	g	19.3	0.31	6.29	0.78	33.6	4.99	0.09
CUMIN									
seed	100.0	g	375	17.8	44.2	168	1790	499	22.3
1 Tbsp Whole	6.0	g	22.5	1.07	2.65	10.1	107	29.9	1.34
NUTMEG									
ground	100.0	g	525	5.84	49.3	16	350	213	36.3
1 tsp	7.0	g	36.8	0.41	3.45	1.12	24.5	14.9	2.54
CLOVES									
ground	100.0	g	274	5.97	65.5	277	1020	104	13
1 tsp	6.5	g	17.8	0.39	4.26	18	66.3	6.76	0.84
PARSLEY									
fresh	100.0	g	36	2.97	6.33	56	554	58	0.79
dried	100.0	g	292	26.6	50.6	452	2680	436	5.48
CORIANDER									
seed	100.0	g	298	12.4	55	35	1270	409	17.8
leaves, raw	100.0	g	23	2.13	3.67	46	521	48	0.52
THYME									
fresh	100.0	g	101	5.56	24.4	9	609	106	1.68
dried	100.0	g	276	9.11	63.9	55	814	201	7.43
LEMON GRASS									
citronella, raw	100.0	g	99	1.82	25.3	6	723	101	0.49

	SERVING QUANTITY	SERVING UNIT	CALORIES (kcal)	PROTEIN (g)	TOTAL CARBOHYDRATES (g)	SODIUM (mg)	POTASSIUM (mg)	PHOSPHORUS (mg)	TOTAL FAT (g)
FENNEL									
Bulb, raw	100.0	g	31	1.24	7.3	52	414	50	0.2
seed	100.0	g	345	15.8	52.3	88	1690	487	14.9
1 Tbsp	5.8	g	20	0.92	3.03	5.1	98	28	0.86
DILL									
weed, fresh	100.0	g	43	3.46	7.02	61	738	66	1.12
weed, dried	100.0	g	253	20	55.8	208	3310	543	4.36
1 Tbsp	3.1	g	7.8	0.62	1.73	6.45	103	16.8	0.13
ANISE									
seed	100.0	g	337	17.6	50	16	1440	440	15.9
1 Tbsp	6.7	g	22.6	1.18	3.35	1.07	96.5	29.5	1.06
CARDAMOM									
spices	100.0	g	311	10.8	68.5	18	1120	229	6.7
1 Tbsp	5.8	g	18	0.63	3.97	1.04	65	10.3	0.39
CAYENNE									
pepper, red or cayenne	100.0	g	318	12	56.6	30	2010	293	17.3
1 tbsp	5.3	g	16.9	0.64	3	1.59	107	15.5	0.91
CURRY POWDER									
	100.0	g	325	14.3	55.8	52	1170	367	14
1 tbsp	6.3	g	20.5	0.90	3.52	3.28	73.7	23.1	0.88
PAPRIKA									
ground	100.0	g	282	14.1	54	68	2280	314	12.9
1 tbsp	6.8	g	19.2	0.96	3.67	4.62	155	21.4	0.87
CELERY									
celery, raw	100.0	g	14	0.69	2.97	80	260	24	0.17

	SERVING QUANTITY	SERVING UNIT	CALORIES (kcal)	PROTEIN (g)	TOTAL CARBOHYDRATES (g)	SODIUM (mg)	POTASSIUM (mg)	PHOSPHORUS (mg)	TOTAL
SAFFRON									
	100.0	g	310	11.4	65.4	148	1720	252	5.8
1 tbsp	2.1	g	6.51	0.24	1.37	3.11	36.1	5.29	0.
PEPPER, BLACK									
ground	100.0	g	251	10.4	64	20	1330	158	3.
1 tbsp	6.9	g	17.3	0.72	4.42	1.38	91.8	10.9	0.
PEPPER, WHITE									
ground	100.0	g	296	10.4	68.6	5	73	176	2.
1 tbsp	7.1	g	21	0.74	4.87	0.35	5.18	12.5	0.
TARRAGON									
dried	100.0	g	295	22.8	50.2	62	3020	313	7.
1 Tbsp, leaves	1.8	g	5.31	0.41	0.90	1.12	54.4	5.63	0.
1 Tbsp, ground	4.8	g	14.2	1.09	2.41	2.98	145	15	0.
HORSERADISH									
	100.0	g	48	1.18	11.3	420	246	31	0.
1 tbsp	15.0	g	7.2	0.18	1.7	63	36.9	4.65	0.

Chapter 5: Flavor Without the Pinch

Low-Sodium Recipe Ideas

Fantastic! Having navigated the essential groundwork of understanding a low-sodium diet for kidney health, including a comprehensive exploration of food lists and items to thoughtfully incorporate or avoid, we now arrive at a truly exciting juncture: putting that knowledge into flavorful practice. This chapter is your personal invitation to step into the kitchen with confidence and discover the delicious possibilities that await. Think of it as your culinary launchpad, providing a curated selection of sample low-sodium recipes meticulously designed to ignite your cooking creativity and nourish your body.

Within these pages, you'll find a diverse array of options, spanning satisfying breakfasts to power-packed lunches, comforting dinners, and guilt-free snacks. Each recipe serves not just as a meal idea, but as a tangible example of how to apply the principles you've learned. We delve beyond mere ingredients and instructions, offering insights into the nutritional profile of each dish, with a keen focus on its low sodium content and how it aligns with the needs of individuals managing kidney disease.

Furthermore, we'll touch upon the sustainability aspects of the ingredients, encouraging choices that are both good for you and the planet. And importantly, we'll highlight any specific precautions to keep in mind, ensuring that your culinary explorations are both safe and beneficial. Consider these recipes as your initial guides, your trusted companions as you begin to experiment and adapt to a low-sodium lifestyle. They are intended to spark your imagination, demonstrating that eating well while managing kidney disease can be a vibrant and enjoyable experience. So, let's turn the page and embark on a delicious adventure, transforming knowledge into truly nourishing and flavorful meals!

BREAKFAST

Low-Sodium Vegetable Omelet

Ingredients

- 2 large egg whites (or 1 whole egg if preferred)
- 1/2 cup fresh spinach (chopped)
- 1/4 cup bell pepper (diced; any color)
- 1/4 cup onion (diced)
- 1/4 cup mushrooms (sliced)
- 1 tablespoon olive oil (for cooking)
- 1/4 teaspoon black pepper (to taste)
- 1/4 teaspoon garlic powder (optional)
- Fresh herbs (such as parsley or chives, for garnish; optional)

Directions

1. Prepare Vegetables: Wash and chop the spinach, bell pepper, onion, and mushrooms.
2. Sauté Vegetables: In a non-stick skillet, heat 1 tablespoon of olive oil over medium heat. Add the diced onion and sauté for about 2-3 minutes until it becomes translucent. Add the bell pepper and mushrooms, and cook for another 3-4 minutes until tender. Stir in the spinach and cook until wilted.
3. Prepare Egg Mixture: In a bowl, whisk the egg whites (or whole egg) with black pepper and garlic powder (if using).
4. Cook Omelet: Pour the egg mixture over the sautéed vegetables in the skillet. Cook on medium-low heat, gently lifting the edges with a spatula to allow uncooked egg to flow to the edges. Cook until the egg is set (about 3-5 minutes).
5. Serve: Carefully fold the omelet in half and slide it onto a plate. Garnish with fresh herbs if desired.

Servings: 1
Preparation Time: Approximately 10 minutes
Cooking Time: Approximately 10 minutes
Total Time: 20 minutes

Nutritional Information per Serving

- Calories: 150 kcal (approximately)
- Carbohydrates: 7 g
- Fat: 10 g
- Protein: 12 g
- Potassium: 400 mg (may vary based on vegetables)
- Phosphorus: 100 mg
- Sodium: 100 mg (depending on added salt and seasoning)

Why is this good for you?

- *This vegetable omelet is low in sodium, making it an excellent option for individuals needing to limit their salt intake. The dish is flavorful due to the combination of fresh vegetables and herbs, allowing for a satisfying meal without the need for added salt.*
- *Sustainability: The Low-Sodium Vegetable Omelet is a sustainable recipe for patients following a low-sodium diet. It utilizes fresh, whole ingredients that are nutrient-dense and can help maintain heart health and weight management. The flexibility of the recipe allows for seasonal vegetables, making it adaptable to different times of the year and reducing environmental impact.*

SPECIAL PRECAUTIONS!

- Monitor portion sizes of vegetables to manage potassium and phosphorus intake, especially for individuals who need to restrict these nutrients.
- Ensure that any additional ingredients, such as cheese or condiments, are low-sodium if added to the omelet.
- Consult with a healthcare provider or dietitian for personalized dietary advice, especially regarding egg consumption if cholesterol is a concern.

Oatmeal with Fresh Fruits

Ingredients

- 1 cup rolled oats (gluten-free if needed)
- 2 cups water or unsweetened almond milk (for cooking oats)
- 1 medium banana (sliced)
- 1/2 cup mixed berries (e.g., strawberries, blueberries, raspberries)
- 1/4 cup apple (diced)
- 1 tablespoon chia seeds (optional, for added fiber and omega-3)
- 1 teaspoon cinnamon (optional, for flavor)
- Honey or maple syrup (optional, adjust based on sweetness preference)

Directions

1. Cook Oats: In a saucepan, bring 2 cups of water or almond milk to a boil. Stir in the rolled oats, reduce the heat to low, and simmer for about 5-7 minutes, stirring occasionally until the oats are tender and the liquid is absorbed.
2. Prepare Fruits: While the oatmeal is cooking, wash and prepare the fresh fruits. Slice the banana, and if using, dice the apple.
3. Mix in Chia Seeds: If using chia seeds, stir them into the cooked oatmeal during the last minute of cooking to allow them to absorb moisture.
4. Add Flavoring: Stir in the cinnamon and any sweetener (honey or maple syrup) if desired.
5. Serve: Divide the oatmeal into bowls and top with sliced banana, mixed berries, and diced apple.

Servings: 2
Preparation Time: Approximately 5 minutes
Cooking Time: Approximately 10 minutes
Total Time: 15 minutes

Nutritional Information per Serving

- Calories: 220 kcal (approximately; varies based on milk and sweetener)
- Carbohydrates: 40 g
- Fat: 5 g (varies with added ingredients)
- Protein: 7 g
- Potassium: 450 mg (may vary based on fruits used)
- Phosphorus: 100 mg
- Sodium: 5 mg (depending on added salt)

Why is this good for you?

- *This oatmeal recipe is naturally low in sodium, making it a great option for individuals who need to limit their salt intake. The addition of fresh fruits adds natural sweetness and flavor without the need for excessive sugar or salt.*
- *Sustainability: Oatmeal with Fresh Fruits is a sustainable recipe for patients on a low-sodium diet. It uses whole, fresh ingredients and can be filled with seasonal fruits, thus promoting a healthy diet while minimizing environmental impact. The oats provide a good source of fiber, which is beneficial for heart health and digestion.*

SPECIAL PRECAUTIONS!
- Monitor portion sizes of oats and fruits to manage potassium and phosphorus intake, especially for individuals who need to restrict these nutrients.
- Adjust sweetness according to individual dietary restrictions and consult with a healthcare provider or dietitian for personalized dietary advice.

LUNCH

Quinoa Salad with Lemon Dressing

Ingredients

- 1 cup quinoa (dry)
- 2 cups water or low-sodium vegetable broth (for cooking quinoa)
- 1 cup cherry tomatoes (halved)
- 1 medium cucumber (diced)
- 1/4 cup red onion (finely chopped)
- 1 medium bell pepper (diced; any color)
- 1/4 cup fresh parsley (chopped, optional)
- 2 tablespoons olive oil
- 2 tablespoons fresh lemon juice (about 1 lemon)
- 1/4 teaspoon black pepper
- Salt to taste (optional, use sparingly)

Servings: 4
Preparation Time: Approximately 10 minutes
Cooking Time: Approximately 15 minutes
Total Time: 25 minutes

Directions

1. Cook Quinoa: Rinse 1 cup of quinoa under cold water. In a saucepan, combine the quinoa with 2 cups of water or low-sodium vegetable broth. Bring to a boil, then reduce heat to low, cover, and simmer for about 15 minutes, or until the quinoa is fluffy and the liquid is absorbed. Remove from heat and let it cool slightly.
2. Prepare Vegetables: While the quinoa is cooking, wash and chop the cherry tomatoes, cucumber, red onion, and bell pepper. If using, chop the parsley.
3. Combine Ingredients: In a large mixing bowl, combine the cooked quinoa, halved cherry tomatoes, diced cucumber, chopped red onion, diced bell pepper, and parsley (if using).
4. Make Lemon Dressing: In a small bowl, whisk together the olive oil, fresh lemon juice, black pepper, and a pinch of salt (if desired).
5. Dress the Salad: Pour the dressing over the quinoa salad and toss gently to combine, ensuring that all ingredients are evenly coated.
6. Serve: Serve immediately or refrigerate for about 30 minutes to allow the flavors to meld.

Nutritional Information per Serving

- Calories: 180 kcal (approximately; varies based on ingredients)
- Carbohydrates: 30 g
- Fat: 7 g (varies with olive oil)
- Protein: 5 g
- Potassium: 300 mg (may vary based on vegetables)
- Phosphorus: 100 mg
- Sodium: 50 mg (depending on added salt and broth)

Why is this good for you?

- *This quinoa salad is naturally low in sodium, especially when using low-sodium broth and controlling added salt. The fresh vegetables add flavor and nutrients without the need for excess salt, making it a heart-healthy option.*
- *Sustainability: The Quinoa Salad with Lemon Dressing is sustainable for patients following a low-sodium diet as it utilizes whole, fresh ingredients that are nutrient-dense and can help maintain heart health. The use of quinoa and seasonal vegetables promotes a plant-based diet, which is beneficial for both health and the environment.*

SPECIAL PRECAUTIONS!

- Monitor portion sizes of quinoa and vegetables to manage potassium and phosphorus intake, especially for individuals who need to restrict these nutrients.
- Adjust sweetness and seasoning based on individual dietary restrictions, and consult with a healthcare provider or dietitian for personalized dietary advice.

Grilled Chicken Salad with Olive Oil Vinaigrette

Ingredients

- 4 oz boneless, skinless chicken breast (grilled and sliced)
- 4 cups mixed salad greens (e.g., romaine, spinach, arugula)
- 1/2 cup cherry tomatoes (halved)
- 1/2 cup cucumber (sliced)
- 1/4 cup red onion (thinly sliced, optional)
- 1/4 cup shredded carrots (optional)

For the Olive Oil Vinaigrette:
- 3 tablespoons olive oil
- 1 tablespoon balsamic vinegar or red wine vinegar
- 1 teaspoon Dijon mustard (optional, check for low-sodium)
- 1/4 teaspoon black pepper
- Salt to taste (optional, use sparingly)

Servings: 1
Preparation Time: Approximately 10 minutes
Cooking Time: Approximately 15 minutes (for grilling the chicken)
Total Time: 25 minutes

Directions

1. Grill Chicken: Preheat your grill or grill pan over medium-high heat. Season the chicken breast with a little olive oil, black pepper, and salt (if desired). Grill the chicken for about 6-7 minutes per side or until fully cooked (internal temperature should reach 165°F or 74°C). Remove from the grill and let it rest for a few minutes before slicing.
2. Prepare Salad Ingredients: While the chicken is grilling, wash and prepare the mixed salad greens, cherry tomatoes, cucumber, red onion, and shredded carrots.
3. Make Vinaigrette: In a small bowl, whisk together the olive oil, balsamic vinegar (or red wine vinegar), Dijon mustard (if using), black pepper, and a pinch of salt (if desired).
4. Combine Salad: In a large mixing bowl, combine the salad greens, cherry tomatoes, cucumber, red onion, and shredded carrots. Drizzle with the vinaigrette and toss gently to combine.
5. Top with Chicken: Arrange the sliced grilled chicken on top of the salad.
6. Serve: Serve immediately, garnished with additional herbs if desired.

Nutritional Information per Serving

- Calories: 350 kcal (approximately; varies based on chicken and vinaigrette)
- Carbohydrates: 15 g
- Fat: 20 g (varies with olive oil)
- Protein: 30 g
- Potassium: 600 mg (may vary based on vegetables)
- Phosphorus: 250 mg
- Sodium: 200 mg (depending on added salt and mustard)

Why is this good for you?

- *This grilled chicken salad is naturally low in sodium, especially when using fresh ingredients and controlling the amount of added salt. The vinaigrette provides flavor without excessive sodium, making it a heart-healthy choice.*
- *Sustainability: The Grilled Chicken Salad with Olive Oil Vinaigrette is a sustainable option for patients on a low-sodium diet. It incorporates lean protein and a variety of fresh vegetables, promoting a balanced and nutritious meal. The use of seasonal vegetables can further enhance sustainability by reducing environmental impact.*

SPECIAL PRECAUTIONS!

- Monitor portion sizes of chicken and any added salt to manage potassium and phosphorus intake, especially for individuals who need to restrict these nutrients.
- Adjust seasoning based on individual dietary restrictions, and consult with a healthcare provider or dietitian for personalized dietary advice.

DINNER

Baked Salmon with Asparagus

Ingredients

- 4 oz salmon fillet (per serving; skinless or skin-on)
- 1 bunch asparagus (about 1 pound; ends trimmed)
- 2 tablespoons olive oil
- 1 tablespoon fresh lemon juice (about 1/2 lemon)
- 1 teaspoon dried dill or parsley (optional)
- 1/4 teaspoon black pepper
- 1/4 teaspoon garlic powder (optional)
- Salt to taste (optional, use sparingly)
- Lemon wedges for serving (optional)

Directions

1. Preheat Oven: Preheat your oven to 400°F (200°C).
2. Prepare Asparagus: Place the trimmed asparagus on one side of a baking sheet. Drizzle with 1 tablespoon of olive oil, and sprinkle with black pepper, garlic powder (if using), and a pinch of salt (if desired). Toss to coat the asparagus evenly.
3. Prepare Salmon: Place the salmon fillet on the other side of the baking sheet. Drizzle with the remaining 1 tablespoon of olive oil and 1 tablespoon of lemon juice. Sprinkle with dried dill or parsley (if using), black pepper, and a pinch of salt (if desired).
4. Bake: Bake in the preheated oven for about 12-15 minutes, or until the salmon is cooked through and flakes easily with a fork, and the asparagus is tender.
5. Serve: Remove from the oven and serve immediately, garnished with lemon wedges if desired.

Servings: 1
Preparation Time: Approximately 10 minutes
Cooking Time: Approximately 15 minutes
Total Time: 25 minutes

Nutritional Information per Serving

- Calories: 300 kcal (approximately; varies based on olive oil and salmon)
- Carbohydrates: 8 g
- Fat: 20 g (varies with olive oil and salmon)
- Protein: 25 g
- Potassium: 700 mg (may vary based on vegetables)
- Phosphorus: 300 mg
- Sodium: 60 mg (depending on added salt)

Why is this good for you?

- *This baked salmon with asparagus recipe is naturally low in sodium, particularly when using fresh ingredients and controlling added salt. The dish is flavorful due to the herbs and lemon juice, allowing for a satisfying meal without excess sodium.*
- *Sustainability: The Baked Salmon with Asparagus recipe is sustainable for patients following a low-sodium diet. It features lean protein from salmon and seasonal vegetables, promoting a balanced and nutritious meal. Choosing wild-caught salmon and locally sourced asparagus can further enhance sustainability by reducing environmental impact.*

SPECIAL PRECAUTIONS!

- Monitor portion sizes of salmon and asparagus to manage potassium and phosphorus intake, especially for individuals who need to restrict these nutrients.
- Adjust seasoning based on individual dietary restrictions, and consult with a healthcare provider or dietitian for personalized dietary advice.

Stir-Fried Tofu with Vegetables

Ingredients

- 14 oz firm tofu (drained and cubed)
- 2 tablespoons olive oil or sesame oil
- 1 medium bell pepper (sliced)
- 1 cup broccoli florets
- 1 medium carrot (sliced into thin rounds)
- 1 cup snow peas or snap peas
- 2 cloves garlic (minced)
- 1 tablespoon fresh ginger (grated)
- 2 tablespoons low-sodium soy sauce or tamari
- 1 tablespoon rice vinegar (optional)
- 1/4 teaspoon black pepper
- Sesame seeds for garnish (optional)

Servings: 2-3
Preparation Time: Approximately 10 minutes
Cooking Time: Approximately 15 minutes
Total Time: 25 minutes

Directions

1. Prepare Tofu: Press the tofu to remove excess moisture. Cut the tofu into cubes.
2. Heat Oil: In a large skillet or wok, heat 2 tablespoons of olive oil or sesame oil over medium-high heat.
3. Cook Tofu: Add the cubed tofu to the skillet and cook for about 5-7 minutes, turning occasionally, until golden brown on all sides. Remove the tofu from the skillet and set aside.
4. Sauté Vegetables: In the same skillet, add the sliced bell pepper, broccoli florets, sliced carrot, and snow peas. Stir-fry for about 5-7 minutes, or until the vegetables are tender-crisp.
5. Add Aromatics: Add the minced garlic and grated ginger to the skillet and cook for about 1 minute until fragrant.
6. Combine Ingredients: Return the cooked tofu to the skillet. Pour in the low-sodium soy sauce and rice vinegar (if using). Stir well to combine and heat through for an additional 2-3 minutes.
7. Garnish and Serve: Remove from heat and garnish with sesame seeds if desired. Serve warm as a main dish or over brown rice or quinoa.

Nutritional Information per Serving

- Calories: 200 kcal (approximately; varies based on oil and tofu)
- Carbohydrates: 18 g
- Fat: 12 g (varies with oil)
- Protein: 12 g
- Potassium: 450 mg (may vary based on vegetables)
- Phosphorus: 180 mg
- Sodium: 200 mg (depending on added soy sauce)

Why is this good for you?

- *This stir-fried tofu with vegetables recipe is suitable for a low-sodium diet, especially when low-sodium soy sauce is used. It offers a flavorful meal without the need for excessive salt, relying on fresh ingredients and spices for taste.*
- *Sustainability: The Stir-Fried Tofu with Vegetables recipe is sustainable for patients following a low-sodium diet. It features plant-based protein from tofu and a variety of colorful vegetables, promoting a balanced and nutritious diet. The use of seasonal vegetables can further enhance sustainability by reducing environmental impact.*

SPECIAL PRECAUTIONS!

- Monitor portion sizes of tofu and vegetables to manage potassium and phosphorus intake, especially for individuals who need to restrict these nutrients.
- Adjust seasoning based on individual dietary restrictions and consult with a healthcare provider or dietitian for personalized dietary advice.

SNACKS

Hummus with Veggies

Ingredients

- 1 can (15 oz) chickpeas (garbanzo beans), drained and rinsed
- 1/4 cup tahini (sesame seed paste)
- 2 tablespoons olive oil
- 2 tablespoons fresh lemon juice (about 1 lemon)
- 2 cloves garlic (minced)
- 1/2 teaspoon ground cumin (optional)
- Salt to taste (optional, use sparingly)
- 1/4 cup water (adjust for desired consistency)
- For the Veggies:
- 1 cup carrot sticks
- 1 cup cucumber sticks
- 1 cup bell pepper strips (any color)
- 1 cup celery sticks
- 1 cup cherry tomatoes (optional)

Directions

1. Make Hummus: In a food processor, combine the drained chickpeas, tahini, olive oil, lemon juice, minced garlic, ground cumin (if using), and a pinch of salt (if desired). Blend until smooth.
2. Adjust Consistency: Add water gradually while blending until you reach your desired creamy consistency. Taste and adjust seasoning as needed.
3. Prepare Veggies: While the hummus is being made, wash and cut the vegetables into sticks or bite-sized pieces.
4. Serve: Transfer the hummus to a serving bowl and arrange the vegetable sticks around it. Drizzle with a little extra olive oil on top of the hummus if desired.

Servings: 4
Preparation Time: Approximately 10 minutes
Total Time: 10 minutes

Nutritional Information per Serving

- Calories: 150 kcal (approximately; varies based on hummus and vegetables)
- Carbohydrates: 20 g
- Fat: 7 g (varies with olive oil)
- Protein: 5 g
- Potassium: 400 mg (may vary based on vegetables)
- Phosphorus: 90 mg
- Sodium: 150 mg (depending on added salt)

Why is this good for you?

- *This Hummus with Veggies recipe is suitable for a low-sodium diet, especially when using low-sodium chickpeas and controlling added salt. Hummus is nutrient-dense, providing protein and fiber, while fresh vegetables add vitamins and minerals without excess sodium.*
- *Sustainability: The Hummus with Veggies recipe is sustainable for patients following a low-sodium diet. It incorporates plant-based ingredients that are nutrient-dense and can help maintain heart health. The use of seasonal vegetables can further enhance sustainability by reducing environmental impact.*

SPECIAL PRECAUTIONS!

- Monitor portion sizes of hummus to manage potassium and phosphorus intake, especially for individuals who need to restrict these nutrients.
- Adjust seasoning based on individual dietary restrictions, and consult with a healthcare provider or dietitian for personalized dietary advice.

Fruit and Nut Energy Bites

Ingredients

- 1 cup mixed nuts (e.g., almonds, walnuts, or cashews; unsalted)
- 1 cup dried fruit (e.g., dates, apricots, or raisins; unsweetened)
- 1/4 cup rolled oats (old-fashioned)
- 2 tablespoons nut butter (e.g., almond butter or peanut butter)
- 1 tablespoon honey or maple syrup (optional, adjust based on sweetness preference)
- 1 teaspoon vanilla extract (optional)
- 1/2 teaspoon cinnamon (optional)

Healthy Substitute Ingredients

- Mixed nuts: Substitute with seeds (e.g., pumpkin seeds or sunflower seeds) for a nut-free option.
- Dried fruit: Use lower-potassium dried fruits, such as apples or pears, if potassium intake needs to be restricted.

Directions

1. Process Nuts: In a food processor, add the mixed nuts and pulse until coarsely chopped (do not over-process into a flour).
2. Add Remaining Ingredients: Add the dried fruit, rolled oats, nut butter, honey (or maple syrup, if using), vanilla extract (if using), and cinnamon (if using) to the food processor. Process until the mixture is well combined and sticky.
3. Form Energy Bites: Using your hands, take small amounts of the mixture and roll them into bite-sized balls (about 1 inch in diameter). If the mixture is too sticky, you can wet your hands with a little water to help form the balls.
4. Chill: Place the energy bites on a baking sheet or plate and refrigerate for at least 30 minutes to firm up.
5. Serve: Enjoy the energy bites as a quick snack or pre-workout boost. Store any leftovers in an airtight container in the refrigerator for up to one week.

Servings: Approximately 12 energy bites (2 bites per serving)
Preparation Time: Approximately 10 minutes
Chilling Time: 30 minutes
Total Time: 40 minutes

Nutritional Information per Serving

- Calories: 200 kcal (approximately; varies based on nuts and sweetener)
- Carbohydrates: 25 g
- Fat: 10 g (varies with nut butter and nuts)
- Protein: 5 g
- Potassium: 300 mg (may vary based on ingredients)
- Phosphorus: 120 mg
- Sodium: 5 mg

Why is this good for you?

- *This Fruit and Nut Energy Bites recipe is suitable for a low-sodium diet, especially when using unsalted nuts and controlling added salt. The natural sweetness from the dried fruit and the healthy fats from the nuts provide a nutritious, satisfying snack without excessive sodium.*
- *Sustainability: The Fruit and Nut Energy Bites recipe is sustainable for patients following a low-sodium diet. It incorporates whole, nutrient-dense ingredients that are beneficial for overall health. The use of nuts and dried fruits promotes a healthy, balanced diet, and the recipe can be tailored to utilize seasonal ingredients, reducing environmental impact.*

SPECIAL PRECAUTIONS!

- Monitor portion sizes of nuts and dried fruits to manage potassium and phosphorus intake, especially for individuals who need to restrict these nutrients.
- Adjust sweetness based on individual dietary restrictions, and consult with a healthcare provider or dietitian for personalized dietary advice.

Chapter 6: Meal Planning for Success

How to Create a Weekly Meal Plan

Creating a weekly meal plan is a powerful tool for anyone looking to manage their diet effectively, focusing on low-sodium options. Here's a step-by-step guide to help you develop a meal plan that works for you:

1. Assess Your Dietary Needs: Consider any specific health goals, dietary restrictions, or preferences. Think about what meals and snacks you enjoy and how you can incorporate kidney-friendly foods into your diet.

2. Choose Your Foods: Refer to the Low-Sodium food list from Chapter 4. Select a variety of foods from different categories, including fruits, vegetables, proteins, whole grains, and healthy fats.

3. Plan for the Week:

    - Breakfast: Include nutritious options such as smoothies, oatmeal, or omelets.

    - Lunch: Think about salads, grain bowls, or wraps filled with lean proteins and veggies.

    - Dinner: Plan meals like baked fish, grilled chicken, or vegetable stir-fries.

    - Snacks: Choose healthy snacks such as fresh fruit, yogurt, or hummus with vegetables.

4. Create a Grocery List: Once you've planned your meals, make a shopping list of all the ingredients you'll need. Organize your list by category to streamline your shopping experience.

5. Be Flexible: Life can be unpredictable, so be open to adjusting your meal plan as needed. If you have leftovers, incorporate them into your next meals to reduce waste.

Tips for Meal Prepping Low-Sodium Meals

Meal prepping can save you time and help you stick to your low-sodium dietary goals. Here are some tips to make meal prep easier and more effective:

1. Cook in Batches: Prepare large quantities of staple items (such as grains, proteins, and vegetables) at once. This allows you to mix and match ingredients throughout the week, making it easier to create balanced meals.

2. Use Clear Containers: Store your prepped meals and ingredients in clear, labeled containers. This makes it easy to see what you have available and simplifies portioning out meals.

3. Incorporate Freezer-Friendly Meals: Prepare and freeze portions of soups, stews, and casseroles. These meals can be a lifesaver on busy days when you need something quick and nutritious.

4. Invest in a Slow Cooker or Instant Pot: These appliances can be incredibly helpful for meal prep. You can throw in ingredients in the morning and come home to a ready meal, or prepare soups and stews that can be easily frozen.

5. Plan for Snacks: Don't forget to prep healthy snacks! Portion out items like cut vegetables, hummus, yogurt, and nuts to have on hand for quick, low-sodium options.

6. Keep It Simple: Focus on simple recipes with fewer ingredients to avoid feeling overwhelmed. Choose meals that can be quickly assembled or require minimal cooking time

Sample One-Week Low-Sodium Meal Plan

Here's a sample one-week low-sodium meal plan. This plan includes breakfast, lunch, dinner, and snacks for each day.

Day 1

- Breakfast: Greek yogurt with mixed berries and a drizzle of honey
- Snack: Apple slices with almond butter
- Lunch: Quinoa salad with cucumber, bell pepper, and lemon vinaigrette
- Snack: Carrot sticks with hummus
- Dinner: Baked salmon with asparagus and brown rice

Day 2

- Breakfast: Smoothie with spinach, banana, and unsweetened almond milk
- Snack: Celery sticks with hummus
- Lunch: Grilled chicken salad with mixed greens, avocado, and olive oil dressing
- Snack: Handful of walnuts
- Dinner: Turkey and vegetable stir-fry with cauliflower rice

Day 3

- Breakfast: Oatmeal made with almond milk, topped with sliced bananas and a sprinkle of cinnamon
- Snack: Cucumber slices with guacamole
- Lunch: Lentil soup with carrots and celery
- Snack: Hard-boiled eggs
- Dinner: Herb-crusted baked cod with roasted broccoli and quinoa

Day 4

- Breakfast: Chia seed pudding made with almond milk, topped with kiwi
- Snack: Mixed berries (strawberries, blueberries, and raspberries)
- Lunch: Stuffed bell peppers with ground turkey and cauliflower rice
- Snack: Rice cakes topped with almond butter
- Dinner: Grilled shrimp tacos with cabbage slaw

Day 5

- Breakfast: Scrambled eggs with sautéed spinach and feta
- Snack: Baby carrots with tzatziki sauce
- Lunch: Mediterranean quinoa salad with chickpeas and feta
- Snack: Sliced bell peppers with hummus
- Dinner: Slow-cooked chicken thighs with garlic and rosemary, served with roasted Brussels sprouts

Day 6

- Breakfast: Smoothie bowl with kale, banana, and almond milk, topped with chia seeds
- Snack: Sliced apples with cashew cream
- Lunch: Grilled vegetable and hummus wrap in lettuce leaves
- Snack: Handful of almonds
- Dinner: Baked chicken breast with roasted sweet potatoes and steamed green beans

Day 7

- Breakfast: Coconut yogurt with sliced strawberries and a sprinkle of flaxseeds
- Snack: Cherry tomatoes and cucumber slices
- Lunch: Turkey and avocado salad with mixed greens and balsamic vinaigrette
- Snack: Rice cakes topped with cream cheese and dill
- Dinner: Cauliflower rice stir-fry with mixed vegetables and grilled shrimp

Summary of Weekly Totals

- Total Calories: Approximately 11,500 (averaging about 1,650 per day)
- Total Protein: Approximately 520g (averaging about 75g per day)
- Total Fat: Approximately 350g (averaging about 50g per day)
- Total Carbohydrates: Approximately 1,000g (averaging about 140g per day)
- Total Fiber: Approximately 180g (averaging about 25g per day)
- Average Sodium: Approximately 700mg (varies based on added salt)
- Average Potassium: Approximately 3,200mg (averaging about 450mg per day)
- Average Calcium: Approximately 200mg (averaging about 30mg per day)

Important Micronutrients and Minerals

- Vitamin C: Essential for immune function; found in fruits and vegetables like bell peppers and citrus.
- Potassium: Important for heart health; abundant in leafy greens, bananas, and sweet potatoes.

- Sodium: Monitor sodium intake, especially from processed foods. Aim for low-sodium options to maintain heart health and manage blood pressure effectively.

- Calcium: Important for maintaining bone health, especially in older adults. Incorporate low-oxalate, calcium-rich foods such as dairy, fortified plant-based milks, and certain leafy greens.

- Fiber: Essential for digestive health and can help manage weight. Aim to include plenty of fruits, vegetables, and whole grains in your meals.

This 7-Day Meal Plan is designed to provide balanced and nutritious meals while adhering to Low-Sodium Dieting. Each day includes a variety of foods to ensure you receive essential nutrients and maintain a satisfying diet.

By following this meal plan, you can simplify your transition into healthy eating, making it easier to adhere to your dietary goals. Remember, meal planning is not just about restriction; it's about finding joy in nourishing your body with wholesome ingredients. Embrace this journey with an open heart, and enjoy the delicious meals along the way!

Chapter 7: Cooking Tips and Techniques

Flavor Enhancement Without Salt

Reducing sodium intake doesn't mean sacrificing flavor in your meals. There are numerous ways to enhance the taste of your dishes without relying on salt. Here are some effective strategies:

1. Herbs and Spices: Fresh or dried herbs and spices can elevate the flavor of your dishes significantly. Experiment with combinations such as rosemary and garlic for meats, or basil and oregano for vegetables and sauces. Some great options include:

    - Garlic and onion: These aromatics add depth and richness to any dish.
    - Citrus zest: Grating lemon, lime, or orange zest can brighten flavors and add a refreshing touch.
    - Chili peppers: For those who enjoy heat, adding fresh or dried chili peppers can provide a kick without sodium.

2. Acidic Ingredients: Adding acidity can enhance flavors and balance dishes. Consider incorporating:

    - Vinegars: Balsamic, apple cider, or red wine vinegar can add complexity to salads and marinades.
    - Citrus juices: Fresh lemon, lime, or orange juice can brighten up vegetables, meats, and sauces.

3. Flavorful Broths: Use homemade or low-sodium vegetable or chicken broth as a base for soups, stews, and sauces. This adds depth without excessive sodium.

4. Umami Sources: Incorporate ingredients that provide umami flavors, such as:

    - Mushrooms: Sautéed mushrooms can add a savory depth to dishes.

    - Tomato products: Use crushed tomatoes or tomato paste to enhance sauces and stews.

    - Nutritional yeast: This can provide a cheesy flavor and is great for seasoning popcorn or pasta.

Cooking Methods that Retain Nutrients

The way you prepare and cook your food can significantly impact its nutritional value. Here are some cooking methods that help retain the maximum amount of nutrients in your meals:

1. **Steaming**: Steaming vegetables is one of the best ways to preserve their vitamins and minerals. This method cooks food quickly without direct contact with water, which can leach nutrients. Steamed vegetables retain their vibrant color and crisp texture, making them both appealing and nutritious.

2. **Sautéing**: Lightly sautéing vegetables in a small amount of healthy oil (like olive oil) allows them to cook quickly while preserving their nutrients. This method also enhances the flavor and texture of the vegetables, making them more enjoyable to eat.

3. **Roasting:** Roasting vegetables in the oven concentrates their flavors and retains nutrients. Tossing them in a little olive oil and seasoning before roasting can enhance their natural sweetness and make them a delicious side dish.

4. **Baking:** Baking proteins, such as fish or chicken, is a healthy cooking method that retains moisture and nutrients while minimizing added fats. Using herbs and spices to season your baked dishes can enhance flavor without salt.

5. **Blanching**: Blanching vegetables involves briefly boiling them and then plunging them into ice water. This method can help preserve color, texture, and nutrients, particularly when preparing vegetables for freezing.

6. **Slow Cooking:** While some nutrients may be lost over long cooking times, slow cooking can be beneficial for tenderizing tougher cuts of meat and allowing flavors to meld in soups and stews. Using fresh herbs and spices can enhance the nutritional profile of slow-cooked dishes.

Quick Cooking Techniques for Busy Lives

For those with hectic schedules, finding time to prepare healthy meals can be a challenge. Here are some quick cooking techniques that can help you create nutritious meals without spending hours in the kitchen:

1. **Batch Cooking**: Prepare large quantities of grains, proteins, and vegetables at the beginning of the week. Store them in portion-sized containers in the refrigerator or freezer. This allows you to mix and match ingredients for quick meals throughout the week. For example, you can cook a big batch of quinoa or brown rice and use it in salads, stir-fries, or as a side dish.

2. **One-Pan Meals:** Simplify cooking by preparing one-pan meals that combine protein, vegetables, and healthy grains. This not only reduces cleanup time but also allows flavors to meld together. For instance, you can roast chicken thighs with seasonal vegetables and quinoa all in one baking dish.

3. **Quick Stir-Fries**: Stir-fries are a great way to whip up a healthy meal in under 30 minutes. Use pre-cut vegetables and lean proteins (like chicken or shrimp) to make a flavorful dish. Toss everything together with a low-sodium sauce and serve it over cauliflower rice or quinoa.

4. **Utilize Frozen Vegetables**: Frozen vegetables are a convenient way to add nutrients to your meals without the need for washing and chopping. They are often flash-frozen at peak ripeness, preserving their nutrients. Simply steam or sauté them for a quick addition to any dish.

5. **Use a Pressure Cooker or Instant Pot:** These appliances can significantly reduce cooking times for grains, beans, and stews. For example, you can cook dried beans in under an hour instead of soaking and simmering them for several hours. This can be a game-changer for meal prep.

6. **Pre-Made Sauces and Dressings**: Prepare or purchase low-sodium sauces and dressings that can enhance the flavor of your meals without added salt. Having these on hand can make it easy to add flavor to simple dishes quickly.

7. **Plan Quick Meals:** Keep a few quick meal ideas in your repertoire for busy nights. Dishes like omelets, salads, or grain bowls can be assembled in minutes. For instance, a simple omelet with leftover vegetables and cheese can be ready in under 10 minutes, providing a nutritious meal without much fuss.

8. **Utilize Slow Cooker**: If you have a busy day ahead, consider using a slow cooker to prepare meals. You can set it up in the morning with your choice of proteins, vegetables, and seasonings, and come home to a warm, fully cooked meal. Slow cookers are perfect for soups, stews, and casseroles.

9. **Make Use of Leftovers**: Plan to make larger portions of meals so you can enjoy leftovers the next day. Leftover grilled chicken can be sliced and added to salads, wraps, or grain bowls, saving you time while ensuring you eat healthily.

10. **Prep Ingredients in Advance:** Spend a little time each week washing and chopping vegetables, marinating proteins, or measuring out grains. Storing prepped ingredients in the fridge makes it easier to throw meals together on busy days.

By implementing these cooking tips and techniques, you can create delicious, nutritious Low-sodium meals while fitting into your busy lifestyle. Meal planning and efficient cooking methods not only save time but also help you maintain a healthy diet that supports your health goals. Remember, the key to success is preparation—when you are prepared, eating well becomes an enjoyable and sustainable part of your life.

Chapter 8: Coping with Dietary Restrictions

Navigating Social Situations with Dietary Needs

Adopting a kidney-friendly low-sodium diet can present unique challenges, especially when attending social gatherings or dining out. However, with thoughtful preparation and open communication, you can navigate these situations with confidence. Here are some strategies to help:

1. Communicate Your Needs: Don't hesitate to inform your friends, family, or hosts about your dietary restrictions. Most people appreciate your honesty and want to accommodate your needs. If you're attending a gathering, offer to bring a dish that fits your dietary requirements, ensuring there's something safe for you to enjoy.

2. Research Restaurants: Before dining out, check the restaurant's menu online. Look for establishments that offer fresh, whole foods, as they are more likely to have low-sodium options. Many restaurants now provide nutritional information, allowing you to make informed choices.

3. Ask Questions: When ordering, feel free to ask your server about how dishes are prepared and what ingredients are included. Inquire about low-sodium options or modifications that can be made to a dish, such as substituting high-sodium ingredients with healthier alternatives.

4. Choose Wisely: Opt for grilled, baked, or steamed items rather than fried or heavily sauced dishes. Focus on meals that highlight fresh vegetables and lean proteins while avoiding high-sodium sauces and dressings.

5. Stay Positive: Focus on the social aspects of dining out rather than just the food. Engage in conversations and enjoy the company of your friends and family, making the experience enjoyable regardless of the menu.

Involving Family in Meal Preparation

Involving family members in meal preparation can create a supportive environment and make following a kidney-friendly diet easier and more enjoyable. Here are some effective ways to engage your family:

1. ***Educate and Inform:*** Share information about the importance of a low-sodium diet and how it benefits your health. When family members understand your dietary needs, they are more likely to support your choices and participate in meal planning.

2. ***Plan Meals Together:*** Encourage family involvement in creating a weekly meal plan. Gather everyone to brainstorm recipes that accommodate your dietary restrictions while still appealing to the whole family. This inclusive approach fosters collaboration and ensures everyone's preferences are considered.

3. ***Cook Together:*** Make cooking a fun family activity. Involve kids, partners, or other family members in preparing meals. Assign specific tasks, such as washing vegetables, measuring ingredients, or stirring pots. This not only teaches valuable cooking skills but also strengthens family bonds.

4. ***Experiment with New Recipes:*** Encourage family members to explore and try new recipes that align with the Low-Sodium Diet. Challenge each other to come up with creative, low-sodium meals that everyone can enjoy. This exploration can introduce new flavors and ingredients into your family's diet.

5. ***Share Responsibilities:*** Assign different family members specific meal preparation tasks, such as chopping vegetables, setting the table, or cleaning up afterward. Sharing responsibilities can make cooking less overwhelming and more enjoyable for everyone.

6. ***Make It Fun:*** Incorporate themes or challenges into your cooking sessions. For example, you could have a "family taco night" where everyone assembles their own low-sodium tacos with safe ingredients. This makes meal preparation more engaging and enjoyable.

Tips for Cooking for Mixed Dietary Needs

Cooking for a family with varying dietary preferences can be challenging, but with some strategies in place, it can also be rewarding. Here are some tips to help you accommodate different dietary:

1. ***Choose Versatile Ingredients***: Select ingredients that can be used in multiple dishes. For example, grilled chicken can be served in salads, wraps, or as a main dish with vegetables. This allows you to prepare a base meal that can be customized according to individual preferences.

2. ***Prepare Components Separately***: Rather than cooking one dish for everyone, consider preparing components of meals separately. For instance, you might cook a batch of quinoa, roast a variety of vegetables, and grill different proteins. Each family member can then assemble their own meal based on their dietary preferences.

3. ***Create Build-Your-Own Meals***: Encourage creativity by setting up a "build-your-own" meal station. For example, for taco night, provide low-sodium tortillas, grilled proteins, various toppings (like lettuce, tomatoes, and avocado), and sauces on the side. This allows everyone to customize their meal according to their dietary requirements.

4. ***Use Low-Sodium Alternatives***: When preparing meals, use low-sodium versions of sauces, broths, and condiments. This ensures that the meals are suitable for those on a low-sodium diet while still appealing to others in the family.

5. ***Incorporate Flavorful Herbs and Spices***: Use fresh herbs and spices to enhance the flavor of dishes without adding salt. This is a great way to keep meals interesting for everyone while adhering to dietary restrictions.

6. ***Communicate and Collaborate***: Keep an open dialogue with family members about their dietary needs and preferences. Understanding each other's requirements can lead to more harmonious meal times and less frustration in the kitchen.

7. ***Meal Prep Together:*** Involve family members in meal prep activities. This not only makes the process more efficient but also helps educate everyone about healthy cooking practices and the importance of dietary choices.

Adopting a new dietary approach can be challenging, but it also presents opportunities for creativity, connection, and shared experiences around food. With the right planning and communication, you can ensure that everyone in your household feels valued and included in the journey toward better health.

Remember, your commitment to a kidney-friendly, low-sodium lifestyle not only benefits you but also sets a positive example for your family and friends. Each step you take toward healthier eating is a step toward enhancing your overall well-being. Embrace the process, share your experiences, and enjoy the journey of nourishing your body with delicious, wholesome meals.

Conclusion

Empowering Your Kidney Health Journey

As we conclude this guide, I want to emphasize the importance of taking charge of your kidney health through informed dietary choices. The **Low-Sodium Food List for Kidney Disease Patients** is not just a collection of foods; it is a pathway to a healthier lifestyle. By understanding the impact of sodium on kidney function and making conscious decisions about what you eat, you can significantly improve your quality of life.

Managing chronic kidney disease (CKD) can be challenging, but you are not alone. With the right knowledge and resources, you can navigate your dietary journey with confidence. Remember that every meal is an opportunity to nourish your body and support your health. With the help of your doctor and nutritionist dietitian, you can work on creating new recipes and ingredients that align with your dietary needs.

Encouragement for Healthy Living

Thank you for allowing me to accompany you on this journey toward better health. Your commitment to following a low-sodium diet reflects a proactive approach to managing your kidney health and enhancing your overall well-being. I commend you for taking this important step, as it can lead to transformative changes in your life.

As you move forward, I encourage you to stay engaged with your health. Continue to educate yourself about kidney disease, seek support from healthcare professionals, and connect with others who share similar experiences. Your journey is unique, and every small change you make contributes to a larger transformation.

May you find joy in preparing and enjoying delicious, kidney-friendly meals that nourish your body and bring happiness to your table. Here's to a vibrant, heart-healthy future filled with satisfying meals and the support of your loved ones!

Thank You For Reading!

I sincerely appreciate you investing your time and energy in *Kidney Friendly Low-Sodium Diet*. My goal in writing this book was to provide you with practical and supportive guidance for navigating Low-sodium dieting for your Kidney Disease.

If you found this book beneficial and feel it could help others, I would be deeply grateful if you would consider leaving a review on Amazon. Your feedback is invaluable and helps spread the word to those who may also be needing some help.

Leaving a review is easy! Simply visit:

https://go.binnovatedigital.com/lowsodiumfoodlist

Or Scan the QR code below to go directly to the review page:

Your support means the world to me. Thank you very much!

Love,

-Janeth

Reference

1. Centers for Disease Control and Prevention (CDC). "Chronic Kidney Disease (CKD)." Available at: CDC - Chronic Kidney Disease.

2. National Kidney Foundation. "Nutrition and Chronic Kidney Disease." Available at: NKF - Nutrition.

3. Mayo Clinic. "Chronic Kidney Disease." Available at: Mayo Clinic - CKD.

4. KDOQI (Kidney Disease Outcomes Quality Initiative). "KDOQI Clinical Practice Guidelines for Nutrition in Chronic Kidney Disease: 2020 Update." Available at: KDOQI Nutrition Guidelines.

5. American Heart Association. "Sodium and Your Health." Available at: AHA - Sodium.

6. American Society of Nephrology. "Dietary Management of Chronic Kidney Disease." Available at: ASN - Dietary Management.

7. Nutrients Journal. "Dietary Recommendations for Chronic Kidney Disease: A Review." Available at: Nutrients - CKD Dietary Recommendations.

8. Kidney Disease: Improving Global Outcomes (KDIGO). "KDIGO Clinical Practice Guidelines for Nutrition in Chronic Kidney Disease: 2020 Update." Available at: KDIGO Nutrition Guidelines.

9. National Kidney Foundation. "Nutrition and Chronic Kidney Disease." Available at: NKF - Nutrition.

10. Mayo Clinic. "Chronic Kidney Disease." Available at: Mayo Clinic - CKD.

11. American Heart Association. "Sodium and Your Health." Available at: AHA - Sodium.

12. Bansal, N., & Katz, R. (2019). "Dietary Management of Chronic Kidney Disease." *The Clinical Advisor*. Available at: Clinical Advisor on CKD.

13. Cleveland Clinic. "Diet and Chronic Kidney Disease." Available at: Cleveland Clinic - CKD Diet.

14. American Society of Nephrology. "Nutrition in Kidney Disease." Available at: ASN - Nutrition.

15. He, F. J., & MacGregor, G. A. (2018). "Reducing Population Salt Intake Worldwide: From Evidence to Implementation." *Progress in Cardiovascular Diseases*, 60(4), 327-332. DOI: 10.1016/j.pcad.2017.09.007.

16. Murray, J. A., & Muir, J. G. (2018). "Dietary Management of Menopausal Symptoms: The Role of Nutrition." *Clinical Reviews in Allergy & Immunology*, 54(1), 68-86. DOI: 10.1007/s12016-017-8651-7.

17. KDOQI (Kidney Disease Outcomes Quality Initiative). "KDOQI Clinical Practice Guidelines for Nutrition in Chronic Kidney Disease: 2020 Update." Available at: KDOQI Nutrition Guidelines.

18. Kidney Disease: Improving Global Outcomes (KDIGO). "KDIGO Clinical Practice Guidelines for Nutrition in Chronic Kidney Disease: 2020 Update." Available at: KDIGO Nutrition Guidelines.

19. National Kidney Foundation. "Nutrition and Chronic Kidney Disease." Available at: NKF - Nutrition.

20. American Heart Association. "Sodium and Your Health." Available at: AHA - Sodium.

21. Mayo Clinic. "Diet for Chronic Kidney Disease: What to Eat." Available at: Mayo Clinic - CKD Diet.

22. Institute of Medicine (IOM). "Dietary Reference Intakes for Water, Potassium, Sodium, Chloride, and Sulfate." Available at: National Academies Press.

23. He, F. J., & MacGregor, G. A. (2018). "Reducing Population Salt Intake Worldwide: From Evidence to Implementation." *Progress in Cardiovascular Diseases*, 60(4), 327-332. DOI: 10.1016/j.pcad.2017.09.007.

24. Bansal, N., & Katz, R. (2019). "Dietary Management of Chronic Kidney Disease." *The Clinical Advisor*. Available at: Clinical Advisor - Dietary Management.

25. American Society of Nephrology. "Nutrition in Kidney Disease." Available at: ASN - Nutrition.

26. National Institute on Aging. "Healthy Eating for Older Adults." Available at: NIA - Healthy Eating.

27. Cleveland Clinic. "Diet and Chronic Kidney Disease." Available at: Cleveland Clinic - CKD Diet.

28. U.S. Department of Agriculture (USDA). "Dietary Guidelines for Americans 2020-2025." Available at: USDA Dietary Guidelines.

29. National Kidney Foundation. "Understanding Sodium and CKD." Available at: NKF - Sodium and CKD

A Great Big Thank You!

From the bottom of my heart, thank you for investing your time and resources in The Complete Kidney Disease Diet & Food List Guide. It's been my privilege to compile these essential renal diet resources, designed to help you avoid dialysis and thrive with kidney disease.

If this collection has made a positive difference in your life—whether by simplifying your food lists, clarifying low potassium options, or easing your low sodium meal planning—I'd be incredibly grateful for your review.

Your honest feedback helps me and my team reach more individuals who can benefit from this information and strengthen our growing community. You can easily leave a review by scanning this QR code:

or by typing **https://go.renaltracker.com/4in1** into your browser.

Thank you for being a part of this journey!

Always grateful and wishing you the best of Kidney Health,

Janeth Kingston, BSN RN

Made in United States
North Haven, CT
08 September 2025

72683661R00368